Cutaneous Manifestations
of Infection in the Immunocompromised Host

Marc E. Grossman • Lindy P. Fox • Carrie Kovarik
Misha Rosenbach

Cutaneous Manifestations of Infection in the Immunocompromised Host

Second Edition

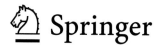 Springer

Authors

Marc E. Grossman, M.D.
Professor of Clinical Dermatology
College of Physicians and Surgeons
Director, Hospital Consultation Service
New York Presbyterian Hospital
Columbia University Medical Center
New York, New York, USA

Lindy P. Fox, M.D.
Associate Professor of Clinical Dermatology
Director, Hospital Consultation Service
University of California, San Francisco
San Francisco, California, USA

Carrie Kovarik, M.D.
Assistant Professor of Dermatology
Dermatopathology, and Infectious Diseases
University of Pennsylvania
Philadelphia, Pennsylvania, USA

Misha Rosenbach, M.D.
Assistant Professor of Dermatology
and Internal Medicine
Director, Dermatology Inpatient Consult Service
University of Pennsylvania
Philadelphia, Pennsylvania, USA

ISBN 978-1-4419-1577-1   e-ISBN 978-1-4419-1578-8
DOI 10.1007/978-1-4419-1578-8
Springer New York Dordrecht Heidelberg London

Library of Congress Control Number: 2011933837

Printed on acid-free paper

Springer is part of Springer Science+Business Media (www.springer.com)

Preface to the Second Edition

Immunocompromised patients are often some of the sickest patients in the hospital. Dermatologists who focus on inpatient consultations and caring for hospitalized patients are often faced with the gravely ill, severely immunocompromised patient who presents with cutaneous lesions that are a mystery to the primary team and the other involved subspecialty consultants. More often than not these lesions are a sign of an infection, typically one that is potentially life-threatening. Infections in the immunocompromised host often lead to rapid demise, making early recognition of the infectious process crucial to the patient's survival. The dermatologist plays a central role in identifying the pathogenic organism, implementing the appropriate therapy and prolonging or saving a life. That is the crux of this book. We have combed the literature carefully and combined what we have read with our experience in caring for these very sick, complex patients to present the cutaneous manifestations of infection in the immunocompromised host.

This textbook centralizes the available literature on the cutaneous manifestations of infection in the immunocompromised host. The book is a collection of well-documented references (confirmed by biopsy and culture) on specific skin lesions of infection that illustrates cutaneous lesions of routine and rare infectious organisms, demonstrates the evolution of skin lesions over time, – with immune reconstitution or with the recovery of neutrophils – and highlights recognizable patterns of infection and likely causes in different clinical settings (human immunodeficiency virus/acquired immune deficiency syndrome [HIV/AIDS] vs. post solid organ transplantation vs. neutropenia post chemotherapy vs. bone marrow recovery post hematopoietic stem cell transplantation).

We have given particular attention to the pattern of disease produced by routine and opportunistic pathogens to simplify the expanding list of infectious disease possibilities and recognize the most likely organism for a given clinical situation (e.g., fever, pneumonia and rash or fever, meningitis and rash). Starting with the skin lesion (e.g., acral hemorrhagic bullae or subcutaneous nodules), we present an evidence-based tiered differential diagnosis based on a literature review, well-documented case reports and the probability of a specific organism manifesting as a specific pattern of infection in the immunocompromised patient. This approach to skin lesions in the immunocompromised host has resulted in a unique textbook with bold illustrations that can be used as a bedside guide for diagnosis.

The text has been thoroughly updated and expanded since the first edition to reflect emerging trends in infectious organisms that cause disease in each subgroup of immunosuppressed patients. A new chapter discussing the role of viruses in potentiating malignancies in the immunocompromised patient has been added. The collection of images presented here is a rare and precious anthology gathered from our work in the "hospital trenches."

This book is written by dermatologists but intended for all physicians who care for immunocompromised patients, including, but not limited to, internists, transplant surgeons, infectious disease specialists, pediatricians, rheumatologists, and hematologist-oncologists. It is intended to be a diagnostic tool for the clinician, as well as a teaching syllabus for medical students and house staff.

Preface to the First Edition

In 1979, after training in internal medicine at the Hospital of the University of Pennsylvania and in dermatology at Columbia-Presbyterian Medical Center, I began performing an in-hospital dermatology consultation service at Columbia. I relished the challenge of treating the sickest patients with the worst rashes. I was often rewarded for a compulsively complete skin examination by finding the subtle skin clue which was the diagnostic solution to an otherwise complex clinical problem. The patients I treated were usually members of the population of immunocompromised patients, a population whose numbers have increased logarithmically over the past 16 years because of major advances in cancer chemotherapy, transplantation, treatment of autoimmune diseases and the AIDS epidemic.

The major problem in these compromised patients was often infection. The inflammatory response to the invasive organism was altered by either the primary disease or its treatment. Thus, routine pathogens presented in disguise, and the patient became a living culture plate for opportunistic microorganisms, some of which had never been previously described as human pathogens. Skin lesions had to be evaluated not by the morphology alone, but by the clinical setting in which they occurred. There were no atlases or textbooks available to help me in these critical situations. Nor were there teachers or specialists to depend on for dermatology knowledge and advice in the acute care hospital setting, although the infectious disease experts or intensive care specialists, Harold C. Neu and Glenda Garvey, were always willing to share their considerable expertise and wisdom with me. To find out more about cutaneous lesions in the immunocompromised host, I (or more often the dermatology resident doing consults with me for the month) had to search the literature for case reports which were scattered in all general and subspecialty medical journals. Similarly, the care of the compromised host has been managed by all types of physicians: surgeons, internists, primary care physicians, oncologists, rheumatologists and specialists in AIDS, transplantation, infectious disease and dermatology.

This book is a first attempt to centralize the information on cutaneous lesions of infection in the immunocompromised host; to collect well-documented references (by biopsy or culture) on specific skin lesions of infection; to illustrate cutaneous lesions of routine and rare infectious organisms; to demonstrate the evolution of skin lesions over time or with the recovery of neutrophils; to recognize patterns of infection and likely causes in different clinical settings; and to provide a list of pathogens that may cause a particular skin lesion when the host is immunocompromised.

Lastly, and perhaps most importantly, this book will be used to teach. I am fortunate to have studied under some of the best physician-teachers, both as a medical student and house officer at the University of Pennsylvania Medical Center and as a dermatology resident at the Columbia-Presbyterian Medical Center. I can only try to do as well as those from whom I have learned.

Scarsdale, New York   Marc E. Grossman, M.D.

Acknowledgments for the Second Edition

Leonard Harber, M.D., former chairman of the department of dermatology at Columbia Presbyterian Medical Center, gave me my start in 1976 by supporting my idea of a dermatology consultation service in the medical center for Presbyterian and Babies Hospital (later renamed NY Presbyterian Hospital and Children's Hospital of NY). Perhaps the first inpatient consultation service of its kind in dermatology, it morphed under the equally supportive and encouraging department chairman, David Bickers, M.D., into hospitalist dermatology as the field of medical dermatology became established. I am grateful to Dr. Bickers who has indulged all of my academic pursuits and my idiosyncratic teaching methods and for a job in the morning that I love.

Phyllis Della Latta, Director of Clinical Microbiology at Columbia Presbyterian Medical Center, her staff and the laboratory technicians were always available to do their work and show off their results to me and the dermatology residents. It was a special educational experience we all appreciated when I brought all the residents through the microbiology laboratory on consultation rounds to see the microbiologic culprit.

David N. Silvers, M.D., my colleague, friend and Columbia Presbyterian Medical Center dermatopathologist, was always willing to go the distance with deeper cuts, extra cuts, special stains and extra time at the microscope to find the causative "bug." He also provided a counterpoint to my ideas and theories from his own perspective.

Alexis Young, M.D., while a dermatology resident at Columbia worked as a research assistant and fact checker in her spare time.

Special thanks goes to Michele Nunez whose computer skills and organizational talent coordinated the four authors working from New York, San Francisco and Philadelphia to assemble the book and illustrations.

With much thanks to my wife, Leslie, whose vision and guidance created the dermatology practice which allowed me the luxury of this book project.

Scarsdale, NY   Marc E. Grossman, M.D.
2011

Under the expert tutelage of Marc Grossman, M.D., and Paul Schneiderman, M.D., at Columbia University Medical Center, I learned inpatient dermatology. Richard Edelson, M.D., at Yale, unconditionally encouraged my early ideas. With the support of Bruce Wintroub, M.D., and Timothy Berger, M.D., at University of California, San Francisco (UCSF), the modern hospitalist dermatology movement began.

A special thank you to the UCSF dermatology residents, without whom the hospitalist dermatology service at UCSF could not succeed.

Thank you to my parents, Cyril and Mignon, and my brother Keith for their unconditional love and support always.

To my partner in life and love, Ken, and our little Zuri Zev.

San Francisco, CA   Lindy Peta Fox, M.D.
2011

William D. James, M.D., Vice Chair and Director of Clinical Practices and Training Program at the University of Pennsylvania, Department of Dermatology, has inspired us to be the best clinicians we can be and to pursue our interests in medical and infectious dermatology.

We would like to thank the Penn dermatology residents for their hard work and dedication, and for diagnosing and caring for so many challenging and complicated patients.

We are extraordinarily appreciative of the fellows and faculty of the Infection Disease Division of Internal Medicine at the University of Pennsylvania for collaborating and consulting with us and helping to diagnose and treat these challenging patients.

Philadelphia, PA
2011

Carrie Kovarik, M.D.
Misha Rosenbach, M.D.

Acknowledgments for the First Edition

Dermatologic Manifestations of Infections in Immunocompromised Patients by the late John S. Wolfson, M.D., Arthur J. Sober, M.D., and Robert M. Rubin, M.D., was one of the first published collected series of clinical experience with skin infection in the compromised host. Their outstanding paper was the stimulus for this book. More importantly, Drs. Rubin and Sober established the approach and some of the principles to the diagnosis of skin lesions in the immunocompromised patient. I am grateful to them for allowing me to reproduce parts of their paper (Medicine 1985;64:115–133).

I am most grateful to the faculty and house staff of Columbia-Presbyterian Medical Center (CPMC) who consulted the dermatology service and allowed us to participate in the care of their patients. I am indebted to the dermatology residents through whose efforts the skin biopsies, couch preparations, cultures, and clinical photographs were obtained. The precise etiologic diagnoses could not have been recorded without the high caliber infectious disease laboratories of Presbyterian Hospital. Jeff Roth, when he was chief resident in dermatology at CPMC, arranged the book contract with the publisher and helped me to get started. He assisted me during the formative phase of the book's development.

And to Leonard Harber, M.D., who supported me in the early years after residency, always encouraged my academic pursuits, and taught me professionalism and a level of excellence in practice that I have tried to emulate and teach, I am thankful.

Special praise goes to Deborah Duffy, whose secretarial skills enabled her to transcribe my illegible handwriting into the computer-printed word and continuously organize and reorder the text from the inception of this project.

My colleagues, Paul Schneiderman and Vincent DeLeo, encouraged this project, and my wife, Leslie, and children, Andrea and Julie, sacrificed family time so I could work on it and bring this book to print.

Some figures are reproduced with the kind permission of colleagues:

Selim Aractingi
M. Arico
Mary Ruth Buchness
Geetinder Chattha
Phillip Cohen
Haig Donabedian
Samuel Dreizen
Stephen A. Estes
E.C. Fehl III
James Fitzpatrick
Robert Greenwald
Hiroshi Hachisuk

Contents

Introduction

The diagnosis of infectious disease complications that occur in the skin of the immunocompromised host poses a formidable challenge to the clinician. The clinician is confounded by the two central characteristics of infection in patients with impaired host defenses: (a) the array of potential pathogens is all inclusive, ranging from rare and exotic fungal or protozoan infections to common bacterial and viral infections; and (b) the clinical presentation and course of even the most common infectious process may be greatly modified or obscured by the impaired inflammatory response associated with the patient's disease or its treatment.

The skin and subcutaneous tissue occupy a central position in any consideration of infection in the immunocompromised host. First, the skin and the mucosal surfaces of the body interface with the environment and are the primary host barriers against infection. These primary barriers assume even greater importance in patients whose secondary host defenses – phagocytosis, cell-mediated immunity, antibody production, etc. – are impaired. Second, the rich blood supply of the skin provides an opportunity for metastatic spread of infection both from the skin as the initial portal of entry and to the skin from other sources. The skin is readily available and easily accessible for examination and biopsy that can provide an "early warning" sign to the clinician that systemic dissemination of infection has occurred. Third, skin infections are common in different immunocompromised patient populations.

The immunocompromised host is an individual with one or more defects in the body's natural defense mechanisms sufficient to predispose that individual to infection. The population of patients at risk has expanded and the etiology of these infections has expanded since the last edition. The principal examples of compromised patients are those with acute leukemia, lymphoma, acquired immune deficiency syndrome (AIDS), solid organ and hematopoietic stem cell transplants, anti-rejection therapy, graft versus host disease, malignancy receiving aggressive and intensive chemotherapeutic regimens, multiple myeloma, or chronic lymphocytic leukemia, and patients with a variety of autoimmune diseases treated with systemic corticosteroids or other immunosuppressant drugs including the newest tumor necrosis factor (TNF) inhibitors, T-cell depleting therapies, and other immunomodulators. Every immunosuppressive regimen that has been devised to prevent rejection increases infection. Excluded from this text are primary immunodeficiency diseases, hyper-IgE syndrome, chronic granulomatous disease, diabetes mellitus, uremia, alcoholism, severe burns, protein/calorie malnutrition, advanced age, premature birth, and asplenic patients.

The most important factors that predispose to infection are: (a) neutropenia, (b) cellular immune dysfunction, (c) humoral immune deficiency, and (d) damage to the anatomic barriers (skin or mucous membranes). Other risk factors for infection include medical or surgical procedures, irradiation, indwelling catheters and medical devices (such as left ventricular assist devices (LVADS) pre-heart transplantation). Broad-spectrum antibiotics, antimicrobial prophylaxis (such as fluconazole for antifungal prophylaxis or ganciclovir for cytomegalovirus [CMV] prophylaxis), and prolonged hospitalization cause alterations in the normal microbial flora and produce the opportunity to acquire new organisms that may be environmental pathogens or resistant to various antibiotics. Other potential sources of infection besides endogenous flora include contaminated air, water, and food, and direct contact with individuals carrying potential pathogens particularly within the hospital environment. The presence or absence of infection with one or more of the known immunomodulating viruses (CMV, Epstein-Barr virus [EBV], hepatitis B or C, human immunodeficiency virus (HIV), and perhaps human herpes virus [HHV] 6 and 7) has been known to accentuate the severity of opportunistic infections.

In addition to the classification of skin infections in the immunocompromised host on the basis of microbial etiology (listed in the Table of Contents), these cases can also be categorized on the basis of the pathophysiologic events that have occurred:

1. Infection originating in the skin and typical of that occurring in immunocompetent patients albeit with the potential for more serious consequences
2. Widespread or extensive cutaneous involvement with organisms that usually produce localized or trivial infection in immunocompetent individuals
3. Infection originating in the skin caused by opportunistic organisms that rarely produce disease in immunocompetent patients but which may produce localized or disseminated infection in immunocompromised individuals
4. Disseminated systemic infection metastatic to the skin from a noncutaneous portal of entry

1. *Typical primary skin infection*

Conventional forms of infections originating in the skin such as cellulitis appear to be increased in incidence and severity in immunocompromised patients. These infections are commonly caused by Gram-positive organisms such as Group A *Streptococcus* and *Staphylococcus aureus*. The cutaneous lesions may be indistinguishable from those of other unusual organisms, making diagnosis difficult from clinical assessment alone. Neutropenic patients appear prone to cellulitis caused by *Pseudomonas* and other Gram-negatives or anaerobes. Individuals with leukemia or other diseases or medications affecting cell-mediated immunity may have cellulitis caused by *Cryptococcus neoformans*. This emphasizes the need for skin biopsy, special stains, and cultures for routine appearing skin infections if there is not an adequate response to what appears to be the appropriate antimicrobial therapy.

2. *Unusually widespread cutaneous infection*

Usually minor skin infections in normal individuals such as human papillomavirus and superficial fungal infections are more common, more extensive, and may be associated with serious systemic consequences in immunosuppressed patients. Although single verruca are common in normal individuals, in patients receiving chronic immunosuppressive therapy, warts may be so numerous as to be disfiguring. Warts (condyloma acuminatum) may be so florid with HIV infection as to cause anal blockage. Unusual clinical presentations such as oral condyloma acuminatum may occur in these patients. Warts in immunosuppressed patients are of more than cosmetic significance, as malignant transformation, particularly in sun-exposed areas, has been well documented.

Unusually widespread cutaneous infection may be due to "nonvirulent fungi" in addition to viruses. The fungi include dermatophytes, which have both an increased incidence and an increased severity of infection. In these patients local disease, especially on the extremities, can provide a potential portal of entry for life-threatening bacterial superinfection.

More extensive skin involvement with organisms usually causing limited local infection may occur with herpes simplex, herpes zoster, molluscum contagiosum, human papilloma virus, *Malassezia* species, and scabies.

These common skin diseases may not respond to the usual therapies at all or may require higher doses of medication for prolonged periods or repeated surgical procedures. Dermatophyte infections may be poorly responsive to topical and oral antifungal medications. In many cases, treatment must be continued indefinitely because, when therapy ceases, prompt recurrence may be seen.

3. *Opportunistic primary skin infections*

In most cases, infections follow some form of injury to the skin that has provided the opportunity for these usually nonvirulent microbes to invade. Then with secondary host defenses impaired, significant local or disseminated disease may result. Important causes of localized disease include the fungi *Paecilomyces*, *Penicillium*, *Alternaria*, *Fusarium*, and *Trichosporon*; the atypical mycobacterium; and the alga *Prototheca wickerhamii*. New organisms have appeared in the immunocompromised patient population. These emerging infections have occurred with increasing frequency.

Dissemination and systemic disease followed primary skin infection with *Aspergillus*, *Candida*, and *Rhizopus* species.

Both invasive aspergillosis and disseminated candidiasis with the skin as the primary site of infection have been observed in patients whose skin has been injured by intravenous therapy. Fungal spores of *Rhizopus* contaminating Elastoplast (Beiersdorf UK Limited, Birmingham, United Kingdom) tape used for occlusive dressings resulted in both locally invasive and disseminated infection.

4. *Disseminated infection metastatic to the skin*

Hematogenous dissemination to the skin and subcutaneous tissues from a distant primary site may be the first clinical sign of a widespread life-threatening infection. Three groups of organisms are responsible for this category of cutaneous infection in the immunocompromised host: (a) *Pseudomonas aeruginosa* and to a lesser extent other bacteria; (b) the endemic or endogenous infections such as the so-called geographically restricted fungi *Histoplasma capsulatum*, *Coccidioides immitis*, and *Blastomyces dermatitidis* or the parasites in patients from endemic areas such as *Strongyloides stercoralis*; and (c) the opportunistic organisms *Nocardia* species, *Aspergillus* species, *Cryptococcus neoformans*, *Candida* species, *Scedosporium*, hyaline and black molds, and Mucoraceae.

An important aspect of dermatologic diagnosis in the normal host is the gross morphologic appearance of the skin lesion. In the immunocompromised patient, this approach is limited because the variety of organisms causing infection in this population is greater than in normals, and the inflammatory response to the microbe is altered. Even the most banal appearing skin lesion may represent an unusual infection. The physician must consider the "zebras," or the rare infections, as well as the routine ones in disguise. Common entities may assume unusual or bizarre presentations while serious opportunistic infections may be nondescript clinical lesions. The clinician must keep a high index of suspicion that the innocuous skin lesion or the "harmless" laboratory contaminant represents a devastating pathogen in the compromised host. For these reasons, the differential diagnosis of any skin lesion is large and skin biopsy most useful in making a diagnosis.

An infectious process should always be considered in an immunocompromised patient with skin lesions even though fever may not be present. Just as the clinical manifestations of an infectious disease may be unusual, so too may the histologic appearances be bizarre. An inflammatory response may be absent on a skin biopsy specimen. The inability of an immunosuppressed patient to mount an inflammatory response may account for the absence of neutrophils, plasma cells, multinucleated giant cells, or granulomas, usually found with an infection. The pathologist must not be fooled by an unimpressive infiltrate. If the pathologist reads a biopsy specimen as showing panniculitis or vasculitis, the clinician must consider an infectious panniculitis or vasculitis and request appropriate special stains or cultures. Even if a pathogen is identified histologically or by culture from a skin biopsy specimen, the possibility of more than one pathogen or pathologic process should be considered. Complex combined infections may present in the same lesion.

To maximize the chance of identifying the invading organism by skin biopsy, appropriate stains and cultures should be obtained. A wedge excision is preferred, half of which is sent to the pathology laboratory for both routine processing and special stains (for fungi, mycobacteria, and conventional bacteria). The other half is sent to the microbiology laboratory for aerobic and anaerobic bacterial, fungal (at 25°C and 37°C), and mycobacterial culture, and Gram, acid-fast, and fungal stains of touch preparations, ground material from biopsied tissue, or both.

Any unexplained skin lesion in an immunocompromised patient should be biopsied for culture and histologic examination. The skin biopsy is inexpensive, relatively noninvasive, without contraindication, and may avoid the performance of more serious invasive procedures such as open lung biopsies and liver biopsies. Early diagnosis may be made by skin biopsy, as blood cultures and other diagnostic studies (such as antibody tests) may be negative or delayed despite disseminated disease.

1

Subcutaneous and Deep Mycoses

ASPERGILLOSIS

Invasive aspergillosis is the most common opportunistic fungal infection in the hematopoetic stem cell transplant patient. Prior to the regular use of antifungal prophylaxis, invasive fungal infections caused by *Candida* were the most common infection, followed by infection by *Aspergillus*.[1] In the 1990s, 90% of *Aspergillus* infections were due to *A. fumigatus*; however *A. flavus, A. terreus, A. niger,* and *A. versicolor* are all potential causes of invasive aspergillosis. *A. flavus,* followed by *A. niger,* is the most common cause of primary cutaneous disease while *A. fumigatus* more commonly causes disseminated disease.[2] *A. glaucus, A. chevalieri,* and *A. ustus* are rare causes of cutaneous disease.[3]

Invasive aspergillosis occurs in the settings of severe or prolonged neutropenia due to cytotoxic therapy for leukemia or lymphoma, high-dose systemic corticosteroids for transplants or collagen vascular disease, a functional neutrophil defect, long-term immunosuppression for graft versus host disease (GVHD), chronic granulomatous disease, neonates, and burn wounds. It is less common, but not infrequently reported, in organ transplant recipients and human immunodeficiency virus (HIV)-positive patients. In HIV-positive patients, low CD4 counts, cytomegalovirus infection, and neutropenia either due to HIV disease, antiretroviral therapy, or ganciclovir are risk factors for cutaneous aspergillosis.[4] Emerging data also implicate polymorphisms in innate immunity genes as a risk factor for *Aspergillus* infection.[5] In patients status post stem cell transplant (SCT), invasive aspergillosis is now more common in the post engraftment phase, often due to immunosuppression for GVHD, than in the neutropenic period.[6]

Aspergillus infection can involve the skin of an immunocompromised patient as either a primary or secondary process. Primary cutaneous aspergillosis is rare in the immunocompe-tent host and should prompt an evaluation for compromised immune status when the diagnosis is made.[7] In immunocompromised patients, primary cutaneous aspergillosis is classically associated with nosocomially induced infection via contaminated intravenous cannulas, Hickman catheters, non-sterile gauze, adhesive tape, arm boards, or, rarely, in a surgical wound. Occasionally, a clear history of cutaneous injury may not be elicited.[8] Hematogenous dissemination from the skin may occur. Secondary cutaneous aspergillosis is most common in bone marrow transplant recipients and leukemic patients. It arises either from direct invasion of skin from an underlying infected structure such as the nose, sinus, or orbit, or as disseminated lesions from hematogenous spread of infection. In secondary cutaneous aspergillosis, the lungs are usually the initial site of infection.

Aspergillus is a ubiquitous fungus readily isolated from soil, plants, decaying vegetation, food, and water. Nosocomial epidemics of invasive aspergillosis in susceptible patients occur in the hospital environment when large numbers of spores are widely dispersed in the air during construction, renovation, and fire-proofing. This release of spores, coupled with both the interruption of primary host defenses (i.e., the skin and mucosal barrier) and impairment by the underlying disease and chemotherapy of secondary host defenses (i.e., neutrophils and macrophages), allow for nosocomial primary cutaneous aspergillosis to occur.

The lesions of primary cutaneous aspergillosis begin as tender erythematous or purpuric macules or papules that progress to violaceous edematous plaques, often with hemorrhagic bullae. Lesions tend to be large (centimeters) and single or a few grouped lesions if multiple. Lesions then develop dark centers and maintain a peripheral brightly purpuric rim. They may then ulcerate or form black necrotic eschars. The bullous phase of invasive aspergillosis is important to recognize, as potassium hydroxide (KOH) preparation of the hemorrhagic blister roof can provide an

M.E. Grossman et al., *Cutaneous Manifestations of Infection in the Immunocompromised Host,*
DOI 10.1007/978-1-4419-1578-8_1, © Springer Science+Business Media, LLC 2012

immediate presumptive diagnosis.[9] Cutaneous aspergillosis should be suspected when a hemorrhagic bulla or necrotizing plaque develops in an immunocompromised host, particularly if the patient is receiving broad-spectrum antibiotic therapy. The initial erythematous phase of invasive aspergillosis can be mistaken for a cellulitis or an irritant contact dermatitis to an arm board or tape. The straight borders of a hemorrhagic bulla would suggest a contact dermatitis in a thrombocytopenic leukemic patient. Erythematous to violaceous, sometimes suppurative, plaques studded with pustules, occasionally mimicking *Candida*, are an emerging clinical presentation of cutaneous aspergillosis.[10-12]

Less common presentations or morphologies of primary cutaneous aspergillosis include otomycosis[13]; nodules[14]; necrotic, zosteriform lesions followed by widespread eschars and death[15]; subcutaneous tumor with mild purple color to the overlying skin[16]; tender nodule with a dusky, necrotic center[7]; ulceration with overlying gray necrosis of the dorsum of the tongue[17]; infiltrated plaque on the nares and nasal skin[18]; retronuchal erythematous swelling[18]; sporotrichoid nodules with a fluctuant ipsilateral mass[19]; and a dehisced surgical wound with black necrotic margins in a heart transplant patient.[20]

Primary cutaneous aspergillosis in HIV-positive patients is most commonly due to *A. fumigatus*.[4] Lesions near catheter insertion sites and under adhesive tape are characteristic. Secondary cutaneous disease is exceptionally rare in this patient group.[4,21] Unusual presentations of *Aspergillus* in HIV-positive patients include Majocchi's granuloma presenting as a red brown plaque with surrounding pustule[22]; a violaceous plaque covered in a yellow-brown crust with adjacent follicular papules[23]; umbilicated papules resembling molluscum contagiosum[24]; nodules, fluctuant papules, deep seated pustules, vesicopustular plaques, and nonhealing ulcers[4]; and penile papules and ulcerated plaques under a condom catheter.[25]

Skin manifestations of secondary or disseminated aspergillosis are uncommon and occur in less than 10% of patients with invasive aspergillosis. However, cutaneous lesions may be the presenting sign of disseminated disease.[26] They appear as erythematous macules, papules, or nodules that become purpuric, hemorrhagic, necrotic, or ulcerate[27,28]; a hemorrhagic bulla; or subcutaneous nodules or abscesses. Other presentations include a cellulitic plaque on the leg with erythematous, firm, subcutaneous nodules within the plaque and violaceous firm nodules on the axilla and elbow[29]; verrucous lesions in addition to typical erythematous to violaceous papules and nodules with central necrosis[28]; extension from underlying sinus infection to overlying skin presenting with vegetative plaques with crusts on the nares, hemorrhagic bullae overlying the eyelid, and hemorrhagic plaques on the face[28]; or linear suppurative and ulcerative nodules.[30] Transmission of invasive aspergillosis from an infected donor to a host, who presented with *Aspergillus* endocarditis and periorbital and skin lesions, has been reported.[31]

Skin biopsy specimens from *Aspergillus* infected patients demonstrate acute angle, regularly septate, dichotomously branching hyphal elements that may be angioinvasive. The histopathologic differential diagnosis includes several other opportunistic fungi including *Fusarium*, *Scopulariopsis*, *Pseudallescheria*, and *Penicillium* which appear identical to *Aspergillus* in tissue. In primary cutaneous disease, the inflammatory infiltrate is superficial or superficial and deep. In secondary cutaneous aspergillosis, the infiltrate is in the deep dermis and subcutaneous fat; intravascular thrombosis with masses of hyphae may be seen.[3] While a skin biopsy is needed to prove invasive disease, isolation in culture of the organism from tissue specimens is needed for definitive identification of the fungus.

Enzyme linked immunoassay (ELISA) testing for the galactomannan antigen may aid in the diagnosis of invasive aspergillosis. Galactomannan is a carbohydrate component of the *Aspergillus* cell wall that is released during hyphal growth. It requires angioinvasion of the organism to be detected and can be tested in serum, brocheoalveolar lavage fluid, or cerebral spinal fluid. The sensitivity of the test ranges from 65% to 90% and the specificity is ≥90%; thus, a negative result rules out disease while a positive result requires a second positive to confirm true infection. False negatives occur if patients are tested while on antifungal agents or if there is limited angioinvasion. False positives occur with loss of integrity of gastrointestinal mucosa (mucositis, neonates, GVHD, cytotoxic chemotherapy) or with the use of piperacillin-tazobactam.[32] The β-D-glucan assay is a nonspecific marker for invasive fungal infection as it detects the β-D-glucan component of the cell wall of various fungi including *Aspergillus*, *Fusarium*, *Trichosporon*, and *Candida*. Its sensitivity is 70% while its specificity is 87–94%.[32] It is not as widely used as the galactomannan ELISA.

Primary cutaneous aspergillosis has a more favorable prognosis than secondary or disseminated disease. Surgical excision in addition to systemic antifungal therapy may be beneficial for primary cutaneous aspergillosis. Systemic treatment is with antifungal therapy such as amphotericin B, itraconazole, voriconazole, or an echinocandin. Fluconazole is not an effective treatment for aspergillosis.

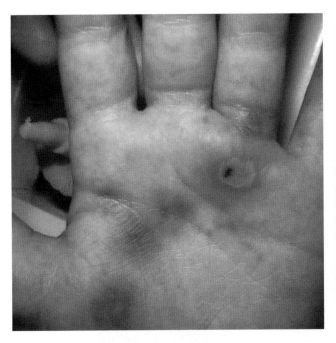

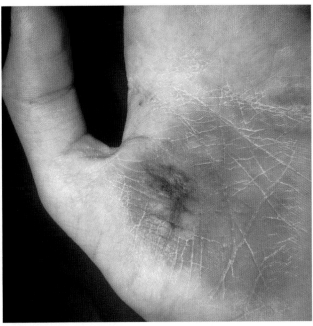

Figure 1.1. Purpuric papules and a gray flat bullae due to *Aspergillus flavus* on the palm of a 7-year-old with acute lymphocytic leukemia (ALL) on the 15th day of chemotherapy, febrile with an absolute neutrophil count of 60 on triple antibiotics

Figure 1.3. A 4 × 6-cm erythematous patch with a central hemorrhagic bulla on the palm of a 13-year-old with ALL on her 11th day of antibiotics for *Staphylococcus aureus* sepsis and osteomyelitis with an absolute neutrophil count of 42

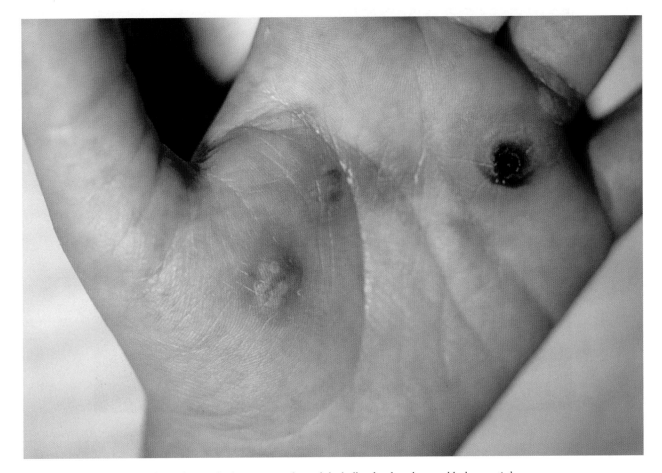

Figure 1.2. Forty-eight hours later, the papules became pustular and the bullae developed a gray-black necrotic base

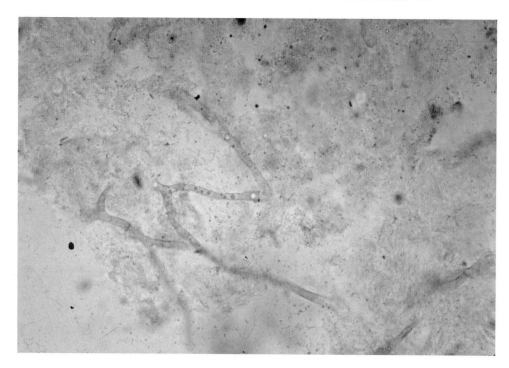

Figure 1.4.   A wet mount of a blister with potassium hydroxide and Parker blue-black ink, which stains the *Aspergillus* hyphae. The characteristic broad hyphae dichotomously branched with acute angles are present. Fungal cultures confirmed the diagnosis of aspergillosis

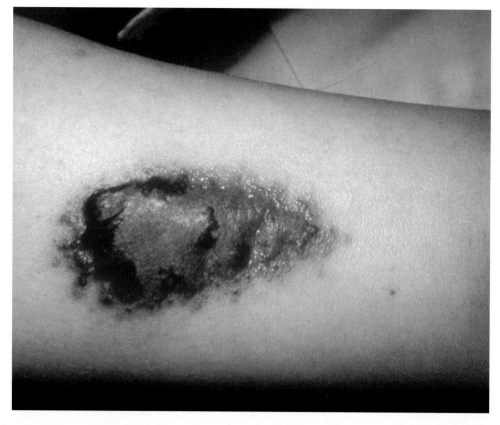

Figure 1.5.   A hemorrhagic bulla with linear vesicular borders on the forearm of a 9-year-old with ALL. Potassium hydroxide (KOH) preparation, biopsy, and culture demonstrated *Aspergillus fumigatus*

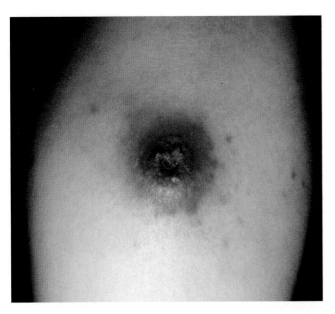

Figure 1.6. A 3×3-cm hemorrhagic nodule with a black necrotic eschar was surgically excised from a 7-year old with ALL. A touch preparation of the biopsy revealed typical hyphae of *Aspergillus. A. flavus* was confirmed by culture

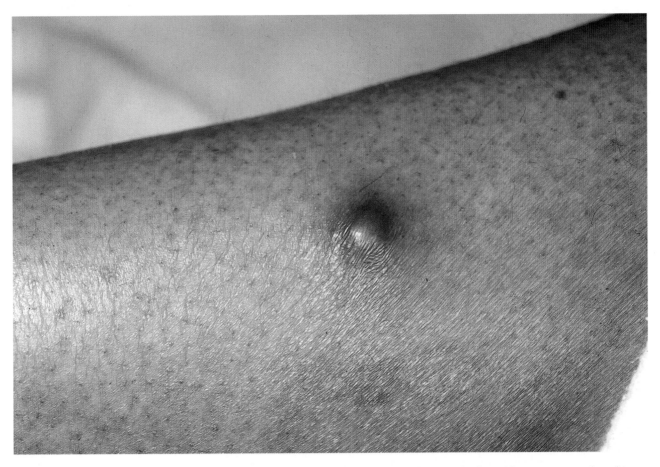

Figure 1.7. Four months after cardiac transplantation, a new non-tender subcutaneous nodule was noted on the anterior thigh of a 50-year-old man. An "iceberg lesion" was surgically excised and *A. flavus* was demonstrated on biopsy and culture. After a negative workup, this was felt to be primary cutaneous aspergillosis

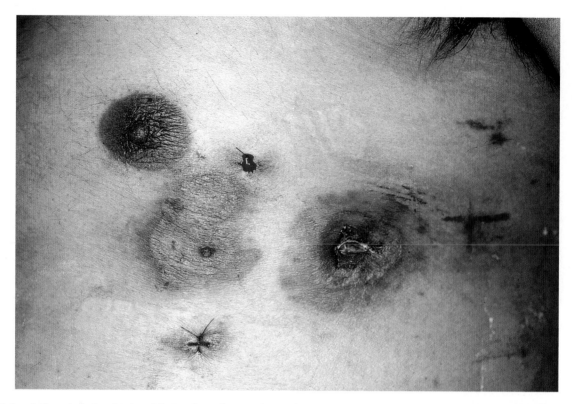

Figure 1.8.   *A. flavus* infection developed during chemotherapy where a chest tube had been in a 24-year-old with Hodgkin's disease

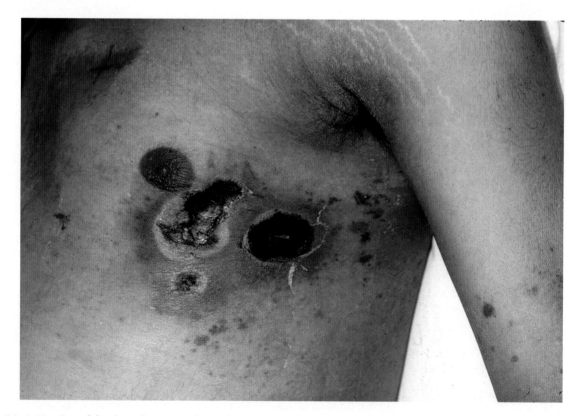

Figure 1.9.–1.11.   Several days later, the purpuric hemorrhagic plaques became necrotic black eschars

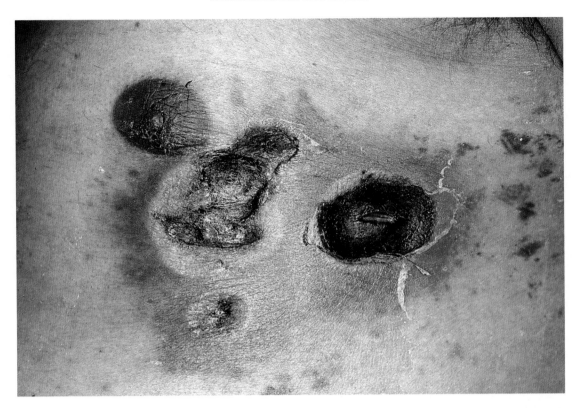

Figure 1.10.

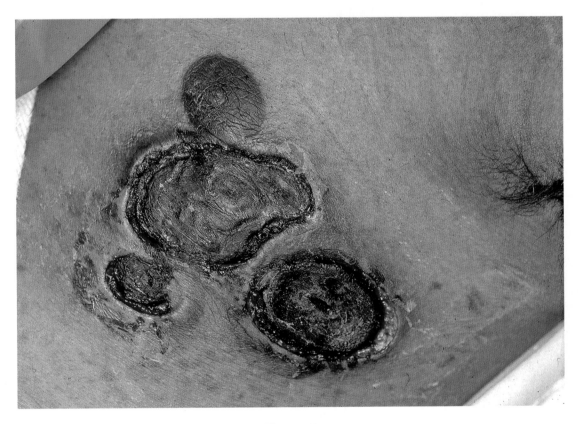

Figure 1.11.

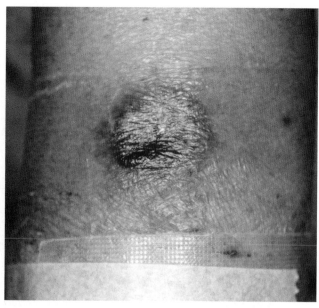

Figure 1.13.   Close-up of the black necrotic bulla

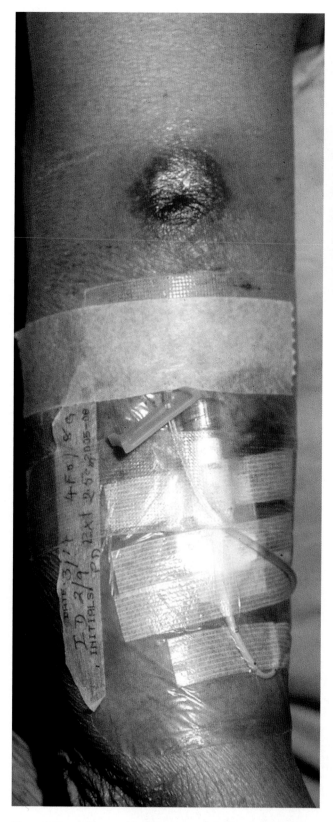

Figure 1.12.   A 73-year-old with neutropenic fever post chemotherapy for AML developed a hemorrhagic necrotic bulla above the peripherally inserted central catheter (PICC) line on her arm due to *Aspergillus flavus*

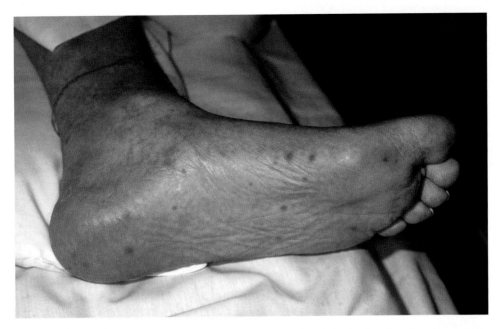

Figure 1.14. Fatal disseminated *A. fumigatus* in multiple myeloma. Purpuric papulonodules developed on the palms and soles

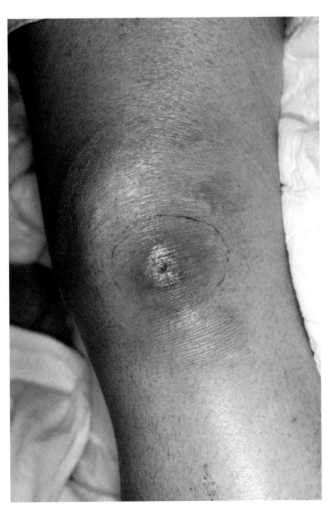

Figure 1.15. A 44-year-old man with peripheral T cell lymphoma developed neutropenic fevers post chemotherapy and a hemorrhagic necrotic knee bulla due to *Aspergillus* species

BLASTOMYCOSIS

Blastomyces dermatitidis is a dimorphic fungus endemic to the Mississippi and Ohio River valleys and the Great Lakes region in the USA, the central provinces of Canada that border the Great Lakes, in the areas of New York and Canada adjacent to the St. Lawrence Seaway, and wide portions of Africa. India is a newly recognized endemic focus.[33] Dogs may transmit the fungus to humans through a bite wound.[34] Blastomycosis may present as pulmonary, disseminated, or primary cutaneous disease, with cutaneous disease secondary to dissemination accounting for approximately 60% of cases involving the skin.[35] Human infection usually occurs through inhalation and most commonly leads to asymptomatic infection. Inhalation disease may be associated with erythema nodosum. Primary cutaneous inoculation blastomycosis is rare, but presents as a solitary chancre-like ulcer with associated lymphangitis, lymphadenitis, and nodules along lymphatics.[36]

Clinically, lesions typical of blastomycosis present either as a plateau-like ulcerated or verrucous plaque with a scarred center and edges that are studded with pustules or a pustule that develops into an ulcer with a granulating base and heaped up borders.[36,37] Skin lesions in immunosuppressed patients tend to be more pustular and ulcerative than the typical heaped-up chronic lesions seen in patients who are not immunosuppressed.[38] Less common presentations include disseminated papulopustules which may demonstrate the yeast on potassium hydroxide staining of the exudate[37,39] and subcutaneous nodules.[35] Histopathology of blastomycosis reveals 8–15 μm thick-walled, broad-based budding yeasts that stain well with Gomori methenamine-silver stain. In immunocompromised patients, larger yeasts (greater than 40 μm in diameter) and hyphal elements have been reported.[40] Cultures take several weeks but provide definitive proof of infection with *B. dermatitidis*.

While blastomycosis most often affects immunocompetent patients, data suggest that up to 25% of patients with blastomycosis have preceding immunosuppression.[41] Severe immunosuppression, including HIV disease, chronic corticosteroid use, hematologic malignancies, organ transplantation, pregnancy, chemotherapy, and end-stage renal or liver failure, may predispose to more severe or disseminated disease[35]; however this is not substantiated by all reports.[41] Blastomycosis is an uncommon infection in solid organ transplant patients.[42] The skin, bone, genitourinary system (especially the epididymis and prostate), and central nervous system (in order of decreasing frequency) are the most common sites of disseminated disease.[34] Central nervous system (CNS) involvement occurs rarely in immunocompetent patients.[43] In solid organ transplant recipients, blastomycosis may progress rapidly and may be complicated by acute respiratory distress syndrome, dissemination and opportunistic co-infection with organisms such as cytomegalovirus, varicella zoster virus, and *Aspergillus*. Solid organ transplant recipients are less likely than HIV patients to have CNS involvement.[42]

The treatment of choice for disseminated blastomycosis is initial therapy with amphotericin B followed by itraconazole. Lifelong antifungal therapy may be required particularly in those who are profoundly immunosuppressed, have multiple opportunistic infections, experience relapse despite appropriate therapy, or have persistently positive *B. dermatitidis* cultures.[42] The mortality rate of blastomycosis in the immunocompromised is 29–40%.[35]

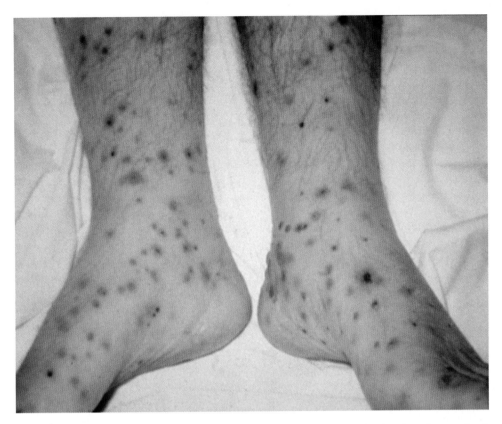

Figure 1.16. A 66-year-old man with well-differentiated lymphocytic lymphoma on chlorambucil and prednisone developed disseminated papulopustules of *Blastomyces dermatitidis* (From Pappas PG, et al. Blastomycosis in immunocompromised patients. Medicine 1993;72:311–325)

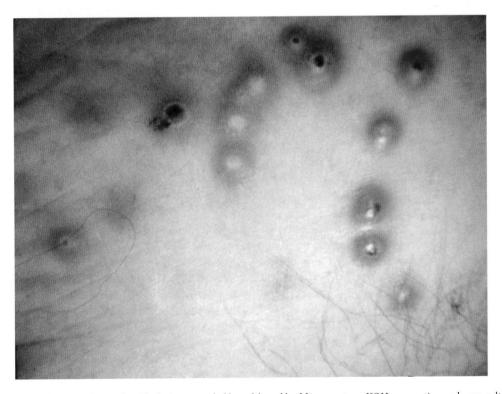

Figure 1.17. Close-up of the papulopustules. The lesions revealed broad-based budding yeasts on KOH preparation and were culture-positive for *B. dermatitidis* (From Pappas PG, et al. Blastomycosis in immunocompromised patients. Medicine 1993;72:311–325)

Candidiasis

Prior to the use of antifungal prophylaxis, candidiasis was the most common invasive fungal infection complicating patients with hematologic malignancies. Over the past two decades, *Candida* has emerged as the second most common invasive fungal infection (second to *Aspergillus*) in the patient with hematologic malignancy, status post hematopoietic stem cell transplant, and status post lung transplantation. All solid organ transplant patients taken together, *Candida* is the most common cause of invasive fungal infections.[1] The spectrum of infection includes localized forms (thrush), which usually indicate superficial colonization by the fungus, gastrointestinal infections, which may be superficially erosive and invasive (candida esophagitis), invasive visceral infections, and widespread dissemination. Conditions most strongly predisposing to disseminated candidiasis include hematologic malignancies, chemotherapy, neutropenia, radioablative therapy, immunosuppressive medications such as corticosteroids and cyclosporine, prolonged use of broad-spectrum antibiotics, heroin use, and diabetes mellitus.[44] Disseminated candidiasis is rare, but reported, in HIV-positive patients.[45,46] The source of infection is endogenous (gastrointestinal [GI] tract), nosocomial (intravenous catheter, etc), or may be transferred to the patient in a transplanted organ.[47]

In the 1980s, *Candida albicans* was the species responsible for 75% of disseminated candidal infections. Currently, however, *C. albicans* is responsible for 40–60% of cases[48] while non-*C. albicans* species such as *C. glabrata*, *C. tropicalis*, *C. krusei*, and *C. parapsilosis* now account for more than 50% of systemic candidal infections.[49] *C. tropicalis* causes 7–18%[48] and *C. krusei* 2.3%[50] of disseminated infections. In disseminated *Candida* with skin lesions, however, *C. tropicalis* is the causative species in 60%,[48] *C. krusei* in 4–61%,[50] and *C. albicans* in only 4–10%.[48]

The rise in incidence of fluconazole-resistant *C. krusei* and *C. glabrata* can be explained by the prophylactic use of azole antifungal agents[49]; in fact, the use of prior antifungal therapy has been shown to be a risk factor for developing *C. krusei* fungemia.[50] *C. ciferrii* and *C. dubliniensis* are both emerging fluconazole-resistant organisms that have been associated with systemic infection with skin lesions.[51,52] The observation that *C. tropicalis* and *C. krusei* are less frequent colonizers but more frequent pathogens suggests that both *C. tropicalis* and *C. krusei* are more pathogenic.

The high mortality of disseminated candidiasis relates to the delay in diagnosis because the clinical manifestations are usually not specific, positive blood cultures occur in only 25% of cases (often not reported until the patient is moribund or dead), cultures from other body sites may not distinguish colonization from infection, and serological tests are not uniformly reliable. The skin is involved in 10–13% of patients with disseminated candidiasis.[53] In these patients, recognition of the characteristic skin lesions may allow earlier diagnosis, treatment, and improved survival.

Skin lesions of disseminated candidiasis develop at a time the patient is febrile, neutropenic, clinically deteriorating, and failing to respond to multiple antibiotics.[54] The lesions are single, multiple, localized, or diffuse. They involve the trunk and proximal extremities with less involvement of the head and neck. There are erythematous papules and 0.5– 1 cm papulonodules, most with pale centers. Less often the papules are purpuric with necrotic centers. With recovery of the neutrophil count, the pale centers may become a distinct flat gray pustule.

Other morphologic forms of disseminated candidiasis include necrotic eschars; necrotic pustules and ulcerative plaques mimicking ecthyma gangrenosum; nodular subcutaneous abscesses; nodular folliculitis in hair-bearing areas with fever, ocular and osteoarticular lesions in heroin addicts using brown sugar heroin diluted with lemon juice or white heroin[45]; cellulitis-like, purpuric lesions in thrombocytopenic patients; "nummular brown lesions" on the legs of a leukemic patient with myelodysplastic syndrome and lethal disseminated *C. tropicalis*[55]; necrotizing *C. albicans* fasciitis three months post-op in the renal transplant surgical incision scar of an obese 64-year-old diabetic with Wegener's granulomatosis[56]; disseminated infection with skin lesions and multifocal osteomyelitis due to *C. dubliniensis*[52]; 0.5 mm erythematous papulonodules on the legs due to *C. tropicalis* sepsis 1 year after a bone marrow transplant for chronic myelogenous leukemia (CML)[44]; purpuric macules, papules, and vesicles resembling leukocytoclastic vasculitis in a 53-year-old renal transplant with candida sepsis[57]; and unilateral erythematous papules with central purpura and necrosis on the leg of an 84-year-old man with acute myelogenous leukemia with neutropenia and candida arthritis.[58]

Other clues to the diagnosis of disseminated candidiasis include ocular, musculoskeletal, and visceral involvement. Candida endophthalmitis, which can be seen on funduscopic examination, clinically presents with blurred vision, ocular pain, scotomas, or loss of visual acuity, or it may be asymptomatic. Candida muscle abscesses present as a triad of fever, papular skin rash, and diffuse muscle tenderness. The muscle pain is maximal in the lower extremities, elicited by gentle palpation, and often so severe that the patients may refuse to move his/her legs. Dissemination to the liver and spleen, hepatosplenic candidiasis with *Candida* microabscesses, is also characteristic of systemic candidiasis.

The histopathologic findings of candidiasis may be variable, ranging from a leukocytoclastic vasculitis to a sparse perivascular mononuclear cell infiltrate. Organisms are found mainly in and around dermal blood vessels, but may or may not be present in large number. Identification of *Candida* is difficult on routine hematoxylin and eosin (H&E) stained sections. Either periodic acid-Schiff (PAS) or Gomori methenamine-silver staining along with examination of step sections of the specimen may facilitate arriving at the diagnosis. Skin biopsy for culture will be positive in 50% of patients.[53] Potassium hydroxide examination or Gram stain of a touch preparation of a punch biopsy specimen may allow for rapid diagnosis.[59]

The mortality rate of *C. tropicalis* fungemia approaches 70%,[48] that of *C. albicans* 49%,[50] and that of *C. krusei* 38%.[50] The treatment of disseminated candidiasis may include amphotericin B, fluconazole, voriconazole, an echinocandin (caspofungin, micafungin), and/or flucytosine. Fluconazole is the empiric treatment of choice in a non-neutropenic and hemodynamically stable patient, unless infection with an azole-resistant, non-*C. albicans* species is suspected.[60] Echinocandins or amphotericin are preferred as empiric therapy for patients who are hemodynamically unstable or neutropenic, or if infection with a fluconazole-resistant species is suspected.[60] Antifungal therapy should then be tailored based on the sensitivity profile of the identified organism.

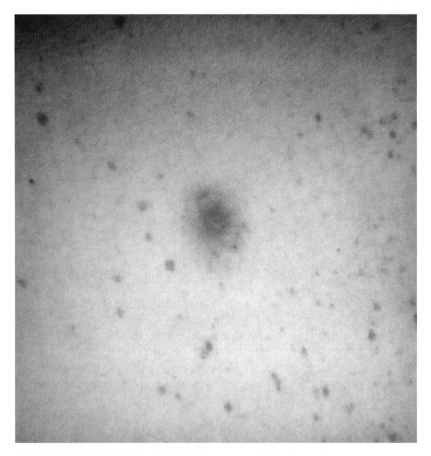

Figure 1.18. Purpuric papule with a pale center due to *Candida tropicalis* is surrounded by petechiae on the trunk of a woman with acute myelogenous leukemia (AML) in blast crisis

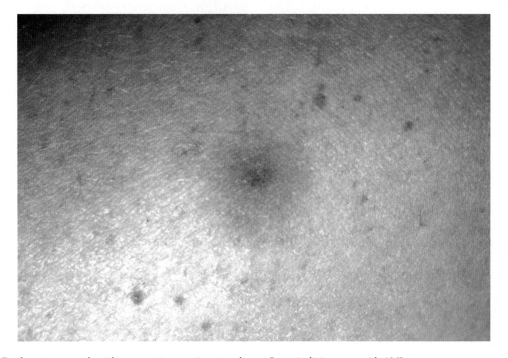

Figure 1.19. Erythematous papule with a purpuric necrotic center due to *C. tropicalis* in a man with AML

Figure 1.20. An erythematous papulonodule with a pale center due to *Candida albicans* in a patient with AML

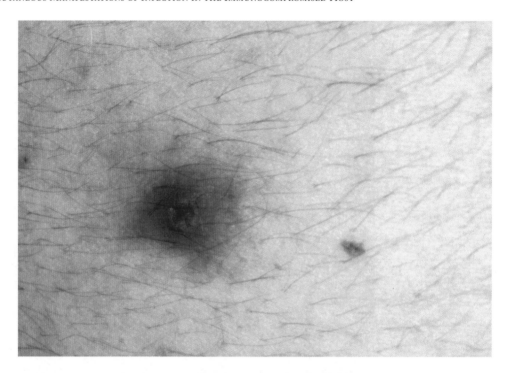

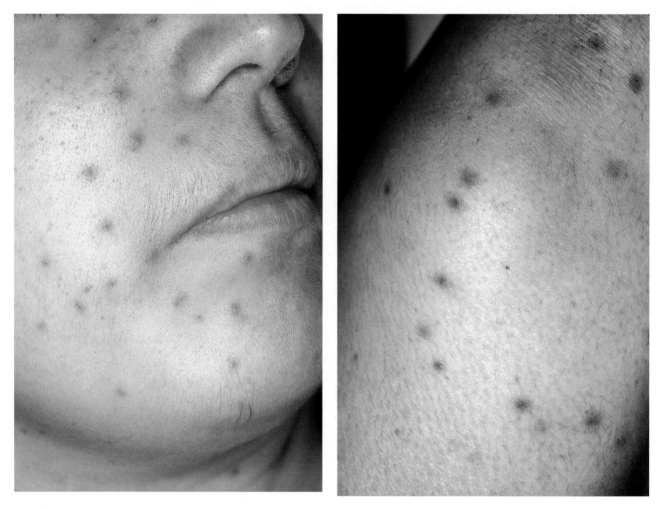

Figure 1.21. and 1.22. Disseminated erythematous papules with central erosions and crusts due to *Candida parapsilosis* in AML. Multiple lesions on the face and extremities

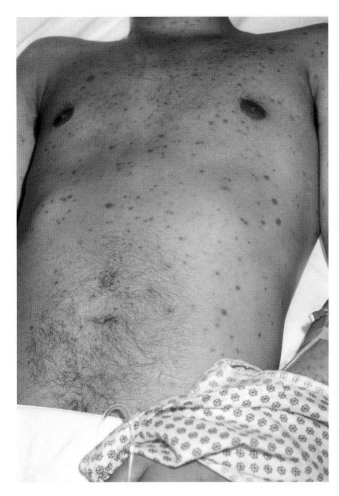

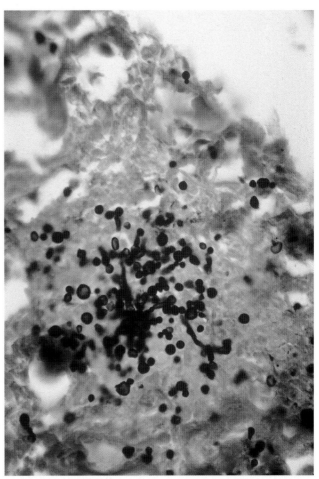

Figure 1.23. Widespread purpuric papules of *C. tropicalis* fungemia in a patient with human T cell lymphotrophic virus type I (HTLV-I)-associated leukemia

Figure 1.24. Pseudohyphae and spores of *C. tropicalis* seen in the dermis with Gomori methenamine-silver stain. A large number of organisms were limited to 20–30 μm (four to six tissue sections) of a 4-mm biopsy specimen

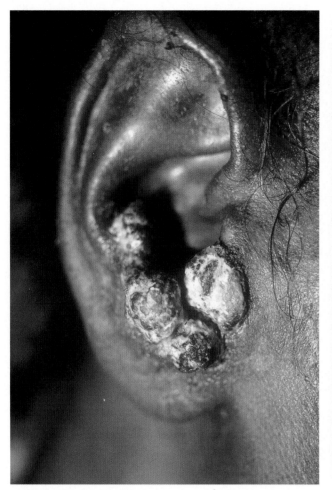

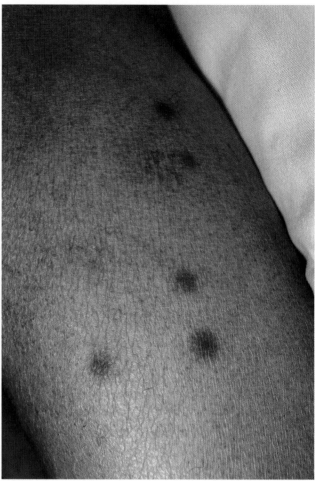

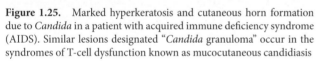

Figure 1.25. Marked hyperkeratosis and cutaneous horn formation due to *Candida* in a patient with acquired immune deficiency syndrome (AIDS). Similar lesions designated "*Candida* granuloma" occur in the syndromes of T-cell dysfunction known as mucocutaneous candidiasis

Figure 1.26. Purpuric papules of *C. tropicalis* in a patient with ALL in blast crisis

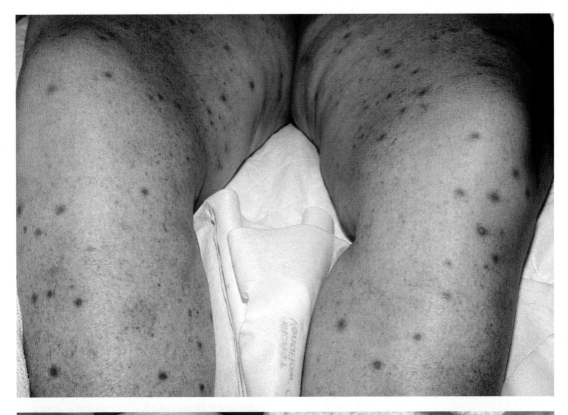

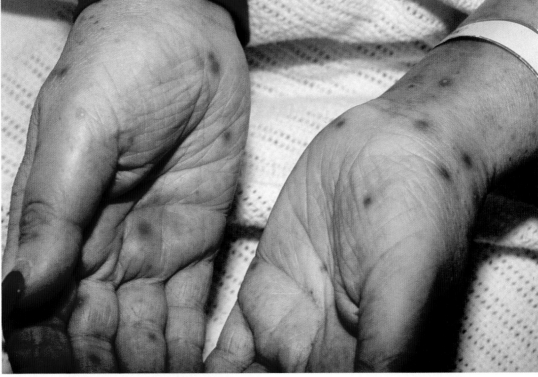

Figure 1.27. and 1.28. A 57-year-old woman with acute erythroblastic leukemia (AML, M6) developed neutropenic fever post-chemotherapy. While on broad-spectrum antibiotics, scattered purpuric papules with gray-white centers developed on the trunk, extremities, and palms. Skin biopsy and culture confirmed *Candida tropicalis* sepsis

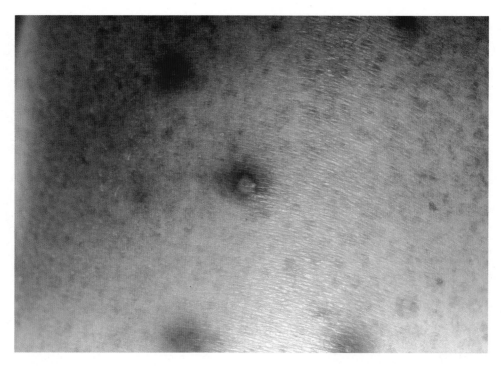

Figure 1.29. Close up of purpuric papules with pale centers due to *C. tropicalis*

Figure 1.30. A 56-year-old man with severe steroid dependent rheumatoid arthritis with extra-articular involvement including scleritis, neuropathy, and constrictive pericarditis presented with increasing joint pain and a pustular eruption. Aspiration of the joint fluid from his olecranon bursitis was positive for *Candida albicans*. Skin biopsy revealed budding yeast, and skin tissue culture and superficial pustule swab were also positive for *Candida albicans*

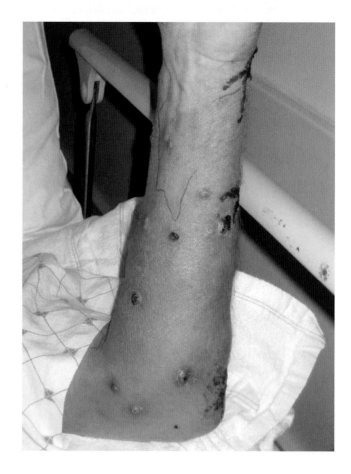

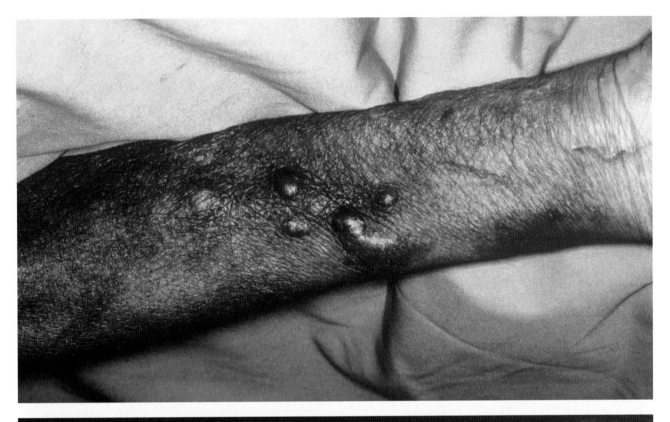

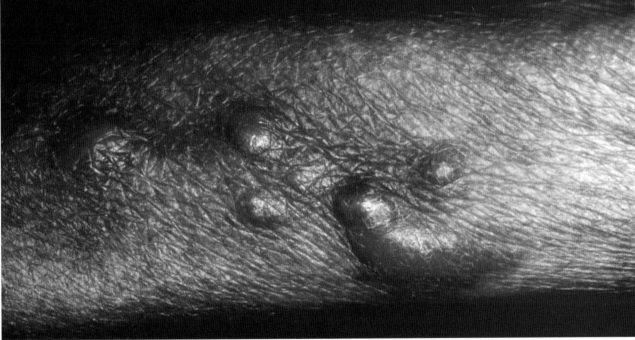

Figure 1.31. and 1.32. A 61-year-old smoker post lung transplant for chronic obstructive pulmonary disease (COPD) developed sporotrichoid nodules due to *C. albicans*

COCCIDIOIDOMYCOSIS

Coccidioides immitis, the causative agent of coccidioidomycosis, is a dimorphic soil-dwelling (saprophytic) fungus that is endemic to the San Joaquin Valley of California, southern Arizona, southern New Mexico, western Texas, Mexico, and Central and South America. In endemic areas, there is a high incidence of exposure to the fungus by inhalation of arthroconidia, but illness, when it occurs, is usually restricted to self-limited and subacute respiratory symptoms. Exposure to dust and soil, such as after dust storms, earthquakes, or droughts, or during archeological work are environmental risk factors for infection.[61] There are several groups of patients with increased risk of fulminant respiratory disease and dissemination, including pregnant women, those of African and Filipino ancestry, patients with diabetes mellitus with serum glucose ≥220 mg/dL,[62] and immunocompromised individuals such as those with hematologic malignancy, transplants, and HIV infection. New data suggest that biologic agents, such as the tumor necrosis factor-α inhibitors infliximab and etanercept, may also predispose to acute, symptomatic disease that typically presents as pneumonia.[63] Although those who recovery from self-limited infections are thought to develop lifelong immunity to the organism, there is evidence to suggest that following exposure, the organism is contained by the immune system but not eradicated, so that immunosuppression later in life may lead to reactivation of the disease.

The cutaneous manifestations of coccidioidomycosis can be divided into two categories: reactive, which includes erythema nodosum, acute generalized exanthem (toxic erythema), erythema multiforme-like eruptions, Sweet syndrome, and reactive interstitial granulomatous dermatitis; and due to the organism itself, either secondary to dissemination to the skin or, rarely, primary inoculation.[61]

There is a large clinical experience with concurrent exposure to *Coccidioides* and immunosuppressive states since densely populated areas of the USA, such as southern California and parts of Arizona, are endemic for the fungus and areas where immunosuppressed (by illness or iatrogenically) patients may be found. Coccidioidomycosis is an acquired immune deficiency syndrome (AIDS) defining disease, with CD4 counts less than 250/μL predisposing to active infection.[61] Despite this, reports of skin lesions of coccidioidomycosis in immunocompromised hosts are rare. This may be true because disseminated coccidioidal infection in immunosuppressed conditions is often rapidly fatal, leaving no time for skin lesions to develop. Erythema nodosum and toxic erythemas, which may represent cutaneous hypersensitivity reactions to coccidioidal infection, are also rare in the immunocompromised patient, but for a different reason: they depend on cell-mediated (type IV) hypersensitivity, which is deficient in most immunosuppressed states.

Disseminated coccidioidomycosis presents with systemic symptoms such as fever, cough, and night sweats. Dissemination to the skin, meninges, bones, and joints is common.[61] Skin lesions of disseminated coccidioidomycosis, most commonly verrucous plaques (usually facial), subcutaneous cold abscesses, and ulcerations, are rarely seen in immunocompromised hosts. Specific skin lesions described in immunosuppressed patients include papulopustules[64]; morbilliform eruption; an indurated, erythematous plaque on the thigh and erythema and edema of distal fingers after fomite transmitted coccidioidomycosis in an immunosuppressed child (skin biopsy not performed)[65]; abscess[66]; necrotizing cellulitis[67]; erythematous masses on the buttocks at the site of pentamidine injections in an HIV-positive patient (*locus minoris resistentiae*)[68]; a cellulitic plaque that developed into an ulcerated nodule on the cheek in a patient with rheumatoid arthritis on infliximab and methotrexate[69]; verrucous, infiltrated nodule, then multiple nodules, and later with lymph node involvement in a patient with mycosis fungoides on isotretinoin and prednisone who then developed adenocarcinoma of the lung[70]; ulcerated eyelid nodule with central ulceration and multiple microabscesses on the palpebral conjunctiva that disseminated into indurated nodules on chest, arms, and scalp in a patient on prednisone for febrile illness that was presumed (incorrectly) to be giant cell arteritis but was actually coccidioidomycosis[71]; and raised, red, ulcerating lesions.[72]

The diagnosis of coccidioidomycosis is made via culture of the organism, demonstration of the organism in biopsy tissue specimens, or serologic testing via enzyme immunoassay, immunodiffusion, and complement fixation. Quantitative testing with IgG complement-fixing antibodies will be positive after 2–3 weeks of symptoms. A positive titer strongly suggests true infection and levels tend to correlate with disease severity. False negative serologic results are uncommon, but may occur in immunosuppressed patients. On skin biopsy specimens, the 10–80 μm spherules are visible on H&E as well as by fungal stains. When sending a specimen for culture to the laboratory when the suspicion for coccidioidomycosis is high, it is imperative to alert the laboratory, as the organism is extremely infectious in the mycelial form and may infect unprotected laboratory workers.[61]

While the need for antifungal therapy for the immunocompetent patient without disseminated coccidioidomycosis is controversial, treatment of the immunocompromised patient with antifungal therapy with amphotericin B, fluconazole, or itraconazole is indicated. Continued therapy (for duration of immunosuppression in transplant patients[73] and lifelong in HIV-positive patients[74]) with an azole such as fluconazole is recommended after the initial infection has been treated.

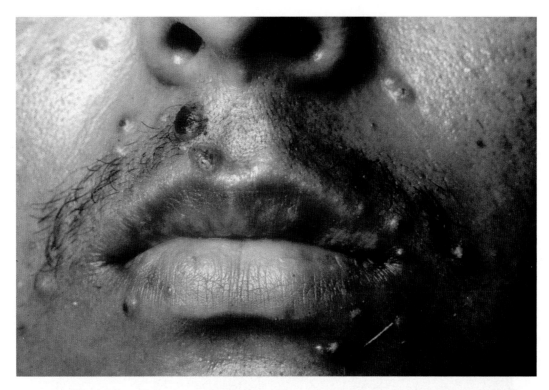

Figure 1.33. Perioral crusted papules of disseminated coccidioidomycosis in a renal transplant recipient (Courtesy of Peter Phillips, M.D.)

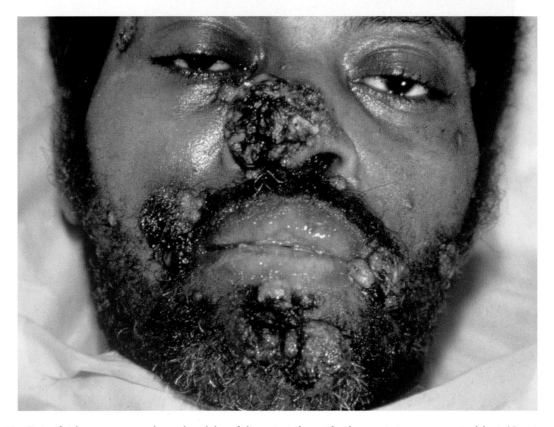

Figure 1.34. Periorificial verrucous papules and nodules of disseminated coccidioidomycosis in a compromised host (Courtesy of Victor Newcomer, M.D.)

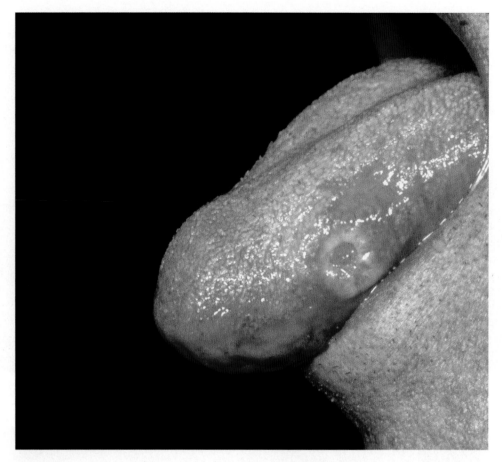

Figure 1.35.   Lateral tongue ulcer due to coccidioidomycosis in an immunocompromised patient

CRYPTOCOCCOSIS

Cryptococcus neoformans is an encapsulated yeast that may be found in soil and wood contaminated with pigeon or other bird excreta and decaying wood, fruits, and vegetables. *C. neoformans* serotype D has been shown to have a predilection for the skin over serotypes A, B, or C. Non-neoformans species, such as *C. albidus*, have rarely been associated with cutaneous disease, most often in immunocompromised patients.[75] *Cryptococcus* is usually acquired following inhalation of spores with primary pulmonary involvement, either obvious or occult. The most common site of disseminated infection is the central nervous system. The skin is the most common extraneural site of infection.[76] In the immunocompromised patient, hematogenous dissemination to the meninges, skin, bone, and kidney occurs. An HIV-positive patient who presents with fever, headache (or other meningeal or craniobulbar manifestations), and skin lesions should be suspected of cryptococcal infection. Most cases of disseminated *Cryptococcus* infection represent reactivation of latent infection.[77]

Although there are some reports of primary cutaneous cryptococcosis, more often cryptococcal skin disease is a sentinel of disseminated disease, with skin lesions presenting in some cases up to 8 months before other signs of systemic infection. Therefore, when cutaneous cryptococcal infection has been diagnosed, a careful search for extracutaneous disease is warranted.

Immunocompromise by HIV/AIDS, systemic corticosteroids, hematologic or solid organ malignancy, CD4+ lymphopenia, chemotherapy, immunosuppression after solid organ transplantation, sarcoidosis, diabetes mellitus, and, rarely, cirrhosis,[78] all predispose to cryptococcal infection. In non-HIV related immunosuppression, the most frequent skin manifestations are cellulitis, subcutaneous nodules, and ulcers. Cellulitis is the most common presentation of cryptococcal infection in solid organ transplant (SOT) recipients.[79] Patients with SOT who receive a calcineurin inhibitor (tacrolimus or cyclosporine) are less likely to develop disseminated or CNS cryptococcal infection and are more likely to manifest skin, soft tissue, osteoarticular or lung involvement.[77-81] Both cyclosporine and tacrolimus suppress growth of *C. neoformans* in vitro by inhibition of the calcineurin pathway at 37°C but not at 24°C, which suggests that this pathway is essential to the fungus only at higher environmental temperatures.[80] Tacrolimus crosses the blood brain barrier better than cyclosporine. It has been suggested that temperature dependent inhibition of *Cryptococcus* species by tacrolimus may prevent CNS infection but allow viability at cooler body sites such as the skin and subcutaneous tissues.[79-82] Tumor necrosis factor-α inhibitor therapy (with and without concomitant methotrexate) has been associated with cryptococcosis.[83,84] In AIDS, the polymorphic cutaneous presentations have included cutaneous lesions resembling herpes simplex, molluscum contagiosum, and ulcerations. However, any morphology may be seen in the immunosuppressed patient.

Disseminated *Cryptococcus neoformans* to the skin in the immunocompromised host occurs in 10–15% of patients with cryptococcal infection. The cutaneous manifestations of disseminated cryptococcosis are protean. More than one morphology may be present simultaneously. In HIV-positive patients, lesions most commonly present on the head and neck as multiple molluscum contagiosum-like umbilicated papules with a central hemorrhagic crust.[85] These lesions often vary in size and may be as large as 3 cm.[86] Cutaneous cryptococcosis resembling molluscum contagiosum has also been reported as a manifestation of the immune reconstitution syndrome.[87] A more acute onset of numerous papules, variation in size, and a central hemorrhagic crust may help the clinician distinguish cryptococcal lesions from molluscum contagiosum.

Cryptococcal cellulitis, more often a sign of disseminated disease than primary cutaneous infection, presents with the same erythema, warmth, and tenderness as bacterial cellulitis. Therefore, cellulitis worsening despite intravenous antibiotics in the immunocompromised host should raise the suspicion for cutaneous cryptococcosis. Lesions typically present on an extremity in a single location, but, in the immunocompromised host, multiple sites of cellulitis may be present. Vesicles, bullae, or subcutaneous abscesses may develop. Bullae may rupture to produce areas of ulcerations. An erysipelas-like lesion that initially grew *S. aureus* and *E. cloacae*, but on skin biopsy and culture of the ulcer base demonstrated *Cryptococcus* has been reported in a patient on chronic systemic corticosteroids, again highlighting the need for a high index of suspicion for fungal infection in the immunosuppressed patient.[88] Necrotizing fasciitis with necrosis of the skin, fat, fascia, and superficial muscle has been documented in a patient with pemphigus vegetans controlled with cyclophosphamide pulse therapy and systemic corticosteroids.[89] Other cases of necrotizing fasciitis and necrotizing cellulitis due to cryptococcal infection have been reported in renal and cardiac transplant recipients.[90,91] The lower extremities are the most common site of infection and, in contrast to bacterial necrotizing fasciitis, bilateral disease is common. Multiple site involvement is likely a reflection of disseminated infection.[91]

Cystic or firm subcutaneous nodules that may ulcerate either spontaneously or after incision may be signs of systemic cryptococcosis. The nodules may be red, warm, and resemble staphylococcal abscesses or erythema nodosum.[92] Disseminated cryptococcosis may simulate the erythema nodosum-like lesions in Behçet's disease treated with systemic steroids. When the nodules fail to resolve with antibiotics, develop a bruised appearance, or ulcerate a deep fungal infection should be suspected.

Disseminated cryptococcosis may also present as palpable purpura; single or multiple ulcers (cutaneous and mucosal, including the penis) due to *C. albidus* in a 70-year-old with Sezary syndrome[75] and vulva of a 60-year-old renal transplant recipient[93]; pustules; a maculopapular eruption mimicking a drug rash; papules, subcutaneous nodules or abscesses[94]; papulonodules[95]; pustular-ulcerative lesions[95]; an ulcerated solitary subcutaneous nodule on the forearm in a patient with AIDS and a CD4 count of 5 cells/mm^3; scattered crusted papules and plaques and a verrucous exophytic nodule on the nose of a 49-year-old HIV-positive man with a CD4 count of

9 cells/mm[396]; vesicles that develop into suppurative erythematous nodules[88]; linear sclerotic scaly plaques,[92] and a tender oval plaque on the penis of a 39-year-old with AIDS.[97]

The cutaneous lesions of *Cryptococcus* may mimic other primary dermatologic disorders in addition to molluscum contagiosum such as pyoderma gangrenosum, rhinophyma, herpes simplex, Kaposi sarcoma, follicular or nummular eczema,[85] ulcerated squamous cell carcinoma of the vulva,[93] keratoacanthoma,[96] keloid,[98] and basal cell carcinoma.[99,100] Acneiform papules and pustules with a predilection for the face and neck due to disseminated *Cryptococcus* may enlarge, ulcerate, and coalesce. Facial papules with central necrosis and vesicles can simulate varicella. Simultaneous involvement of a single lesion with both Kaposi sarcoma and *Cryptococcus* has been reported. Concomitant infection of the same lesion with both *Cryptococcus* and another organism such as *Leishmania*,[86] molluscum contagiosum,[101] or histoplasmosis[102] may occur. Most simultaneous infections with multiple organisms in skin lesions occur in AIDS patients with low CD4 counts (<100 cells/mm³).

Primary cutaneous cryptococcosis as an entity is controversial.[103] In the immunocompromised host, it is much less common than disseminated disease and should be considered a diagnosis of exclusion, i.e., a thorough evaluation for systemic involvement is required to rule out systemic disease in all immunosuppressed patients. When it occurs, primary cutaneous *Cryptococcus* is more common in non-HIV related immunosuppression. The route of infection may be via inhalation or inoculation. A history of trauma, contact with birds or bird droppings, or outdoor occupation may be present. Patients are rarely febrile or ill-appearing. Lesions tend to be single, and if multiple are confined to one area of the body. Exposed areas such as the hands are more commonly affected.[82,103] Regional lymphadenopathy may or may not be present.[103] The most common lesions of primary cutaneous cryptococcosis are ulcers, nodules, cellulitis, and a whitlow with or without phlegmon.[103] Specific lesions described in immunocompromised patients in the literature include a verrucous plaque on the wrist; an ulcer on the dorsum of the hand and sporotrichoid nodules on the forearm; a forearm ulcer with surrounding cellulitis; ulcers on the chin and scalp; an erythematous plaque with peripheral scale and central erosion on the lateral second digit after a splinter injury[83]; rapidly progressive cellulitis with soft tissue and muscle necrosis requiring amputation of the right hand after a cat scratch in a renal transplant recipient on prednisone and cyclosporine[104]; a pustule on an erythematous base that slowly progressed to an ulcer on the thigh post liver transplant[105]; a painless thigh nodule that drained and ulcerated in a 57-year-old lung transplant recipient employed at a lawn care service[106]; a tender, ill-defined, boggy, crusted, fluctuant plaque with overlying alopecia with associated posterior occipital lymphadenopathy mimicking dissecting cellulitis or kerion due to *C. albidus* in a 14-year-old after 5 months of anti-tumor necrosis factor-α inhibitor therapy (etanercept) for psoriasis[84]; painful ulcers on the arm and a subcutaneous nodule on the abdomen in a patient with chronic essential dermatitis treated with azathioprine and systemic corticosteroids[107]; a 2-cm nodule with central hemorrhagic

crust on the neck in a patient with non-Hodgkin's lymphoma receiving chemotherapy[108]; and bullous "erysipelas" on the arm of a 62-year-old woman on systemic steroids for sarcoidosis.[109] Although controversial, some argue that serum cryptococcal antigen testing may be positive in primary cutaneous disease[103] while others argue that a positive serum test implies disseminated disease.

Once suspected and looked for, the diagnosis of cutaneous cryptococcosis is relatively easy to make. A Tzanck smear prepared from the base of vesicles, pustules, acneiform lesions, or ulcers may demonstrate the budding yeasts of *Cryptococcus*. India ink preparations can be diagnostic when prepared from vesicle fluid, ulcer exudates, aspirates from cellulitis, or touch preparations from skin biopsies.

The skin biopsy of *Cryptococcus* can demonstrate both granulomatous (histiocytes phagocytozing budding yeasts surrounded by clear halos[85]) and gelatinous (infiltrates are filled with masses of spores whose nonstaining capsules (H&E stain) provide an edematous, foamy, or gelatinous appearance) findings. Both may be seen in the immunocompromised host.[85] An inflammatory reaction is often absent. The large numbers of spores may be mistaken for a lymphocytic infiltrate. A newly described histopathological finding includes an inflammatory pseudotumor with a storiform arrangement of spindle cells containing yeasts of *Cryptococcus* within and between vacuolated spindle cells in HIV patients previously treated for disseminated *Cryptococcus*.[77] Molluscum contagiosum-like lesions of cryptococcosis have been shown to demonstrate transepidermal and transfollicular elimination of the organism, which may serve as a source of transmission of the infection.[110]

Special stains of skin biopsy specimens can help identify the organism. The spores of *Cryptococcus* will stain pink with PAS stain, black with Gomori methenamine-silver, and dark brown with Fontana-Masson. The capsule will not stain with either H&E or PAS stains, but will stain purple with methylene blue, blue with alcian blue and colloidal iron, and red with mucicarmine.[96] *Cryptococcus* can be isolated from a skin biopsy taken for culture.

After the diagnosis of cutaneous cryptococcosis is made, a search for pulmonary, CNS and disseminated disease is indicated. Serum testing for cryptococcal antigen titer by latex agglutination will always be positive in disseminated disease. It is a helpful diagnostic tool while cultures and skin biopsy results are pending, and may serve as an early marker for disseminated disease when no extracutaneous site of infection is obvious. Cryptococcal antigen titers can also be performed on cerebral spinal fluid.

Untreated, disseminated cryptoccosis is lethal. Cryptococcal infection is best treated with amphotericin B, alone or in combination with flucytosine, or fluconazole. Lifelong maintenance antifungal therapy, often with fluconazole, is recommended. The echinocandin class of antifungals is inactive against cryptococcal species and does not have a role in treatment. Reduction in the dose of immunosuppression may be life saving in transplant patients despite loss of the grafted organ. Surgical excision or debridement of cutaneous *Cryptococcus* may be used to remove localized or bulky areas of disease and certainly for the purpose of establishing a diagnosis.

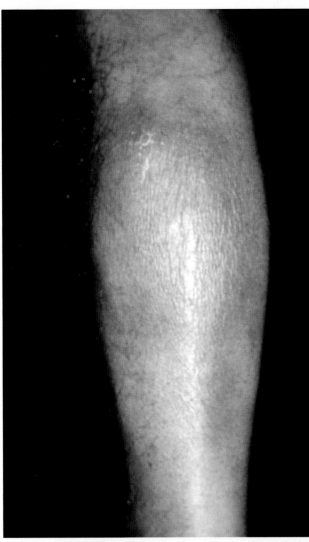

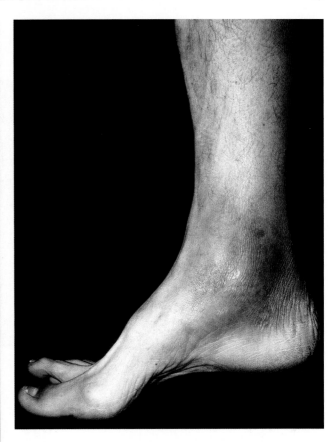

Figure 1.37. Cryptococcal cellulitis involving the ankle of a renal transplant

Figure 1.36. Cryptococcal cellulitis involving the calf of a renal transplant

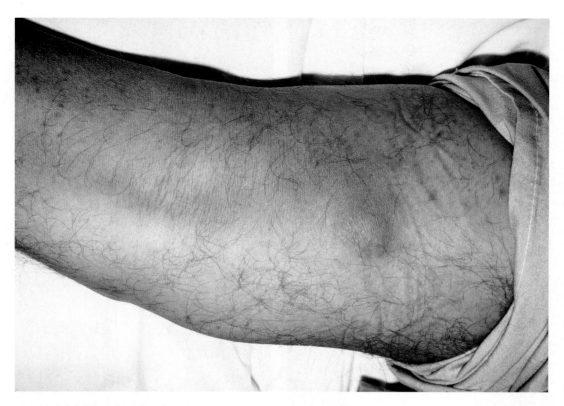

Figure 1.38. One of multiple tender red nodules due to *Cryptococcus* in a renal transplant

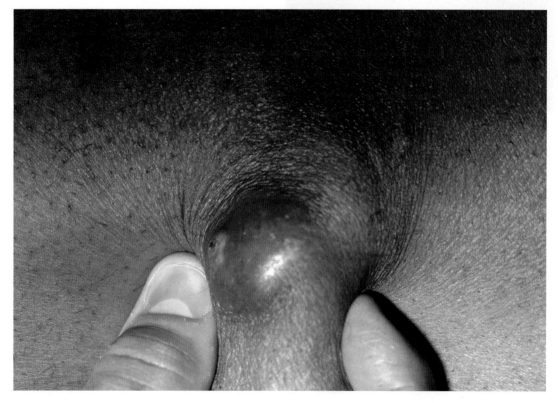

Figure 1.39. A 6-cm iceberg-like subcutaneous nodule of *Cryptococcus neoformans* on the lateral thigh of a renal transplant. The lesion was completely surgically excised and the patient cured with amphotericin

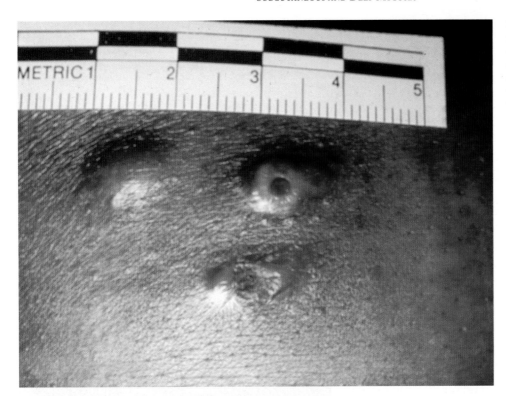

Figure 1.40. Three subcutaneous nodules on the chest wall of a 45-year-old woman on systemic steroids for a decade for her systemic sarcoidosis. Initially thought to be cutaneous sarcoid until one draining lesion cultured *Cryptococcus*

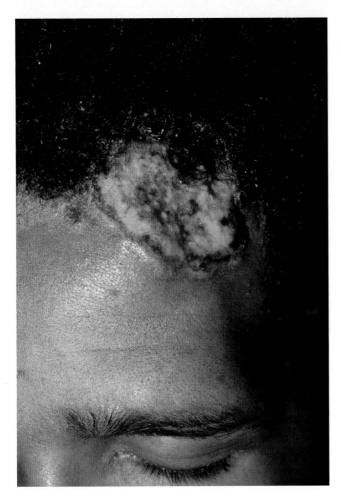

Figure 1.41. A vegetative ulcerated plaque on the forehead of a human immunodeficiency virus (HIV)-positive intravenous drug abuser with fever and headache

Figure 1.42. Tzanck smear of the ulcer base demonstrates multiple thin-necked budding yeast cells with large (8–20-µm) capsules of *Cryptococcus neoformans*

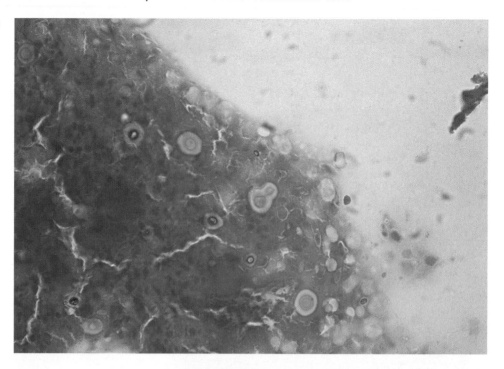

Figure 1.43. A 60-year-old HIV-negative Jamaican man with spastic paraparesis treated with systemic steroids had an ear ulceration for 6 months and a productive cough and fever for 2 months. Multiple cavitary lung lesions and biopsy of the ear demonstrated *Cryptococcus neoformans*

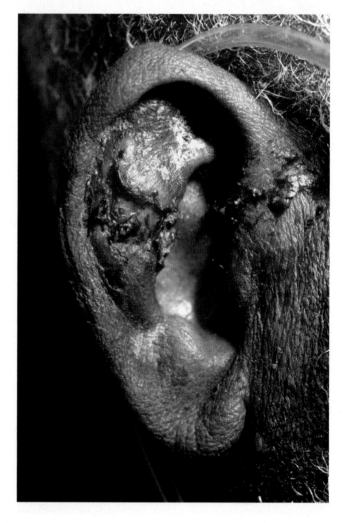

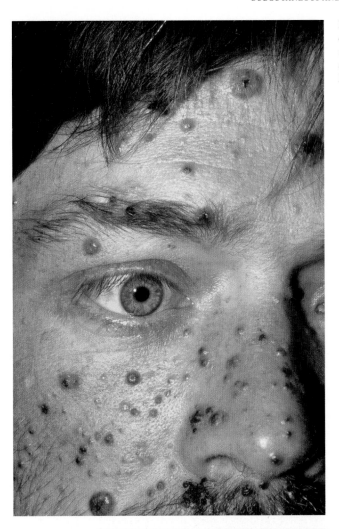

Figure 1.44. A 36-year-old HIV-positive man presented with fever, cough, and molluscum contagiosum-like skin lesions. *Cryptococcus neoformans* was demonstrated histologically and by culture from his skin, lungs, central nervous system, and bone marrow (Courtesy of Mary Gail Mercurio, M.D.)

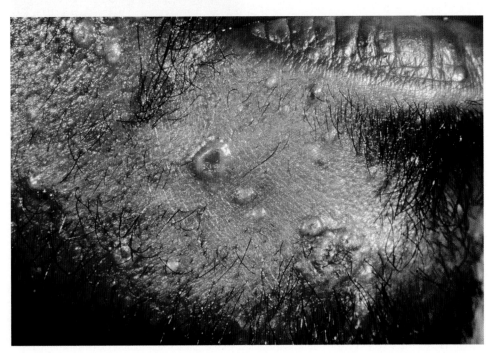

Figure 1.45. Molluscum contagiosum-like lesions on the chin of an AIDS patient due to disseminated cryptococcosis (Courtesy of Mary Ruth Buchness, M.D.)

Figure 1.46. Chronic forehead ulcer of disseminated cryptococcosis in a patient with AIDS (Courtesy of Peter Phillips, M.D.)

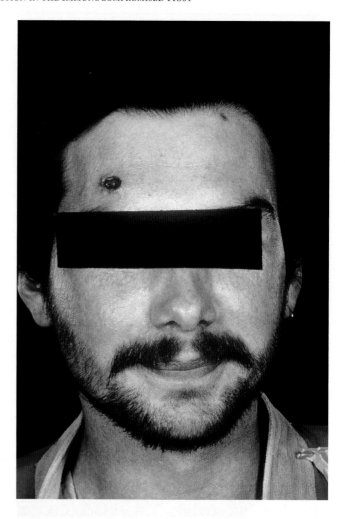

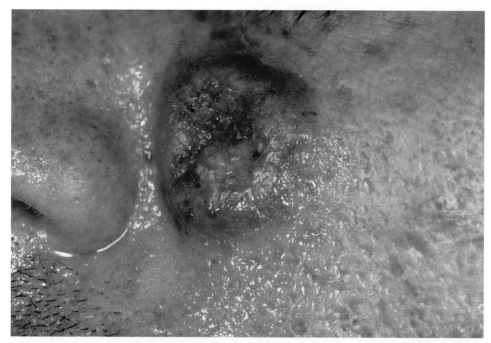

Figure 1.47. A lesion of disseminated cryptococcosis mimicking a cutaneous malignancy in a homosexual man with AIDS

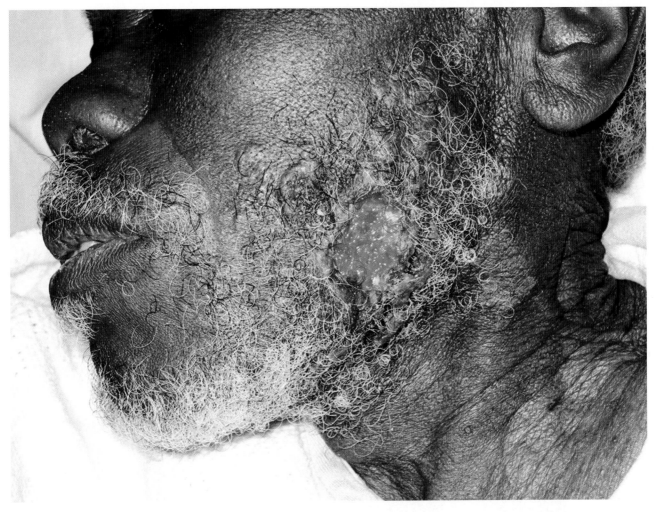

Figure 1.48. An 83-year-old man admitted with presumed dementia and centrally ulcerated plaque on the face was found to have *Cryptococcus* on skin biopsy. This led to the diagnosis of HIV infection and cryptococcal meningitis. His mental status improved with treatment

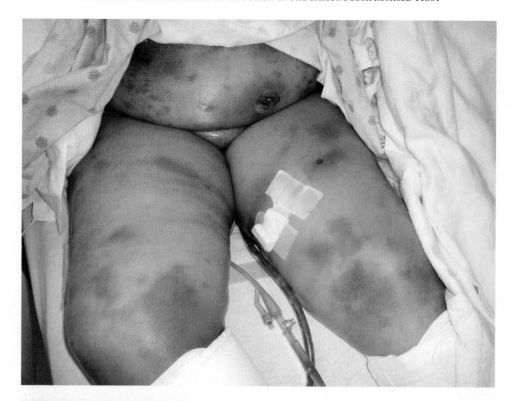

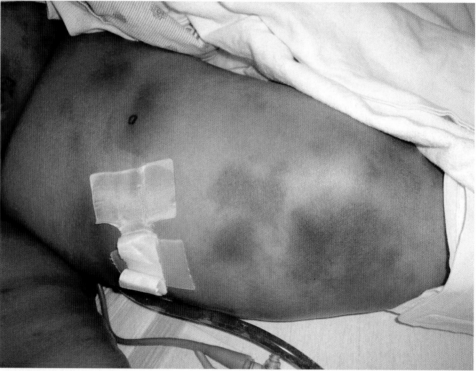

Figure 1.49. and 1.50.   A 29-year-old woman with vertically-acquired hepatitis C with a persistently high viral load presented 2 years after an orthotopic liver transplantation with fever, abdominal pain, nausea, and a painful nodular rash with ulceration on her abdomen and lower extremities. Her skin exam revealed several purpuric subcutaneous firm nodules across the abdomen with one lesion draining purulent fluid. Overlying the right medial knee was a large indurated purpuric plaque. Several firm, purpuric nodules were present over the bilateral thighs. Blood, urine, wound culture swab, skin biopsy, and culture were positive for *Cryptococcus neoformans*

HISTOPLASMOSIS

Histoplasmosis is caused by a dimorphic soil fungus, either *Histoplasma capsulatum* var. *capsulatum*, endemic to the Mississippi and Ohio River Valleys, Puerto Rico, parts of Central and South America, Sub-Saharan Africa, Australia, and East Asia, or *Histoplasma capsulatum* var. *duboisii*, endemic to Central Africa. Almost all cases seen in the USA are due to *Histoplasma capsulatum* var. *capsulatum*. Histoplasmosis is usually seen in rural dwellers exposed to chicken coops, cane fields, pigeons, and other bird or bat droppings. The demolition of old buildings and the excavation of earth at construction sites are the most common causes of the disease in urban dwellers. Inhalation of the 2–5 μm diameter spores is the usual route of infection.

Three types of systemic disease occur: (1) acute pulmonary (self-limited asymptomatic or "flu-like" syndrome); (2) chronic cavitary; and (3) disseminated. Progressive disseminated disease is a complication of depressed cellular immunity and may occur as a primary infection, reinfection, or reactivation. In the past, disseminated histoplasmosis was seen in young children, patients receiving corticosteroids or chemotherapy, or patients with Hodgkin's lymphoma. Currently, disseminated histoplasmosis is generally seen in patients with AIDS. It is considered an AIDS defining illness and occurs in 5% of AIDS patients living in non-endemic areas and in 27% living in endemic areas.[111]

The initial presentation and clinical manifestations of disseminated histoplasmosis are variable. Fever, respiratory complaints, weight loss, hepatosplenomegaly with an elevated alkaline phosphatase, and bone marrow suppression are frequent findings. Dissemination often involves the lungs, bone marrow, liver, spleen, lymph nodes, and adrenal glands. The presence of mucocutaneous lesions has been shown to correlate positively with the presence of pulmonary involvement and negatively with lymph node involvement.[112]

Mucocutaneous lesions of histoplasmosis present in one of three forms: primary cutaneous inoculation (rarest), reactive erythema (erythema nodosum or erythema multiforme), or mucosal and/or cutaneous lesion(s) of disseminated disease.[113-115] Primary cutaneous histoplasmosis presents as a nodule or chancriform ulcer with or without lymphangitis or lymphadenopathy.[113] Mucocutaneous lesions of disseminated histoplasmosis are present in 11–25% of HIV-infected patients in the USA and up to 80% of HIV-infected patients in Latin America. Although the distribution of the lesions is variable, the face, extremities, and trunk are the most frequently affected sites. The morphologic appearance of the skin lesions in the immunosuppressed patient is protean, and more than one morphologic lesion may be present in the same patient. The lower the CD4 count, the more atypical the morphology. Uncommonly, mucocutaneous lesions present only after the initiation of anti-retroviral therapy and may be due to the immune reconstitution syndrome.[116] Rarely mucocutaneous histoplasmosis may be transmitted between HIV-infected partners.[117] Mucocutaneous lesions most commonly present as papules, nodules, or ulcers, but may also present as papules with or without necrotic centers[118]; erythematous macules and patches; maculopapular eruption[119]; follicular, pustular, rosacea-like, or acneiform lesions[115]; vesicular herpeti-form lesions[112,115]; fistulae; verrucous, crusted, or vegetative plaques; pyoderma gangrenosum-like ulcers[120]; molluscum contagiosum-like papules[111]; erythema multiforme-like lesions[121]; exfoliative dermatitis[121]; vasculitic lesions[121]; psoriasiform exanthematous eruptions[122]; nodular purpuric lesions[111]; panniculitis[123]; cellulitis[124]; papules with transepidermal keratin elimination; and violaceous plaques mimicking Kaposi sarcoma.[112] Disseminated histoplasmosis may present as a widespread morbilliform eruption mimicking a drug rash and examination of a peripheral blood smear for intracellular yeast forms can lead to a rapid diagnosis (M.E.G., personal observation). *H. capsulatum* has also been demonstrated in a lesion of Kaposi sarcoma in a patient with AIDS.[125] Co-infection of histoplasmosis and cryptococcosis in the same skin lesion has been described in an AIDS patient.[126]

Mucosal lesions, present in 26–58% of patients with disseminated disease,[112,116] may be the presenting manifestation of disseminated histoplasmosis. Patients frequently have hoarseness, weight loss, painful ulcers, and sore throat. The most common locations include the tongue, palate, buccal mucosa, lips, gingiva, and oropharynx, but the epiglottis, nasal vestibule, submandibular salivary gland, perianal area, and genitalia may also be affected. Lesions described include ulcerated nodules[127] and papules; deep or vegetating ulcers mimicking squamous cell carcinoma[112]; palatal perforation; necrosis with heaped up margins[128]; hemorrhagic plaques on the tongue[112]; perianal and penile herpetiform lesions[129]; painful, well-demarcated penile ulcers with yellow exudates with or without inguinal lymphadenopathy[130]; and perforation of the prepuce.[130]

The most direct route for diagnosis of disseminated disease is skin biopsy if a lesion is present. Specimens should be sent for culture, H&E, and special stains. Culture is the gold standard for confirming the diagnosis. On histopathologic examination of H&E stained sections, the spores of histoplasmosis may be readily visualized. Because the fungal organisms may be so abundant that they are initially mistaken for nuclear debris, disseminated histoplasmosis should be included in the differential diagnosis of atypical vasculitis. The organism has also been found in cutaneous nerves on skin biopsy[131] and may correlate with painful lesions.[121] *H. capsulatum* is easily demonstrated within the cytoplasm of histiocytes in the dermis with PAS and Gomori methenamine-silver stains. Other diseases with intracellular organisms (leishmaniasis, granuloma inguinale, Chagas' disease, *Penicillium marneffei* infection, and rhinoscleroma) should be considered in the histopathologic differential diagnosis. These conditions can be ruled out rapidly because they are not stained by PAS. *Histoplasma* antigen detection by radioimmunoassay in the urine is positive in up to 90% of patients with disseminated histoplasmosis.[132]

Untreated, the mortality rate of disseminated histoplasmosis is 95%.[111] Treatment for disseminated histoplasmosis is 12 weeks of amphotericin B or liposomal amphotericin. In HIV-positive patients, lifelong maintenance therapy with itraconazole is recommended. Prophylaxis with itraconazole may be used for patients who live in endemic areas and have CD4 counts <150/μL. Immune reconstitution syndrome has been described in patients with disseminated histoplasmosis who are started on antiretroviral therapy.[133]

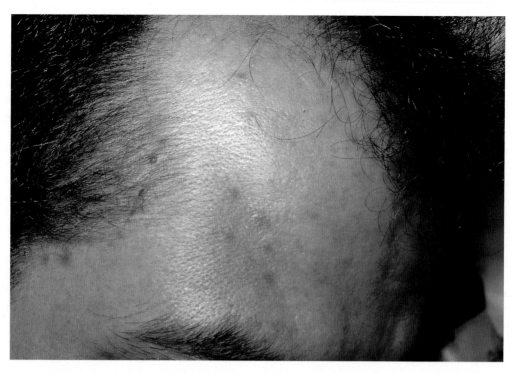

Figure 1.51. A 34-year-old Puerto Rican man presented to the hospital with fever, weight loss, pancytopenia, cough, and bilateral pulmonary infiltrates. He had hepatosplenomegaly and multiple discrete erythematous papules on his face, upper extremities and trunk. Skin biopsy and bronchoalveolar lavage fluid demonstrated many yeast forms confirmed on culture to be *Histoplasma capsulatum*. The patient was seropositive for HIV

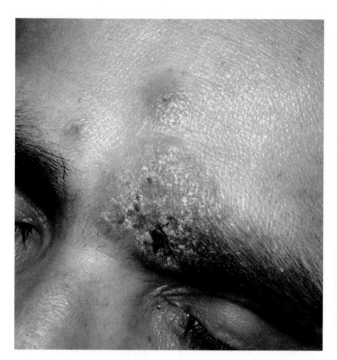

Figure 1.52. A 33-year-old homosexual Puerto Rican man with recent onset fever, lymphadenopathy, hepatomegaly, and a pulmonary infiltrate had skin lesions for 6 weeks. An erythematous vegetative plaque measuring 3–6 × 2.4 cm with superficial scale and central ulceration was located on the nasal bridge and medial left eyebrow. Smaller erythematous papules with and without ulceration were on the forehead

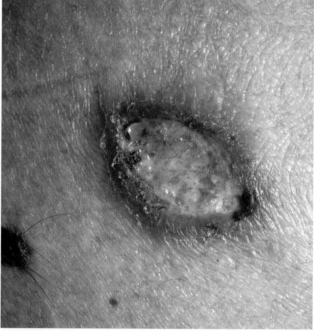

Figure 1.53. A 3.0 × 1.8-cm granulation-based ulcer with raised hyperpigmented borders was on the back of the patient in Fig. 1.52. Skin biopsy and cultures of both lesions demonstrated *H. capsulatum*

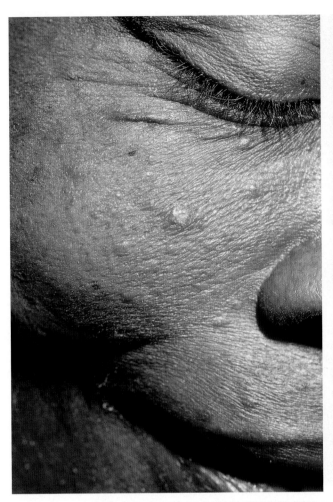
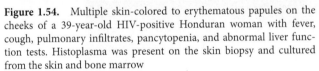

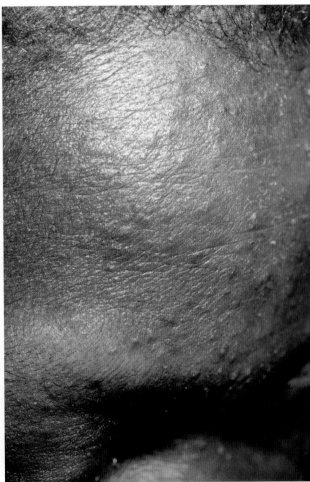

Figure 1.54. Multiple skin-colored to erythematous papules on the cheeks of a 39-year-old HIV-positive Honduran woman with fever, cough, pulmonary infiltrates, pancytopenia, and abnormal liver function tests. Histoplasma was present on the skin biopsy and cultured from the skin and bone marrow

Figure 1.55. Innumerable papules on the forehead of the patient in Fig. 1.54 due to skin biopsy-proven histoplasmosis

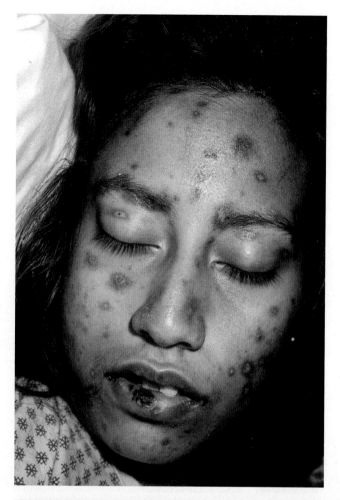

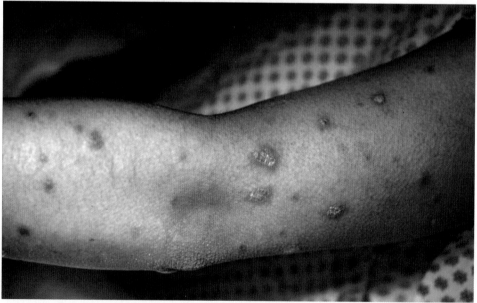

Figure 1.56. and 1.57. A 20-year-old Ecuadorian woman presented with fever, cough, and a widespread skin eruption. Her previous male sexual partner died of AIDS-associated Kaposi's sarcoma. There were 75–100 erythematous-to-dusky brown firm papules with scale crust on the face and extremities. Skin biopsy showed intracellular spores. Cultures from skin biopsies, bronchoscopy, and blood all grew *H. capsulatum*

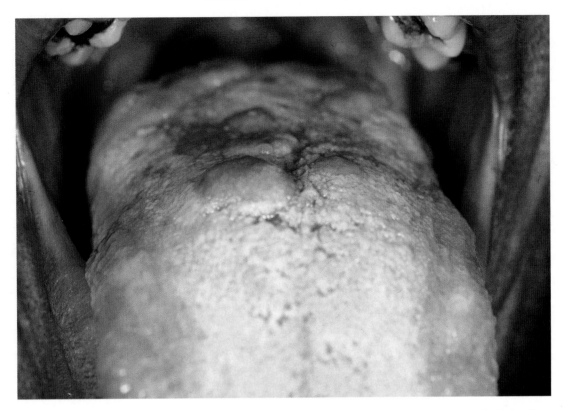

Figure 1.58. A 39-year-old HIV-positive intravenous drug abuser from Louisiana presented with odynophagia, fever, cough, weight loss, and cervical lymphadenopathy. Several firm 0.5–1-cm erythematous papules on the dorsum of the tongue were loaded with yeast forms of *Histoplasma* on biopsy

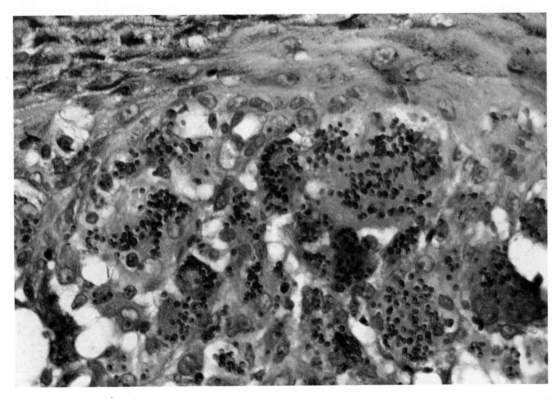

Figure 1.59. Periodic acid-Schiff (PAS) stain of the tongue biopsy revealed 2–4 μm round, oval, or budding bodies surrounded by a halo within parasitized macrophages. Each organism contained a large vacuole and a deeply stained cup-shaped mass at one end

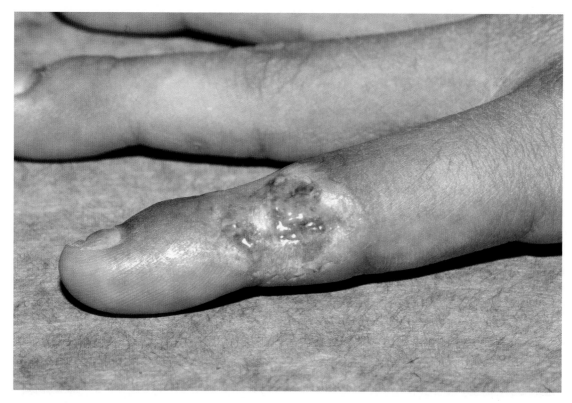

Figure 1.60.   Skin ulceration on the index finger of an HIV-positive man with an abnormal chest x-ray due to histoplasmosis (Courtesy of Mary Gail Mercurio, M.D.)

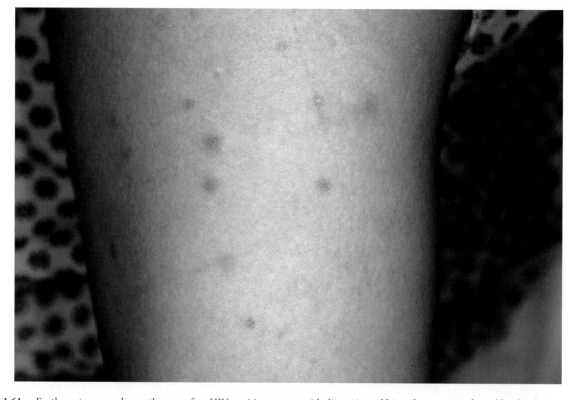

Figure 1.61.   Erythematous papules on the arm of an HIV-positive woman with disseminated histoplasmosis confirmed by skin biopsy

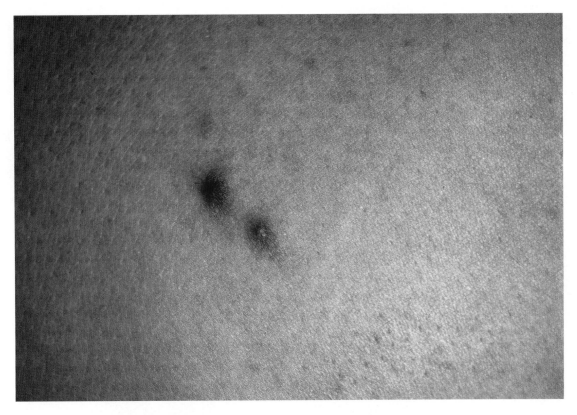

Figure 1.62. Erythematous papulopustules of biopsy-proven disseminated histoplasmosis in an HIV-positive patient

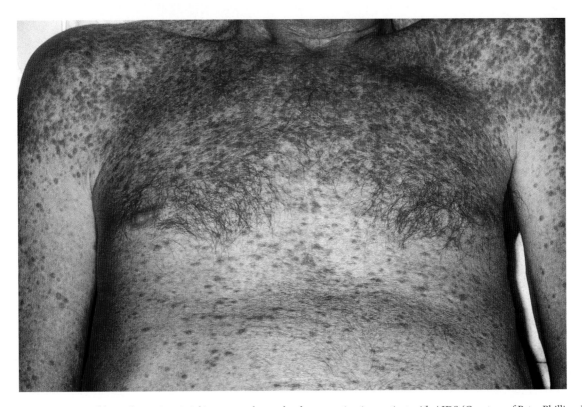

Figure 1.63. Disseminated histoplasmosis mimicking a maculopapular drug eruption in a patient with AIDS (Courtesy of Peter Phillips, M.D.)

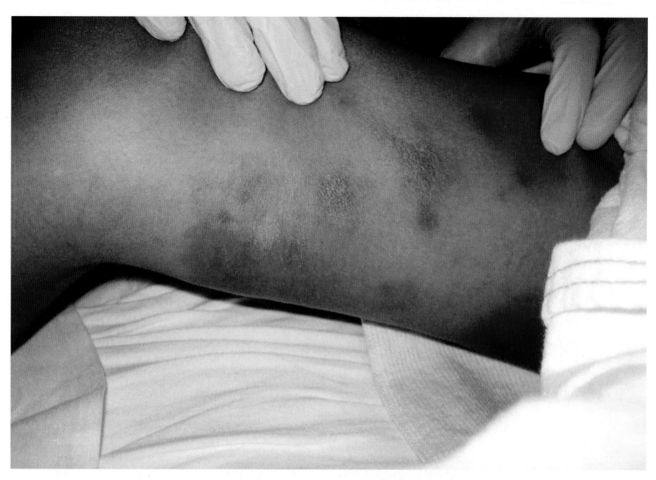

Figure 1.64. A 38-year-old Mexican woman presented with a 1-month history of fevers, generalized weakness/myalgias, weight loss, shortness of breath, abdominal pain, and increased abdominal girth. She was pancytopenic and treated with prednisone, cyclophosphamide, and IVIg for suspected autoimmune hemolytic anemia versus idiopathic thrombocytopenic purpura. Dermatology was consulted to evaluate painful ecchymotic nodules on her lower extremities that had developed following immunosuppressive therapy. Skin biopsy and tissue cultures were positive for *Histoplasma capsulatum* var. *capsulatum*

PHAEOHYPHOMYCOSIS

Phaeohyphomycoses (from the Greek "phaeo," meaning dark) are a diverse group of mycotic infections caused by dematiaceous (pigmented or black) fungi that in tissue form either yeast-like cells, branched or unbranched septate hyphae, or a combination of these forms. The pigmentation due to melanin or melanin-like material is visible in H&E stained or unstained sections and is highlighted by melanin stains such as the Fontana-Masson stain. The melanin is integral to the survival of the organism in its host, as it is thought to function as a virulence factor that protects the organism from destruction by host phagocytic cells. Although some of the same etiologic agents produce chromoblastomycosis (clinically presents with verrucous, nodular, or tumorous plaques with pseudoepitheliomatous hyperplasia and histopathologically demonstrates large, pigmented, round, thick-walled cells with septation called fungoid cells, copper pennies, chlamydospores, or sclerotic or medlar bodies in tissue) or mycetoma (tumefaction with draining sinuses and granules in the abscesses), these clinical entities are considered distinct from phaeohyphomycosis in that they are limited to the skin while phaeohyphomycosis may infect any organ system.

The etiologic agents of phaeohyphomycosis are numerous and increasing as more opportunistic infections are reported in immunocompromised patients. More than 100 species from 60 genera of phaeohyphomycoses have been identified. Common offenders include *Exophiala*, *Phialophora*, *Cladophialophora*, *Fonseca*, *Cladosporium*, *Alternaria*, *Bipolaris*, *Curvularia*, *Wangiella*, *Scedosporium prolificans*, and *Exserohilum* species. The diagnosis of phaeohyphomycosis requires proof of tissue invasion. A positive culture alone cannot confirm the diagnosis, as many dematiaceous organisms are contaminants rather than pathogens. However, identification of the organism in culture can be difficult; if the isolate does not sporulate, it may not be identified.

Infection usually results from accidental inoculation into the skin of organisms found in soil, plant material, vegetable debris, or wood. In immunocompromised patients, cutaneous disease may present during immunosuppression, but many years after the inoculating event occurred.[134] Often, no clear history of inoculation can be obtained. Dematiaceous fungi in the immunocompromised host present as primary subcutaneous phaeohyphomycosis, localized inoculation cutaneous infection, and systemic or invasive phaeohyphomycosis with secondary or metastatic cutaneous lesions. The skin lesions of secondary or metastatic phaeohyphomycosis are the result of hematogenous dissemination rather than of cutaneous inoculation. One fungal organism may produce several different cutaneous lesions, and one specific lesion may be caused by more than one organism.

Subcutaneous phaeohyphomycosis (also referred to as phaeomycotic cyst or abscess) usually presents as a painless solitary subcutaneous firm or cystic nodule or abscess. Multiple, poorly encapsulated, or fistulizing lesions and satellite papules or nodules are more often seen in immunocompromised patients. The nodules are often present for months or years before coming to medical attention which explains why the precipitating trauma is unrecognized. The lesions are usually on areas of the body exposed to trauma, such as the hands, feet, arms, and legs. Phaeomycotic abscesses often lack local or systemic signs of inflammation or associated lymphadenopathy or hematogenous spread of infection, and are attached to the skin, but not underlying muscle or bone. Unusual presentations in immunocompromised patients include tendon involvement with *Exophiala jeanselmei* in a heart transplant recipient and the diagnosis of both phaeohyphomycosis due to *Wangiella dermatitidis* and acute lymphocytic leukemia (ALL) (prior to receiving chemotherapy) by lymph node biopsy in a patient with no cutaneous lesions.[135] Unless surgical incision or spontaneous rupture occurs, the overlying skin is usually intact. Rupture of the cyst onto the skin surface infrequently results in drainage of pus, ulceration, small sinus tracts, or verrucous plaques. When a purulent discharge is present or extracted from a lesion, direct microscopy with potassium hydroxide can reveal light brown spores and hyphae.[136]

Primary cutaneous phaeohyphomycosis in the immunocompromised patient most often presents as one or more, occasionally grouped, nodules that may be suppurative and often have a verrucous or ulcerating surface. The lesions are usually painless, with chronic indolent courses and smolder for weeks to months before being brought to medical attention.[137] Iatrogenic inoculation from a wooden armboard[138] and after intravenous catheter insertion[139] have been reported. Sporotrichoid nodules are uncommon, but have been reported.[140] Other presentations include a subcutaneous cyst; a boggy verrucous plaque; a crusted erythematous nodule studded with pustules; superficial brown keratotic papules that resemble seborrheic keratoses; subcutaneous abscesses with sinus tracts, dermatomal hemorrhagic vesicles, and crusts; a fluctuant abscess with surrounding cellulitis; a necrotic ulcerated plaque with surrounding erythema resembling ecthyma gangrenosum; 0.5–1.5 cm multiple erythematous-to-violaceous asymptomatic nodules on the leg due to *Alternaria alternata* in a renal transplant recipient[141]; an erosive and necrotic plaque with overlying crust and exudates due to *Exserohilum rostratum* and cutaneous T cell lymphoma in the same lesion[142]; a painless verrucous violaceous plaque on the dorsal hand due to *Alternaria infectoria* in a renal transplant recipient[143]; linear erythematous crusted plaques and tiny pustules on the right foot due to *Exophiala jeanselmei* in a patient on systemic corticosteroids[144]; 2-cm poorly demarcated abscess-like lesions with an off-white content on the arms and buttocks due to *Exophiala jeanselmei* in a patient on chronic corticosteroids for polymyositis with pulmonary involvement[144]; painless erythematous nodule on the foot due to *Alternaria infectoria* in a renal transplant patient[145]; multiple ulcerating nodules on the elbow due to *Alternaria tenuissima* in a gardener with pemphigus vulgaris on systemic corticosteroids[146]; widespread ulceronecrotic granulomatous papules, plaques, and draining sinuses on the hands, forearms, and anterolateral legs due to *Alternaria longipes* in a patient with refractory squamous cell carcinoma of the sinuses on palliative systemic corticosteroids[147]; an enlarging nonhealing leg ulcer with adjacent erythematous nodules in a lung transplant recipient due to *Exophilia spinifera*[148]; disseminated crusted papules and plaques on an elbow and contralateral knee due to *Alternaria infectoria* in a patient on systemic corticosteroids for myasthenia[149]; exophytic ulcerating nodules with a surrounding cellulitis on the leg due to *Alternaria alternata* in a renal transplant recipient[150]; a verrucous crusted nodule with surrounding hyperpigmentation on the finger, mobile subcutaneous nodules on the forearm and a nodule with surrounding hypopigmentation in the antecubital fossa due to *Exophiala jeanselmei* in a renal transplant patient with concomitant systemic infection with *Nocardia asteroides*[151]; multiple painful nodules on the back due to *Cladophialophora bantiana* in a patient with lupus and rheumatoid arthritis who had been struck with flying debris during a tornado[152]; an erythematous tender papulonodule with central pustulation and crusting on the arm due to *Colletotrichum coccodes* in a patient with non-Hodgkin's lymphoma status post chemotherapy[153]; a friable, hypertrophic ulcerated, infiltrated mass on the foot mimicking squamous cell carcinoma due to *Alternaria alternata* in a liver transplant patient on tacrolimus[154]; a painless granulomatous nodule on the knee mimicking granuloma annulare due to *Alternaria alternata* in a renal transplant recipient[155]; and ulcers with surrounding cellulitis on the leg due to *Exserohilum longirostratum* in a patient with idiopathic thrombocytopenia treated with systemic corticosteroids.[156] *Veronaeae botryosa* may present with widespread cutaneous disease such as bilateral arm erythematous-to-brown crusted nodules and plaques in a retired farmer on chronic corticosteroids[157] and painless dermal nodules that spontaneously yield pus on the feet, wrists, and arms in a farmer status post liver transplantation.[134]

Secondary or disseminated cutaneous phaeohyphomycosis occurs almost exclusively in the immunosuppressed patient. Immunosuppression due to chemotherapy-induced neutropenia, bone marrow transplantation, systemic corticosteroid use, AIDS, malignancy (hematologic greater than solid organ), and organ transplantation all increase susceptibility to disseminated phaeohyphomycosis.[158] Although many dematiaceous fungi are virulent enough to produce systemic infection in the immunocompromised host, the most reported invasive dematiaceous pathogens are in the genera *Alternaria*, *Exophiala*, *Wangiella*, *Curvularia*, *Bipolaris*, and *S. prolificans*. *S. prolificans*, the most common cause of disseminated phaeohyphomycosis, is particularly virulent, producing fungemia with positive blood cultures in up to 80% of patients, is highly resistant to antifungal therapy, and has a mortality rate approaching 100%.[158] Most patients have known pulmonary or other visceral involvement before hematogeneous spread to the skin, although dissemination from the skin has been reported.[153] Clinical presentations of disseminated phaeohyphomycosis vary and include tender erythematous subcutaneous nodules of *Bipolaris*; ulcerated papules of *Alternaria*; hemorrhagic pustules of *Alternaria*; scaly hyperpigmented plaques of *Curvularia*; hyperpigmented buttock nodules with a purulent exudate and fistula formation of *Phialophera* (suspected disseminated infection)[159]; a nonhealing wound on the shoulder with hyperpigmented borders due to *Cladophialophora bantiana* in a heart transplant recipient[160]; and ecthyma gangrenosum on the thigh and calf due to *Exserohilum* in a child with acute leukemia.[161]

Surgical excision, if feasible, is the treatment of choice for subcutaneous phaeohyphomycosis. Antifungal therapy may include amphotericin b, 5-fluorocytosine, ketoconazole, itraconazole, voriconazole, and terbinafine alone or in combination. Reduction in immunosuppression may be required in disseminated disease.

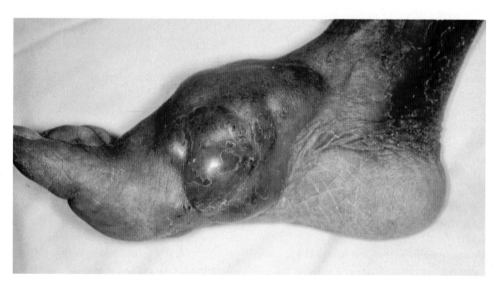

Figure 1.65. Subcutaneous phaeohyphomycosis. A 10 × 10-cm nontender multilobulated subcutaneous mass was present for 2 years on the foot of a 62-year-old man with a renal transplant

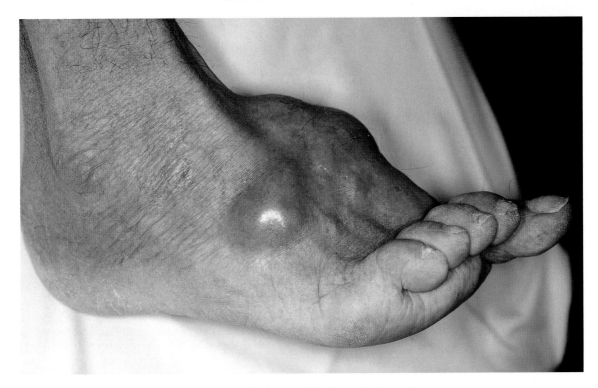

Figure 1.66. The nodules extended from the instep across the dorsum of the foot to the lateral side

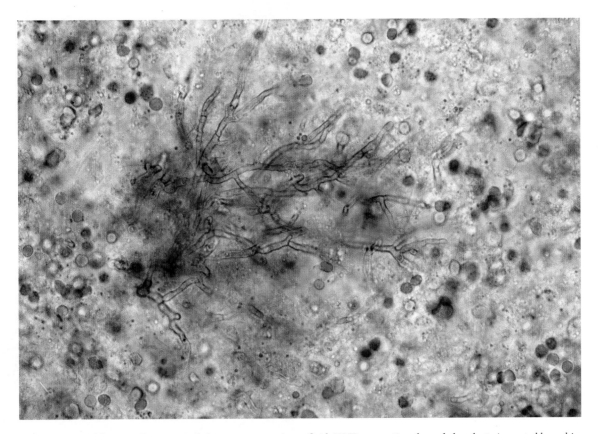

Figure 1.67. Aspirate of the mass demonstrated viscous serosanguinous fluid. KOH preparation showed abundant pigmented branching septate hyphae. Fungal culture grew black colonies. Sporulation could not be induced by multiple mycologic specialists

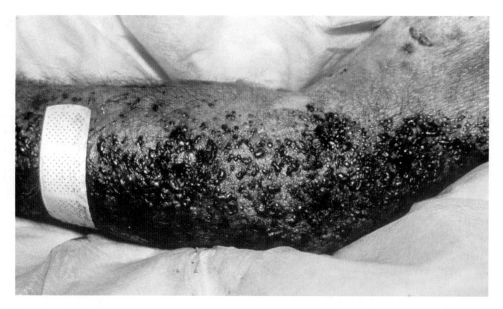

Figure 1.68. Hemorrhagic vesicles in a dermatomal distribution due to *Exserohilum rostratum* at the site of a previous intravenous line infiltration in a 74-year-old man with steroid-dependent chronic obstructive pulmonary disease (From Tieman JM, Furner BB. Phaeohyphomycosis caused by *Exserohilum rostratum* mimicking herpes zoster. J Am Acad Dermatol 1991;25:852–853)

Figure 1.69. The hemorrhagic crusted vesicles caused by *E. rostratum* mimicked herpes zoster in the immunocompromised host

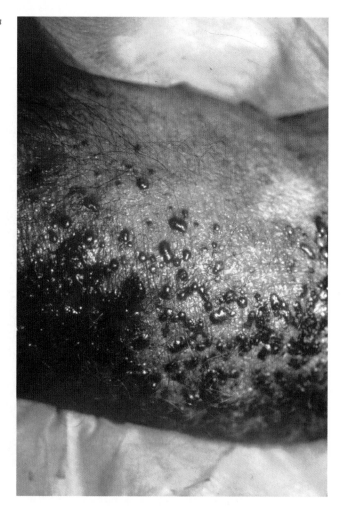

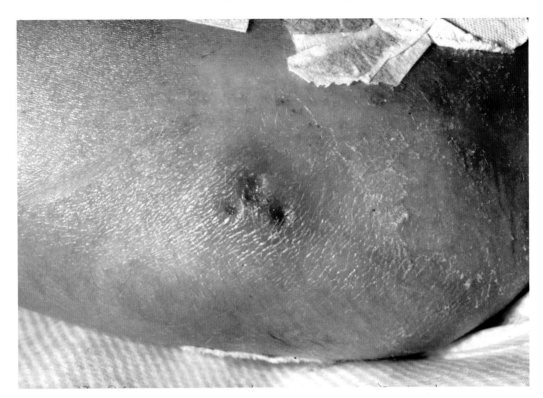

Figure 1.70. A neutropenic 5-year-old receiving chemotherapy for acute lymphocytic leukemia developed an erythematous plaque in an area abraded by adhesive tape securing an intravenous catheter. Three necrotic ulcerations rapidly developed. The lesion was completely excised. Biopsy and culture demonstrated *Bipolaris* (*Drechslera*) *spicifera* as the cause (From Estes SA, Merz WG, Maxwell LG. Primary cutaneous phaeohyphomycosis caused by *Drechslera spicifera*. Arch Dermatol 1977;113:813–815. Copyright 1977, American Medical Association)

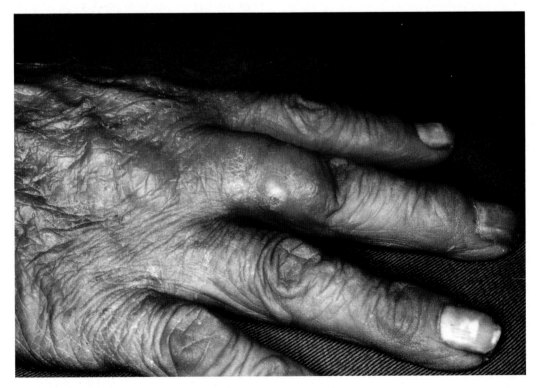

Figure 1.71. A 60-year-old Japanese man with a renal transplant developed a 1.5 × 1-cm nodule on the dorsum of his middle finger over 5 months. Cutaneous phaeohyphomycosis caused by *Exophiala jeanselmei* was confirmed by biopsy and culture (From Hachisuka H, et al. Cutaneous phaeohyphomycosis caused by *Exsophilia jeanselmi* after renal transplantation. Int J Dermatol 1990;29:198–200)

Scedosporium and Pseudallescheria

Pseudallescheria boydii, Scedosporium apiospermum, and *Scedosporium prolificans* (first described as *Scedosporium inflatum* in 1984) are related organisms that are all soil saprophytes. Although *Scedosporium apiospermum* was once considered to be the asexual form of *Pseudallescheria boydii,* recent sequence analysis has determined that the two are indeed unique species. However, since much of the literature to date discusses *P. boydii* as the anamorph of *S. apiospermum,* they are considered together here. *Scedosporium prolificans* is a dematiaceous fungus that may cause phaeohyphomycosis.

Infection is typically acquired through inhalation or inoculation. In immuncompetent hosts, infection with *Scedosporium* spp. is traditionally associated with mycetoma, onychomycosis, and sinopulmonary infections in patients with a history of prior pulmonary compromise (Job syndrome, sarcoidosis, tuberculosis, etc.).[162] However, infections with both *Scedosporium apiospermum* and *Scedosporium prolificans* are emerging in immunosuppressed patients and may account for approximately 25% of non-*Aspergillus* mold infections in organ transplant recipients.[163] Presentations in immunocompromised hosts may include pneumonia, cutaneous lesions, meningitis, endocarditiis, osteomyelitis, septic arthritis, keratitis, endophthalmitis, and thyroid gland involvement. *S. prolificans* is more virulent than *S. apiospermum.*

In general, infection with *Scedosporium* is reported in association with hematopoietic stem cell transplants, organ transplants, hematologic malignancies, and HIV disease. *S. prolificans* is more common in patients with a hematologic malignancy and neutropenia while *S. apiospermum* is more common in organ transplant recipients and in patients undergoing systemic corticosteroid therapy.[163] More than 50% of immunocompromised patients infected with these organisms will present with disseminated disease (69% in hematopoietic stem cell transplant; 55% in organ transplant; 86% in hematologic malignancy; 57% in HIV).[163] Two thirds to three quarters of infections in transplant patients occur within 6 months of transplantation.[163] The mortality rate of all transplant patients infected with *Scedosporium* is as high as 58%.[163]

Thirty three percent of patients with *Scedosporium* infection have skin lesions.[162] Like infection with other deep fungal organisms, cutaneous infection with *Scedosporium* can be localized or disseminated, with localized infection being the most common. Localized disease may be due to cutaneous inoculation, but in most cases patients do not recall obvious injury. Localized *Scedosporium apiospermum* or *Pseudallescheria boydii* may present as a plaque of miliary pustules on the arm in a heart transplant recipient[164]; cysts; tender sporotrichoid subcutaneous nodules within a boggy erythematous plaque on the arm in a patient on systemic corticosteroids for idiopathic pulmonary fibrosis[165]; non-inflammatory subcutaneous nodules on the elbow in a patient on prednisone for sarcoidosis[166]; a postsurgical sternal wound infection in a heart transplant patient[167]; subcutaneous abscesses on the leg and foot in a farmer on methylprednisolone for microscopic polyangiitis[168,169]; ulcerated nodules on the hand and forearm in a heart transplant recipient[170]; a 10-cm annular lesion with an elevated erythematous border with draining satellite papules and pustules on the forearm in a patient with rheumatoid arthritis on cyclosporine and methylprednisolone[171]; tender pustules and draining ulcers on the dorsal foot and shin of a bilateral lung transplant recipient[172]; erythema and papules that progressed to purpura, induration, and necrotic ulcers on the hand with a proximal subcutaneous forearm nodule in a patient with asthma undergoing systemic corticosteroid therapy[173]; and in-hospital post-traumatic erythema and edema on the medial base of the first toe that progressed to a necrotic bulla with secondary ulceration in a patient with acute myelogenous leukemia (AML) undergoing induction chemotherapy.[174] Sporotrichoid spread of subcutaneous, suppurative nodules with a honey-colored exudate is characteristic.[165,173,175,176] *Scedosporium prolificans* may also cause localized disease, although reports are less common than with *S. apiospermum.*

Dissemination of *Scedosporium* usually occurs secondary to a primary pulmonary infection. Most cases of disseminated infection have been reported from Spain or Australia. Disseminated disease to the skin is rare, but may present as target lesions[170]; a 3.5 × 4 cm eschar at a Hickman catheter site accompanied by erythematous nodules with dusky, light-gray centers on the forehead, back, and upper extremity, among widespread erythematous macules and papules due to *P. boydii* in a Cambodian man with relapsed AML[177]; "multiple blackened skin lesions" due to *S. prolificans* in relapsed ALL[178]; and widespread papules, pustules, or nodules.[162,177] Acral hemorrhagic bullae due to *S. apiospermum* was diagnosed post mortem in a 69-year-old Texan woman with systemic lupus erythematosus (SLE) on systemic steroids.[179] Disseminated disease beginning in the skin and spreading to other organs is less common, but has been reported.

Diagnosis is based primarily on culture of infected tissue. Infection with *Scedosporium* spp. must be differentiated by fungal culture from other deep fungal organisms, especially sporotrichosis clinically and *Aspergillus* and *Fusarium* histologically. All can appear as nonpigmented, slender, thick-walled septate hyphae 2–4 μm in diameter. All can show angioinvasion. Culture is the gold standard for identification of *Scedosporium* from tissue specimens. Unlike in many other disseminated fungal infections, blood cultures may be useful in making the diagnosis of *Scedosporium* infection, as blood cultures have been reported to be positive in up to 75% of patients with disseminated disease, especially with *S. prolificans.*[180] However, blood cultures are more likely to be positive toward the end stage of disease, which is often fatal.[181]

Scedosporium apiospermum is more responsive to antifungal therapy than is *S. prolificans,* which is considered resistant to almost all available antifungals. The azole antifungals, specifically itraconazole and voriconazole, may be effective in the treatment of *S. apiospermum.* Surgical debridement may also be required. The mortality rate of *S. prolificans* approaches 100%.

SPOROTRICHOSIS

Sporothrix schenckii, the causative agent of sporotrichosis, is a dimorphic fungus found commonly on plant material, wood, and soil. Infection is acquired through direct inoculation or inhalation of spores. Cutaneous inoculation may occur from scratches from rose thorns, salt meadow hay, cactus plants, carnations, conifer needles, splinters, cuts from barbs, brushing against infected tree bark or contaminated mine timbers, sphagnum moss (especially associated with bonsai trees),[182] or handling of certain animals (especially cats, armadillos, and fish). Predisposed to infection are farmers, florists, gardeners, forestry workers, veterinarians, and carpenters.

Sporothrix schenckii causes disease in both the immunocompetent and immunocompromised patient. The clinical presentations of sporotrichosis include lymphocutaneous (70%), fixed cutaneous (20%), disseminated (including disseminated cutaneous), and extracutaneous[183,184] disease. Disseminated sporotrichosis is rare, but more common in (although not limited to) immunosuppressed patients. It is due to hematogenous dissemination from a primary cutaneous or pulmonary inoculation site or sites. Extracutaneous disease also occurs primarily in the immuncompromised host and is due to hematogenous dissemination from a pulmonary source or deep inoculation site without a primary skin focus.[185] Types of immunosuppression associated with disseminated or extracutaneous disease include severe malnutrition, sarcoidosis, malignancy, diabetes, alcoholism, and immunosuppression from HIV infection, organ transplantation, corticosteroid use, hematologic malignancy, and chemotherapy. Although not an AIDS defining illness, disseminated sporotrichosis as the initial presentation of HIV infection has been reported.[186-188]

The classic cutaneous lesion of sporotrichosis begins at the inoculation site as a painless papule or pustule that develops into a nodule that ultimately enlarges, softens, ulcerates, and drains purulent fluid. Neighboring asymptomatic nodules develop, extend along lymphatics, and may or may not be accompanied by lymphangitis or lymphadenopathy.[183] Fixed cutaneous sporotrichosis is a solitary lesion or group of lesions that remains localized to the inoculation site and may present as facial cellulitis (children), pyodermatous erosions, verrucous or psoriasiform plaques, pyoderma gangrenosum-like ulcers,[183] or an erythematous ulcerated nodule with rolled translucent borders and central eschar, mimicking a basal cell carcinoma.[189] Reactivation of localized, previously treated disease after intralesional corticosteroids[189] has been reported.

Cutaneous lesions of disseminated sporotrichosis tend to be widely distributed, but the morphology is protean: necrotic ulcers; painful, ulcerated papules with a seropurulent exudate[190]; ulcers with rolled erythematous borders; nodules that may be umbilicated, ulcerated, crusted, irregular, or suppurative; ulcerating grayish black smooth papulonodules; psoriasiform plaques; erythematous to violaceous papules; large, tender, ulcerated, and necrotic plaques[191]; erysipeloid plaques in a patient with Cushing's disease[192]; ulcerative sarcoidosis-like lesions[184]; acneiform or furunculosis-like lesions[193]; phagedenic ulcers[193]; and scrotal ulcers[193] have all been described.

Mucosal lesions are rare, but laryngeal, conjunctival, pharyngeal, oral, and nasal involvement have been reported.[190,194] Lesions in the oral or nasal mucosa may present as ulcerations with a thin overlying granulomatous surface and erythematous borders[194] or gingival hyperplasia with painful, erythematous, proliferative papules and plaques on the alveolar process or gingiva.[195] Unusual manifestations in alcoholics, such as ethmoid sinusitis with facial swelling and severe eye pain with periorbital swelling and ecchymosis, may mimic mucormycosis.

Dissemination to other organs including the lung, bones, joints, liver, spleen, pancreas, intestine, meninges, testes, epididymis, and bone marrow may occur.[196,197] Involvement of the bones and joints is characteristic of disseminated sporotrichosis, occurs in 80% of patients, and presents with an indolent, suppurative arthritis and/or osteolytic bone lesions most commonly affecting the joints of the forearms, wrists, hands, ankles, and knees.[185,198] Skin lesions classically precede joint disease. Reports of meningeal involvement are rare, but increasing, especially in HIV-positive patients with CD4 counts below 200 cells/mL.[185,198-200] Skin lesions are often present at the time of presentation of CNS disease. Signs of sporotrichosis affecting the meninges include headache, seizures, confusion, and coma.[197]

The diagnosis of sporotrichosis may be made on skin biopsy, although the cigar-shaped bodies are typically difficult to demonstrate and tissue cultures are usually more productive in establishing the diagnosis. Organisms may be more readily apparent in specimens from immunocompromised patients or from local immunosuppression in patients with fixed cutaneous sporotrichosis treated with intralesional steroids.[201] The yeast cells in these cases may be unusual with many large oval and round organisms (up to 8 μm) in diameter that are difficult to distinguish from cryptococcosis. In fact, the organisms may be so large that they "appear as an amorphous mass that simulates diffuse cutaneous necrosis."[202] Fungal culture of a skin biopsy is essential, not only because the organism (although present) may not be identified on routine or special stains, but also to differentiate sporotrichosis from other mycoses such as cryptococcosis.

Treatment of localized cutaneous disease may be achieved with potassium iodide or itraconazole. Disseminated disease and patients with HIV are best treated with amphotericin B. Lifelong therapy with itraconazole is recommended for patients with HIV. Intra-articular amphotericin B or surgical debridement may be required if joint disease is present. Fatal disseminated disease is rare, but is more likely to occur in HIV/AIDS.[191]

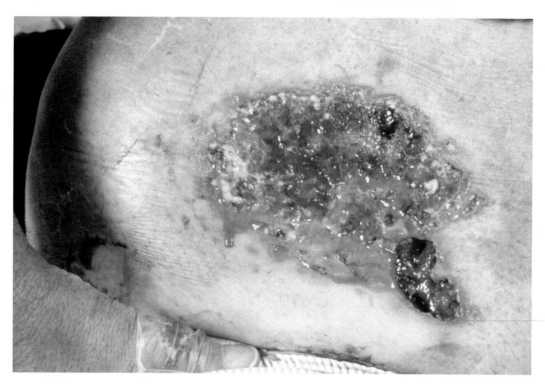

Figure 1.72. Two large confluent ulcers with ragged edges and undermined borders on the abdomen due to *Sporothrix schenckii* masquerading as pyoderma gangrenosum. Treatment with immunosuppression resulted in slowly enlarging ulcers (Courtesy of Sophia J. Hendrick, M.D., and Joseph L. Jorizzo, M.D. From Spiers EM, et al. Sporotrichosis masquerading as pyoderma gangrenosum. Arch Dermatol 1986;122:691. Copyright 1986, American Medical Association)

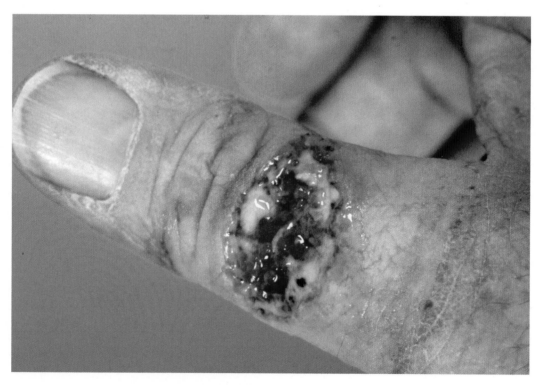

Figure 1.73. Similar ulcer of sporotrichosis on the thumb of the same patient in Fig. 1.72 (Courtesy of Sophia J. Hendrick, M.D., and Joseph L. Jorizzo, M.D. From Spiers EM, et al. Sporotrichosis masquerading as pyoderma gangrenosum. Arch Dermatol 1986;122:691. Copyright 1986, American Medical Association)

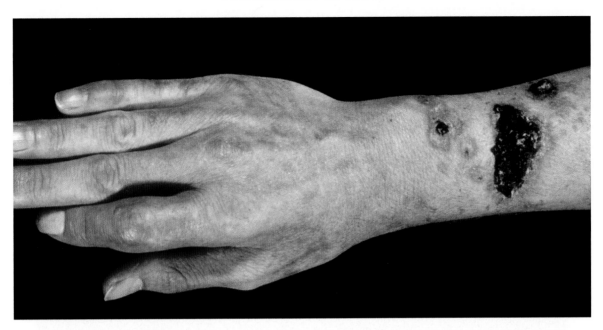

Figure 1.74. Purple subcutaneous nodules and hemorrhagic crusted ulcers due to *Sporothrix schenckii* developed on all four extremities in an AIDS patient. *Sporothrix* synovitis involved the second and third metacarpophalangeal joints and second proximal interphalangeal joint (Courtesy of Robert Greenwald, M.D. From Lipstein-Kresch E, et al. Disseminated *Sporothrix schenckii* infection with arthritis in a patient with acquired immunodeficiency syndrome. J Rheumatol 1985;12:805)

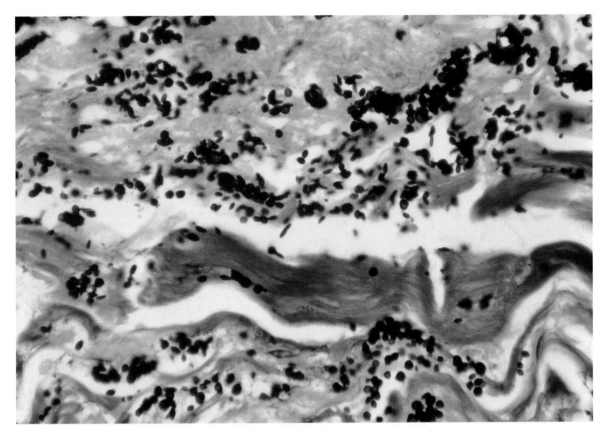

Figure 1.75. Gomori methenamine-silver stain (X 400) demonstrates typical oval to cigar-shaped yeast cells and globose budding cells of sporotrichosis on skin biopsy (Courtesy of Robert Greenwald, M.D. From Lipstein-Kresch E, et al. Disseminated *Sporothrix schenckii* infection with arthritis in a patient with acquired immunodeficiency syndrome. J Rheumatol 1985;12:805)

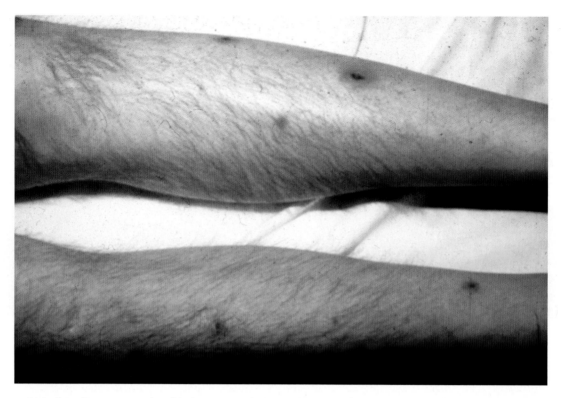

Figure 1.76.   Multiple erythematous papules of the legs, some with ulceration due to *Sporothrix schenckii* in a patient with AIDS (From Fitzpatrick JE, Eubanks S. Acquired immunodeficiency syndrome presenting as disseminated cutaneous sporotrichosis. Int J Dermatol 1988;27:406–407)

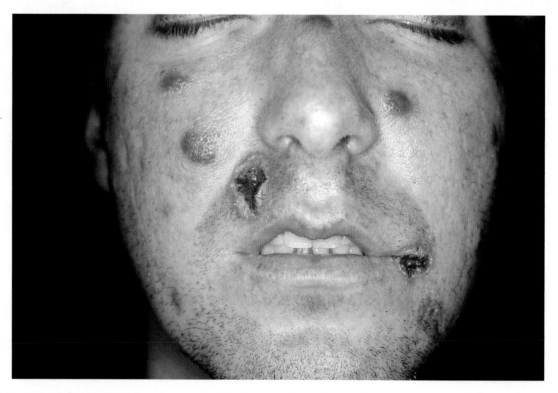

Figure 1.77.   Perioral ulcers with rolled erythematous borders due to *Sporothrix schenckii* with Kaposi's sarcoma on the face of an HIV-positive homosexual (From Shaw JC, Levinson W, Montanaro A. Sporotrichosis with acquired immunodeficiency syndrome. J Am Acad Dermatol 1989;21:1145–1147)

ZYGOMYCOSIS/MUCORMYCOSIS

Zygomycosis describes a group of infectious organisms, of the class Zygomycetes, order Mucorales. Mucormycosis (a term used interchangeably with zygomycosis) describes invasive infection due to the fungi of the genera *Rhizopus*, *Absidia*, *Rhizomucor*, and *Mucor*. Less common organisms include *Cunninghamella bertholletiae*, *Apophysomyces elegans*, *Mortierella*, and *Saksenaea vasiformis*. All organisms of these genera appear morphologically identical in tissue and produce the same disease, but can be differentiated by culture. Spores of the fungi are ubiquitous and are thought to be inhaled frequently. The organisms are found in bread and fruit molds and can be seen in nasal, throat, and stool cultures of healthy subjects. Nosocomial outbreaks of mucormycosis are not as common as hospital-related *Aspergillus* infections but have sometimes been linked to construction or renovation work and contaminated ventilation systems.

The clinical presentations of mucormycosis include rhinocerebral, pulmonary, cutaneous, gastrointestinal, central nervous system, disseminated, and miscellaneous forms.[203] The clinical presentation of cutaneous zygomycosis varies from gradual in onset and slowly progressive to fulminant infection with gangrene and hematogenous dissemination. Infections usually present in the nose and paranasal sinuses or on the palate and then spread rapidly to the central nervous system via the orbit and cribriform plate.

Cutaneous mucormycosis is encountered in several clinical settings: severe burns, poorly controlled diabetes, trauma, leukemia, severe graft vs. host disease, solid organ or hematopoietic stem cell transplantation, HIV infection (especially in those with neutropenia, low CD4 counts, and intravenous drug use),[203-205] prolonged neutropenia, systemic corticosteroid use, prematurity or advanced age , the use of Elastoplast dressings (Beiersdorf UK Limited, Birmingham, United Kingdom), wooden tongue depressors used as splints for intravenous catheters,[206] and as a manifestation of disseminated disease with nodular or infarctive lesions from hematogenous seeding. Iron overload with or without the concomitant use of desferoxamine is also a recognized risk factor. Voriconazole use for fungal prophylaxis or treatment of invasive aspergillosis after transplantation (hematopoietic stem cell or solid organ) is a newly recognized risk factor, as voriconazole does not cover zygomycetes and breakthrough infections with these organisms has been reported.[207] A breakthrough infection with *Rhizopus* has also been reported in a liver transplant patient on caspofungin.[208] In contrast, trauma is the most common predisposing factor leading to zygomycosis in immunocompetent patients.

Cutaneous mucormycosis presents in primary or secondary forms. Primary cutaneous disease is due to direct inoculation of the organism into the skin while secondary cutaneous disease describes hematogenous dissemination to the skin from another primary site of infection, most commonly the sinuses and lungs. Primary cutaneous mucormycosis presents as superficial or gangrenous infection. Superficial infection may develop in wounds dressed with contaminated elasticized adhesive tape. It presents as erythematous plaques with pustules and/or hemorrhagic vesicles and may ulcerate. Infection without a history of trauma may occur.[209] Necrotizing fasciitis and gangrenous lesions develop secondary to entry of the organism through intravenous catheters, injections, macerated skin, burns, and surgical or other types of wounds. Zygomyctes are capable of extending rapidly along tissue planes especially in neutropenic patients. The necrotic eschars are the hallmark of zygomycosis.[210] Systemic dissemination of primary cutaneous lesions has been reported.[211-213]

The typical setting of secondary cutaneous mucormycosis is the patient with late stage leukemia who is febrile with pulmonary infiltrates who then develops skin involvement as a rare complication of dissemination. It has also occurred after bone marrow transplantation. Secondary cutaneous mucormycosis presents as extremely painful, large (2–4 cm diameter, often larger), purpuric areas that may be retiform, and are surrounded by a thin erythematous rim separate from the main lesion. Histologically, thrombosis of the dermal blood vessels is seen with the vasculature occluded by hyphae. As the fungus extends into the vessels and leads to thrombosis, the lesion becomes an ecchymotic nodule or plaque with central necrosis and may resemble ecthyma gangrenosum or necrotizing fasciitis. Lesions may progress to the characteristic "bull's-eye cutaneous infarct of zygomycosis," which describes a central yellow or black eschar with a surrounding thin, purpuric rim.[214]

Presentations of cutaneous mucormycosis that are less common than that described above include swelling and induration with a central area of black blisters[214]; tender, indurated lesions with central necrosis on the vulva[214]; moderate edema and blackish discoloration on the prepuce[214]; annular necrotic punched-out ulcers in a linear array along the cheek at the site of endotracheal tube taping[215]; and an erythematous plaque studded with pustules, necrosis, and ulceration in a dermatomal distribution resembling herpes zoster.[216]

Presentations of primary cutaneous mucormycosis in HIV-positive patients are rare but are similar to those in non-HIV patients. Unusual presentations have included an abscess that became necrotic and ulcerated[204]; pustules that drain and ulcerate[204]; pea-sized intradermal nodules on the chest, forehead, and jaw[204]; co-infection with cytomegalovirus (CMV) and mucormycosis resulting in necrotizing myofascial cellulitis[205]; and palatal and buccal necrosis as a manifestation of rhinocerebral mucormycosis in an HIV-positive patient presenting with Bell's palsy.[204]

Rhinocerebral mucormycosis is the classic, most common presentation of systemic infection. It frequently involves the maxillary sinus, the cavernous sinus, and the brain. Necrotic facial lesions signify aggressive angioinvasive infection. One of the earliest signs of invasive mucormycosis is nasal discharge. The nasal turbinate mucosa may be black and necrotic and easily mistaken for dried, crusted blood (especially in a thrombocytopenic leukemia patient). Invasion inferiorly into the mouth produces a black necrotic eschar or ulcer on the palate due to infarction of tissue. When the infection extends through the nasal turbinates, orbital cellulitis, extraocular muscle paresis, proptosis, chemosis, and eyelid edema with or without necrosis are commonly found. Orbital cellulitis as a manifestation of rhinocerebral mucormycosis is the most common and dramatic presentation of the disease. It occurs most often in association with poorly controlled diabetes, especially in the presence of ketoacidosis. When it has occurred in patients with leukemia or lymphoma, it has been associated with diabetes or the administration of systemic steroids. Rhinocerebral mucormycosis has also complicated organ transplantation. The relationship between invasive mucormycosis and diabetic ketoacidosis can be explained by the ketone reductase system of mucormycosis, which utilizes a high glucose concentration and has a peak activity at a low pH.

The diagnosis of cutaneous mucormycosis is made by confirmation of both infection via culture and tissue invasion via histopathology. Touch preparation of a skin biopsy may allow for rapid confirmation of a fungal infection.[213] Because positive cultures alone only indicate the presence of this ubiquitous saprophyte, tissue invasion by the hyphae of mucormycosis must be seen microscopically to confirm the diagnosis. The biopsy specimen should be taken from the center of the lesion and include subcutaneous fat because zygomycetes invade the blood

vessels of the dermis and the subcutis resulting in an ischemic cone at the skin surface.[217] However, culture is required to identify the fungal species. Histopathologic evaluation will demonstrate the broad, irregularly shaped non-septate hyphae with right-angle branching invading tissue. Organisms can be seen on H&E stained tissue, but are enhanced by periodic acid-Schiff or Gomori methenamine-silver stained specimens. Cytoplasmic inclusions and ameboid terminal expansion are also characteristic. Invasion of blood vessels with thrombosis, hemorrhage, and infarction is a characteristic pathologic manifestation of mucormycosis. Mucormycosis thrives on the matrix of ischemic necrotic tissue and spreads by direct extension along injured blood vessels. Blood cultures in primary cutaneous mucormycosis will always be negative.

The mortality rate of invasive mucormycosis approaches 80%, but depends on the site of infection and underlying disease present.[207] Infection with *Cunninghamella* has a worse prognosis than that of other zygomycetes.[207] The treatment of cutaneous mucormycosis typically requires a combination of surgical debridement, correction of metabolic abnormalities, and antifungal therapy with amphotericin B. Unlike voriconazole, posaconazole is a second generation azole antifungal that does cover the organisms that cause mucormycosis.

Figure 1.78. Periorbital and facial cellulitis due to mucormycosis with proptosis, chemosis, eyelid edema, and loss of full ocular movement. A brain abscess was present on computed axial tomography (CAT) scan

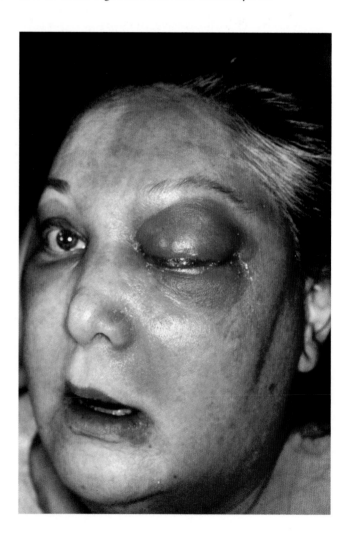

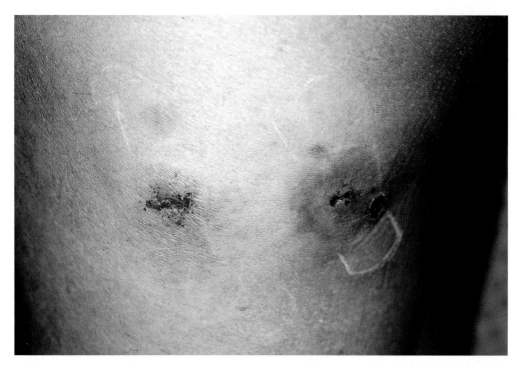

Figure 1.79. Primary cutaneous *Mucor ramosissimus*. Hemorrhagic subcutaneous nodules of the thigh in a woman with aplastic anemia confirmed by biopsy and culture

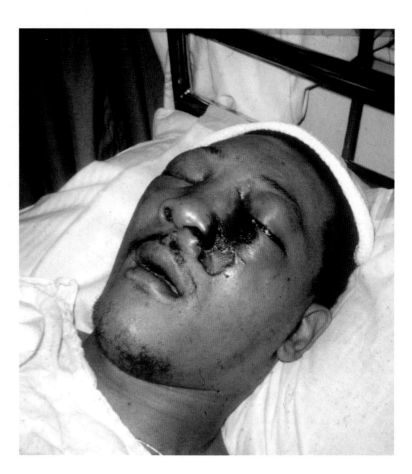

Figure 1.80. Preterminal paranasal cutaneous infarctive lesions of mucormycosis in a leukemic patient (Courtesy of Harold Neu, M.D.)

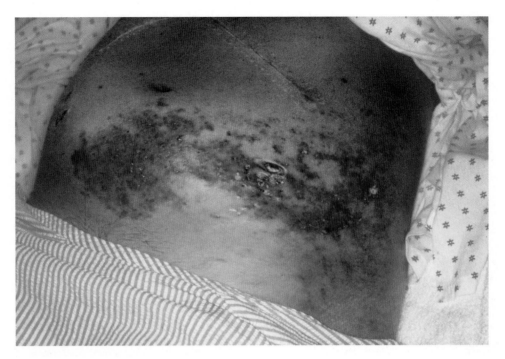

Figure 1.81. A 37-year-old woman with a liver transplant for sclerosing cholangitis developed a broad, red indurated plaque studded with pustules. Within the plaque, extending across the lower abdomen, was a 1-cm ulcer at the site of an abdominal drain. Skin biopsy demonstrated a suppurative granulomatous inflammation with PAS-positive fungal organisms identified as *Rhizopus* species on culture (Courtesy of Mary Gail Mercurio, M.D.)

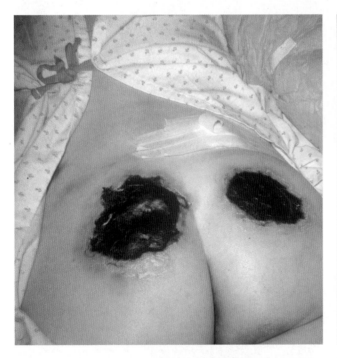

Figure 1.82. Progressive gangrenous cellulitis of the buttocks due to *Mucor* species in a patient with acute myelocytic leukemia. The infection began in areas of chafed skin and then rapidly invaded and successively destroyed the soft tissue to the gluteus muscles (From Dreizen S, et al. Unusual mucocutaneous infections in immunosuppressed patients with leukemia – expansion of an earlier study. Postgrad Med 1986;79(4):287–294)

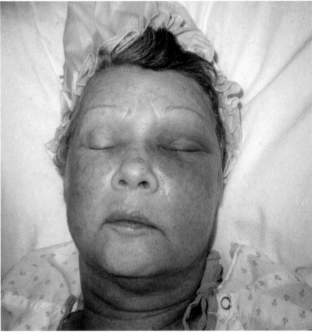

Figure 1.83. Orbital and facial cellulitis due to *Rhizopus oryzae* in a patient with AML (From Dreizen S, et al. Unusual mucocutaneous infections in immunosuppressed patients with leukemia – expansion of an earlier study. Postgrad Med 1986;79(4):287–294)

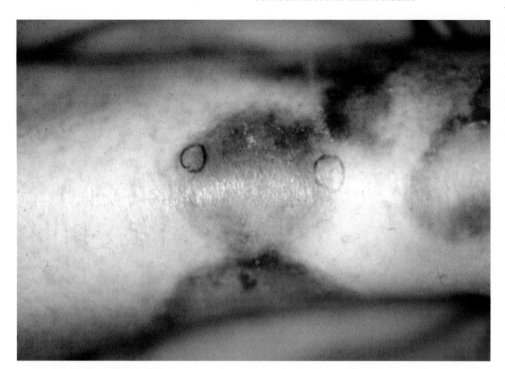

Figure 1.84. Bull's eye cutaneous infarct of zygomycosis. A 77-year-old with leukemic transformation of myelodysplastic syndrome developed neutropenic fever and centrally hemorrhagic necrotic red plaques on her forearm due to *Rhizopus arrhizus* (*oryzae*)

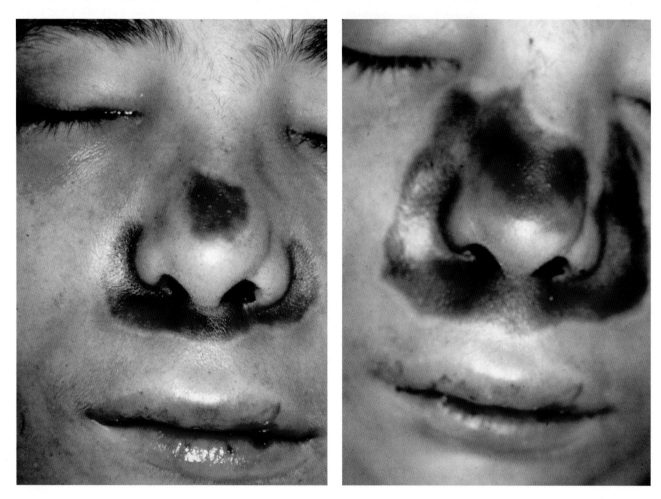

Figure 1.85. and 1.86. Fatal progressive angioinvasive mucormycosis in acute leukemia with central facial infarction

Figure 1.87. Invasive mucormycosis due to nasal oxygen cannula trauma to the cheek of a 90-year-old with diabetic ketoacidosis on high-dose systemic steroids for laryngeal edema

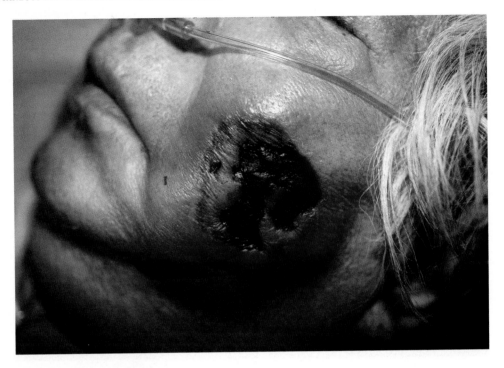

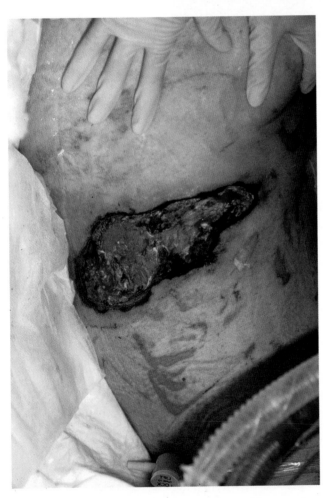

Figure 1.88. Invasive *Rhizopus oryzae* 1 month post heart transplant mimicking a surgical wound dehiscence

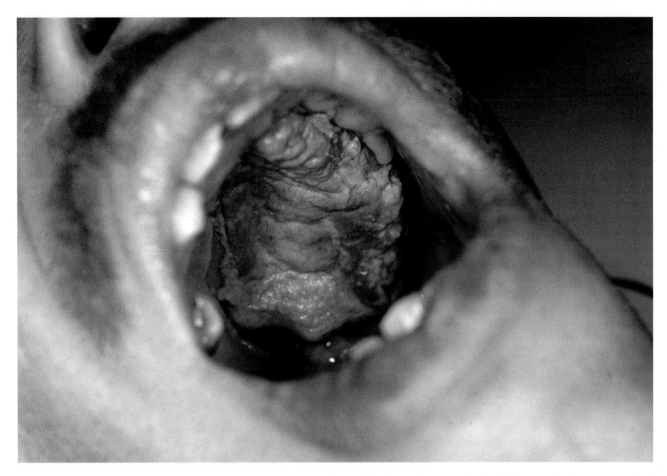

Figure 1.89. A 36-year-old HIV-positive man developed facial numbness, difficulty swallowing, and a facial droop. He had a necrotic palatal eschar due to invasive *Rhizopus* with involvement of peripheral cranial nerve VII and the maxilla

References

Aspergillosis

1. Kriengkauykiat J, Ito JI, Dadwal SS. Epidemiology and treatment approaches in management of invasive fungal infections. Clinical Epidemiology. 2011;3:175–191.
2. Nenoff P, Kliem C, Mittag M, et al. Secondary cutaneous aspergillosis due to *Aspergillus flavus* in an acute myeloid leukaemia patient following stem cell transplantation. Eur J Dermatol. 2002;12:93–8.
3. Roilides E, Farmaki E. Human immunodeficiency virus infection and cutaneous Aspergillosis. Arch Derm. 2000;136:412–4.
4. Murakawa GJ, Harvell JD, Lubitz P, et al. Cutaneous aspergillosis and acquired immunodeficiency syndrome. Arch Derm. 2000;136:365–9.
5. Barnes PD, Marr KA. Risks, diagnosis and outcomes of invasive fungal infection in haematopoietic stem cell transplant recipients. Br J Hematol. 2007;139:519–31.
6. Nucci M, Marr KA. Emerging fungal diseases. Clin Infect Dis. 2005;41:521–6.
7. Walsh TJ. Primary cutaneous aspergillosis – an emerging infection among immunocompromised patients. Clin Infect Dis. 1998;27:453–7.
8. Richards KA, Mancini AJ. A painful erythematous forearm nodule in a girl with Hodgkin disease. Diagnosis: primary cutaneous aspergillosis. Arch Dermatol. 2000;136(9):1165–70.
9. Grossman ME, Fithian EC, Behrens C, et al. Primary cutaneous aspergillosis in six leukemic children. J Am Acad Dermatol. 1985;12:313–8.
10. Munn S, Keane F, Child F, Philpott-Howard J, Du Vivier A. Primary cutaneous aspergillosis. Br J Dermatol. 1999;141:378–80.
11. Ricci RM, Evans JS, Meffert JJ, Kaufman L, Sadkowski LC. Primary cutaneous *Aspergillus ustus* infection: second reported case. J Am Acad Dermatol. 1998;38(5 Pt 2):797–8.
12. Chakrabarti A, Gupta V, Biswas G, Kumar B, Sakhuja VK. Primary cutaneous aspergillosis: our experience in 10 years. J Infect. 1998;37:24–7.
13. Vennewald I, Wollina U. Cutaneous infection due to opportunistic molds: uncommon presentations. Clin Dermatol. 2005;23:565–71.
14. Park SB, Kang MJ, Whang EA, et al. A case of primary cutaneous aspergillosis in a renal transplant recipient. Transplant Proc. 2004;36:2156–7.
15. Thakur BK, Bernardi DM, Murali MR, McClain SA, Clark RA. Invasive cutaneous aspergillosis complicating immunosuppressive therapy for recalcitrant pemphigus vulgaris. J Amer Acad Dermatol. 1998;38:488–90.
16. Mori T, Takae Y, Izaki S, et al. Cutaneous aspergillosis in a patient with follicular lymphoma. Eur J Dermatol. 2003;13:102–3.
17. Correa ME, Soares AB, de Souza CA, et al. Primary aspergillosis affecting the tongue of a leukemic patient. Oral Dis. 2003;9:49–53.
18. D'Antonio D, Pagano L, Girmenia C, et al. Cutaneous aspergillosis in patients with haematological malignancies. Eur J Clin Microbiol Infect Dis. 2000;19:362–5.
19. Palmero ML, Pope E, Brophy J. Sporotrichoid aspergillosis in an immunocompromised child: a case report and review of the literature. Pediatr Dermatol. 2009 ;26(5):592–6.
20. Geyer AS, Fox LP, Rabinowitz A, Grossman ME. Dehisced wound in a heart transplant recipient. Arch Dermatol. 2005;141(8):1037–40.
21. van Burik JA, Colven R, Spach DH. Itraconazole therapy for primary cutaneous aspergillosis in patients with AIDS. Clin Infect Dis. 1998;27:643–4.
22. Saadat P, Kappel S, Young S, Abrishami M, Vadmal MS. Aspergillus fumigatus majocchi granuloma in a patient with acquired immunodeficiency syndrome. Clin Exp Dermatol. 2008;33:450–3.
23. Stanford D, Boyle M, Gillespie R. Human immunodeficiency virus-related primary cutaneous aspergillosis. Australas J Dermatol. 2000;41:112–6.
24. Hunt SJ, Nagi C, Gross KG, Wong DS, Mathews WC. Primary cutaneous aspergillosis near central venous catheters in patients with the acquired immunodeficiency syndrome. Arch Derm. 1992;128:1229–32.
25. Arikan S, Uzun O, Cetinkaya Y, et al. Primary cutaneous aspergillosis in human immunodeficiency virus-infected patients: two cases and review. Clin Infect Dis. 1998;27(3):641–3.
26. Schimmelpfennig C, Naumann R, Zuberbier T, et al. Skin involvement as the first manifestation of systemic aspergillosis in patients after allogeneic hematopoietic cell transplantation. Bone Marrow Transplant. 2001;27:753–5.
27. Nenoff P, Kliem C, Mittag M, et al. Secondary cutaneous aspergillosis due to *Aspergillus flavus* in an acute myeloid leukaemia patient following stem cell transplantation. Eur J Dermatol. 2002;12:93–8.
28. Galimberti R, Kowalczuk A, Hidalgo Parra I, Gonzalez Ramos M, Flores V. Cutaneous aspergillosis: a report of six cases. Br J Dermatol. 1998;139:522–6.
29. Szyfelbein K, Lin JY, Bellucci KS, Williams JM. Tender erythema of the left lower extremity. Disseminated *Aspergillus fumigatus* infection with concurrent active cytomegalovirus infection (CMV). Arch Dermatol. 2007;143:535–40.
30. Chatzipanagiotou S, Takou K, Perogamvros A. Cutaneous purulent aspergillosis in a young man with chronic granulomatous disease. Mycoses. 1998;41(9–10):379–82.
31. Keating MR, Guerrero MA, Daly RC, Walker RC, Davies SF. Transmission of invasive Aspergillosis from a subclinically infected donor to three different organ transplant recipients. Chest. 1996;109:1119–24.
32. Shao PL, Huang LM, Hsueh PR. Invasive fungal infection – laboratory diagnosis and antifungal treatment. J Microbiol Immunol Infect. 2006;39:178–88.

Blastomycosis

33. Hay RJ. Blastomycosis: what's new? J Eur Acad Dermatol Venereol. 2000 ;14(4):249–50.
34. Bradsher RW. Clinical features of blastomycosis. Semin Respir Infect. 1997;12(3):229–34.
35. Pappas PG. Blastomycosis in the immunocompromised patient. Semin Respir Infect. 1997;12(3):243–51.
36. Cohen P, Grossman ME, Silvers DN. Mucocutaneous manifestations of systemic fungal infections in the HIV-seropositive patient. AIDS Read. 1993;3:47–60.
37. Fisher KR, Baselski V, Beard G, et al. Pustular blastomycosis. J Am Acad Dermatol. 2009;61:355–8.
38. Smith JA, Kauffman CA. Endemic fungal infections in patients receiving tumor necrosis factor-alpha inhibitor therapy. Drugs. 2009;69:1403–15.
39. Serody JS, Mill MR, Detterbeck FC, Harris DT, Cohen MS. Blastomycosis in transplant recipients: report of a case and review. Clin Infect Dis. 1993;16(1):54–8.
40. Walker K, Skelton H, Smith K. Cutaneous lesions showing giant yeast forms of *Blastomyces dermatitidis*. J Cutan Pathol. 2002;29:616–8.
41. Lemos LB, Baliga M, Guo M. Blastomycosis: the Great Pretender can also be an opportunist. Initial clinical diagnosis and underlying diseases in 123 patients. Ann Diagn Pathol. 2002;6(3):194–203.
42. Gauthier GM, Safdar H, Klein BS, Andes DR. Blastomycosis in solid organ transplant recipients. Transpl Infect Dis. 2007;9:310–7.
43. Chapman SW, Dismukes WE, Proia LA, et al. Clinical practice guidelines for the management of blastomycosis: 2008 update by the Infectious Diseases Society of America. Clin Infect Dis. 2008;46:1801–12.

Candidiasis

44. Pedraz J, Delgado-Jiménez Y, Pérez-Gala S, et al. Cutaneous expression of systemic candidiasis. Clin Exp Dermatol. 2009;34:106–10.
45. Bougnoux ME, Dupont C, Turner L, et al. Mixed *Candida glabrata* and *Candida albicans* disseminated candidiasis in a heroin addict. Eur J Clin Microbiol Infect Dis. 1997;16:598–600.

46. Kreuter A, Teichmann M, Stuecker M, et al. Generalized fungal infection in a patient with AIDS appearing as skin papules. Eur J Med Res. 2003;8:435–7.

47. Virgili A, Zampino MR, Mantovani L. Fungal skin infections in organ transplant recipients. Am J Clin Dermatol. 2002;3:19–35.

48. Leung AY, Chim CS, Ho PL, et al. Candida tropicalis fungaemia in adult patients with haematological malignancies: clinical features and risk factors. J Hosp Infect. 2002;50:316–9.

49. Nucci M, Marr KA. Emerging fungal diseases. Clin Infect Dis. 2005;41:521–6.

50. Muñoz P, Sánchez-Somolinos M, Alcalá L, et al. *Candida krusei* fungaemia: antifungal susceptibility and clinical presentation of an uncommon entity during 15 years in a single general hospital. J Antimicrob Chemother. 2005;55:188–93.

51. Gunsilius E, Lass-Flörl C, Kähler CM, Gastl G, Petzer AL. *Candida ciferrii*, a new fluconaozle-resistant yeast causing systemic mycosis in immunocompromised patients. Ann Hematol. 2001;80:178–9.

52. Wellinghausen N, Moericke A, Bundschuh S, et al. Multifocal osteomyelitis caused by *Candida dubliniensis*. J Med Microbiol. 2009;58:386–90.

53. Bodey GP. Dermatologic manifestations of infections in neutropenic patients. Infect Dis Clin North Am. 1994;8:655–75.

54. Grossman ME, Silvers DN, Walther RR. Cutaneous manifestations of disseminated candidiasis. J Am Acad Dermatol. 1980;2:111–6.

55. Ruchel R. Clinical presentation of invasive candida mycoses. Mycoses. 1997;40:17–20.

56. Wai PH, Ewing CA, Johnson LB, et al. Candida fasciitis following renal transplantation. Transplantation. 2001;72(3):477–9.

57. Glaich AS, Krathen RA, Smith MJ, Hsu S. Disseminated candidiasis mimicking leukocytoclastic vasculitis. J Am Acad Dermatol. 2005;53(3):544–6.

58. Marcus J, Grossman ME, Yunakov MJ, Rappaport F. Disseminated candidiasis, candida arthritis and unilateral skin lesions. J Am Acad Dermatol. 1992;26:295–7.

59. Held JL, Berkowitz RK, Grossman ME. Use of touch preparation for rapid diagnosis of disseminated candidiasis. J Am Acad Dermatol. 1988;19:1063–6.

60. Spellberg BJ, Filler SG, Edwards Jr JE. Current treatment strategies for disseminated candidiasis. Clin Infect Dis. 2006;42(2):244–51. Epub 2005 Dec 2.

Coccidioidomycosis

61. DiCaudo DJ. Coccidioidomycosis: a review and update. J Am Acad Dermatol. 2006;55(6):929–42.

62. Santelli AC, Blair JE, Roust LR. Coccidioidomycosis in patients with diabetes mellitus. Am J Med. 2006;119(11):964–9.

63. Bergstrom L, Yocum DE, Ampel NM, et al. Increased risk of coccidioidomycosis in patients treated with tumor necrosis factor alpha antagonists. Arthritis Rheum. 2004;50(6):1959–66.

64. Prichard JG, Sorotzkin RA, James III RE. Cutaneous manifestations of disseminated coccidioidomycosis in the acquired immunodeficiency syndrome. Cutis. 1987;39(3):203–5.

65. Stagliano D, Epstein J, Hickey P. Fomite-transmitted coccidioidomycosis in an immunocompromised child. Pediatr Infect Dis J. 2007;26(5):454–6.

66. Braddy CM, Heilman RL, Blair JE. Coccidioidomycosis after renal transplantation in an endemic area. Am J Transplant. 2006;6(2):340–5.

67. Vartivarian SE, Coudron PE, Markowitz SM. Disseminated coccidioidomycosis. Unusual manifestations in a cardiac transplantation patient. Am J Med. 1987;83(5):949–52.

68. Wolf JE, Little JR, Pappagianis D, Kobayashi GS. Disseminated coccidioidomycosis in a patient with the acquired immune deficiency syndrome. Diagn Microbiol Infect Dis. 1986;5(4):331–6.

69. Rogan MP, Thomas K. Fatal miliary coccidioidomycosis in a patient receiving infliximab therapy: a case report. J Med Case Rep. 2007;1:79.

70. Poonawalla T, Diwan H, Duvic M. Mycosis fungoides with coccidioidomycosis. Clin Lymphoma Myeloma. 2006;7(2):148–50.

71. Ugurlu S, de Alba Campomanes AG, Naseri A, Blair JE, McLeish WM. Coccidioidomycosis of the eyelid. Ophthal Plast Reconstr Surg. 2005;21(2):157–9.

72. Gold WL, Campbell I, Vellend H. Disseminated coccidioidomycosis in a Canadian patient with chronic HIV infection – Ontario. Can Commun Dis Rep. 1992;18(19):149–50.

73. Blair JE. Coccidioidomycosis in patients who have undergone transplantation. Ann N Y Acad Sci. 2007;1111:365–76.

74. Ampel NM. Coccidioidomycosis among persons with human immunodeficiency virus infection in the era of highly active antiretroviral therapy (HAART). Semin Respir Infect. 2001;16(4):257–62.

Cryptococcosis

75. Narayan S, Batta K, Colloby P, Tan CY. Cutaneous Cryptococcus infection due to *C. albidus* associated with SeÂzary syndrome. Br J Dermatol. 2000;143:632–4.

76. Cohen P, Grossman ME, Silvers DN. Mucocutaneous manifestations of systemic fungal infections in the HIV-seropositive patient. AIDS Read. 1993;3:47–60.

77. Sing Y, Ramdial PK. Cryptococcal inflammatory pseudotumors. Am J Surg Pathol. 2007;31:1521–7.

78. França AV, Carneiro M, dal Sasso K, Souza Cda S, Martinelli A. Cryptococcosis in cirrhotic patients. Mycoses. 2005;48:68–72.

79. Husain S, Wagener MM, Singh N. Cryptococcus neoformans infection in organ transplant recipients: variables influencing clinical characteristics and outcome. Emerg Infect Dis. 2001;7(3):375–81.

80. Orsini J, Nowakowski J, Delaney V, Sakoulas G, Wormser GP. Cryptococcal infection presenting as cellulitis in a renal transplant recipient. Transpl Infect Dis. 2009;11:68–71.

81. Moe K, Lotsikas-Baggili AJ, Kupiec-Banasikowska A, Kauffman CL. The cutaneous predilection of disseminated cryptococcal infection in organ transplant recipients. Arch Dermatol. 2005;141(7):913–4.

82. Christianson JC, Engber W, Andes D. Primary cutaneous cryptococcosis in immunocompetent and immunocompromised hosts. Med Mycol. 2003;41(3):177–88.

83. Wilson ML, Sewell LD, Mowad CM. Case reports: primary cutaneous Cryptoccocosis during therapy with methotrexate and adalimumab. J Drugs Dermatol. 2008;7:53–4.

84. Hoang JK, Burruss J. Localized cutaneous *Cryptococcus albidus*. Infection in a 14-year-old boy on etanercept therapy. Pediatr Dermatol. 2007;24(3):285–8.

85. Murakawa GJ, Kerschmann R, Berger T. Cutaneous Cryptococcus infection and AIDS. Report of 12 cases and review of the literature. Arch Derm. 1996;132:545–8.

86. Sánchez P, Bosch RJ, de Gálvez MV, Gallardo MA, Herrera E. Cutaneous cryptococcosis in two patients with acquired immunodeficiency syndrome. Int J STD AIDS. 2000;11:477–80.

87. Gasiorowski J, Knysz B, Szetela B, Gładysz A. Cutaneous cryptococcosis as a rare manifestation of the immune reconstitution syndrome in an HIV-1-infected patient. Postepy Hig Med Dosw (Online). 2008;62:1–3.

88. Vandersmissen G, Meuleman L, Tits G, Verhaeghe A, Peetermans WE. Cutaneous cryptococcosis in corticosteroid-treated patients without AIDS. Acta Clin Belg. 1996;51(2):111–7.

89. Adachi M, Tsuruta D, Imanishi H, Ishii M, Kobayashi H. Necrotizing fasciitis caused by *Cryptococcus neoformans* in a patient with pemphigus vegetans. Clin Exp Dermatol. 2009;34(8):751–3.

90. Başaran O, Emiroğlu R, Arikan U, Karakayali H, Haberal M. Cryptococcal necrotizing fasciitis with multiple sites of involvement in the lower extremities. Dermatol Surg. 2003;29(11):1158–60.

91. Baer S, Baddley JW, Gnann JW, Pappas PG. Cryptococcal disease presenting as necrotizing cellulitis in transplant recipients. Transpl Infect Dis. 2009;11(4):353–8.

92. Carbia SG, Chain M, Acuña K, et al. Disseminated cryptococcosis with cutaneous lesions complicating steroid therapy for Behçet's disease. Int J Dermatol. 2003;42:816–8.

93. Blocher KS, Weeks JA, Noble RC. Cutaneous cryptococcal infection presenting as vulvar lesion. Genitourin Med. 1987;63:341–3.

94. Ebara N, Kobayashi N, Asaka H, et al. Localized cutaneous cryptococcosis in a patient with chronic myeloproliferative disease. J Dermatol. 2005;32(8):674–6.

95. Manfredi R, Mazzoni A, Nanetti A, et al. Morphologic features and clinical significance of skin involvement in patients with AIDS-related cryptococcosis. Acta Derm Venereol. 1996;76(1):72–4.

96. Dimino-Emme L, Gurevitch AW. Cutaneous manifestations of disseminated cryptococcosis. J Am Acad Dermatol. 1995;32:844–50.

97. Calista D, Grosso C. Cutaneous cryptococcosis of the penis. Dermatol Online J. 2008;14(7):9.

98. Hecker MS, Weinberg JM. Cutaneous cryptococcosis mimicking keloid. Dermatology. 2001;202:78–9.

99. Murakawa GJ, Mauro TM, Egbert B. Disseminated cutaneous Cryptococcus clinically mimicking basal cell carcinoma. Dermatol Surg. 1995;21(11):992–3.

100. Ingleton R, Koestenblatt E, Don P, et al. Cutaneous cryptococcosis mimicking basal cell carcinoma in a patient with AIDS. J Cutan Med Surg. 1998;3(1):43–5.

101. Annam V, Inamadar AC, Palit A, Yelikar BR. Co-infection of molluscum contagiosum virus and cryptococcosis in the same skin lesion in a HIV-infected patient. J Cutan Pathol. 2008;35 Suppl 1:29–31.

102. Myers SA, Kamino H. Cutaneous cryptococcosis and histoplasmosis coinfection in a patient with AIDS. J Am Acad Dermatol. 1996;34:898–900.

103. Neuville S, Dromer F, Morin O, et al. Primary cutaneous cryptococcosis: a distinct clinical entity. Clin Infect Dis. 2003;36:337–47.

104. Zorman JV, Zupanc TL, Parač Z, Cuček I. Primary cutaneous cryptococcosis in a renal transplant recipient: case report. Mycoses. 2010;53(6):535–7.

105. Hunger RE, Paredes BE, Quattroppani C, Krähenbühl S, Braathen LR. Primary cutaneous cryptococcosis in a patient with systemic immunosuppression after liver transplantation. Dermatology. 2000;200:352–5.

106. Baumgarten KL, Valentine VG, Garcia-Diaz JB. Primary cutaneous cryptococcosis in a lung transplant recipient. South Med J. 2004;97:692–5.

107. Badreshia S, Klepeiss S, Ioffreda M, et al. Cutaneous cryptococcus in an elderly woman with chronic essential dermatitis. Cutis. 2006;78:53–6.

108. Romano C, Taddeucci P, Donati D, Miracco C, Massai L. Primary cutaneous cryptococcosis due to *Cryptococcus neoformans* in a woman with non-Hodgkin's lymphoma. Acta Dermatol Venerol. 2001;8:220–1.

109. Bohne T, Sander A, Pfister-Wartha A, Schöpf E. Primary cutaneous cryptococcosis following trauma of the right forearm. Mycoses. 1996;39(11–12):457–9.

110. Ramdial PK, Calonje E, Sing Y, Chotey NA, Aboobaker J. Molluscum-like cutaneous cryptococcosis: a histopathological and pathogenetic appraisal. J Cutan Pathol. 2008;35:1007–13.

Histoplasmosis

111. Bonifaz A, Chang P, Moreno K, Fernández-Fernández V, et al. Disseminated cutaneous histoplasmosis in acquired immunodeficiency syndrome: report of 23 cases. Clin Exp Dermatol. 2009;34(4):481–6.

112. Couppié P, Clyti E, Nacher M, et al. Acquired immunodeficiency syndrome-related oral and/or cutaneous histoplasmosis: a descriptive and comparative study of 21 cases in French Guiana. Int J Dermatol. 2002;41:571–6.

113. Cohen PR, Grossman ME, Silvers DN. Mucocutaneous manifestations of systemic fungal infections in the HIV-seropositive patient. AIDS Read. 1993;3:47–60.

114. Cohen PR, Grossman ME, Silvers DN. Disseminated histoplasmosis and human immunodeficiency virus infection. Int J Dermatol. 1991;30(9):614–22.

115. Cohen PR, Bank DE, Silvers DN, Grossman ME. Cutaneous lesions of disseminated histoplasmosis in human immunodeficiency virus-infected patients. J Am Acad Dermatol. 1990;23(3 Pt 1):422–8.

116. Cunha VS, Zampese MS, Aquino VR, Cestari TF, Goldani LZ. Mucocutaneous manifestations of disseminated histoplasmosis in patients with acquired immunodeficiency syndrome: particular aspects in a Latin-American population. Clin Exp Dermatol. 2007;32:250–5.

117. Cohen PR, Held JL, Grossman ME, Ross MJ, Silvers DN. Disseminated histoplasmosis presenting as an ulcerated verrucous plaque in a human immunodeficiency virus-infected man. Report of a case possibly involving human-to-human transmission of histoplasmosis. Int J Dermatol. 1991;30(2):104–8.

118. Kucharski LD, Dal Pizzol AS, Fillus J Neto, et al. Disseminated cutaneous histoplasmosis and AIDS: case report. Braz J Infect Dis. 2000;4(5):255–61.

119. Kalter DC, Tschen JA, Klima M. Maculopapular rash in a patient with acquired immunodeficiency syndrome. Disseminated histoplasmosis in acquired immunodeficiency syndrome (AIDS). Arch Dermatol. 1985;121(11):1455–6, 1458–9.

120. Laochumroonvorapong P, DiCostanzo DP, Wu H, et al. Disseminated histoplasmosis presenting as pyoderma gangrenosum-like lesions in a patient with acquired immunodeficiency syndrome. Int J Dermatol. 2001;40(8):518–21.

121. K Ramdial P, Mosam A, Dlova NC, et al. Disseminated cutaneous histoplasmosis in patients infected with human immunodeficiency virus. J Cutan Pathol. 2002;29:215–25.

122. Chaker BM, Cockerell CJ. Concomitant psoriasis, seborrheic dermatitis, and disseminated cutaneous histoplasmosis in a patient infected with human immunodeficiency virus. J Am Acad Dermatol. 1993;29(2 Pt 2):311–3.

123. Abildgaard Jr WH, Hargrove RH, Kalivas J. Histoplasma panniculitis. Arch Dermatol. 1985;121(7):914–6.

124. Rosenberg JD, Scheinfeld NS. Cutaneous histoplasmosis in patients with acquired immunodeficiency syndrome. Cutis. 2003;72(6):439–45.

125. Cole MC, Cohen PR, Satra KH, Grossman ME. The concurrent presence of systemic disease pathogens and cutaneous Kaposi's sarcoma in the same lesion: histoplasma capsulatum and Kaposi's sarcoma coexisting in a single skin lesion in a patient with AIDS. J Am Acad Dermatol. 1992;26(2 Pt 2):285–7.

126. Myers SA, Kamino H. Cutaneous cryptococcosis and histoplasmosis coinfection in a patient with AIDS. J Am Acad Dermatol. 1996;34:898–900.

127. Cole MC, Grossman ME. Disseminated histoplasmosis presenting as tongue nodules in an HIV infected patient. Cutis. 1995;55:104–6.

128. Casariego Z, Kelly GR, Perez H, et al. Disseminated histoplasmosis with orofacial involvement in HIV-1-infected patients with AIDS: manifestations and treatment. Oral Dis. 1997;3:184–7.

129. Barton EN, Roberts L, Ince WE, et al. Cutaneous histoplasmosis in the acquired immune deficiency syndrome – a report of three cases from Trinidad. Trop Geogr Med. 1988;40(2):153–7.

130. de Oliveira EV, Miduati FB, Antonio JR, et al. Histoplasmosis as cause of penile ulcer in acquired immune deficiency syndrome (AIDS): three case reports. Mycopathologia. 2007;164:295–9.

131. Rodríguez G, Ordóñéz N, Motta A. Histoplasma capsulatum var. capsulatum within cutaneous nerves in patients with disseminated histoplasmosis and AIDS. Br J Dermatol. 2001;144(1):205–7.

132. Paul AY, Aldrich S, Scott RS, Ellis MW. Disseminated histoplasmosis in a patient with AIDS: case report and review of the literature. Cutis. 2007;80(4):309–12.

133. Breton G, Adle-Biassette H, Therby A, et al. Immune reconstitution inflammatory syndrome in HIV-infected patients with disseminated histoplasmosis. AIDS. 2006;20(1):119–21.

Phaeohyphomycosis

134. Foulet F, Duvoux C, de Bièvre C, Hézode C, Bretagne S. Cutaneous phaeohyphomycosis caused by Veronaea bothryosa in a liver transplant recipient successfully treated with itraconazole. Clin Infect Dis. 1999;29(3):689–90.

135. Liou JM, Wang JT, Wang MH, Wang SS, Hsueh PR. Phaeohyphomycosis caused by Exophiala species in immunocompromised hosts. J Formos Med Assoc. 2002;101(7):523–6.

136. Umemoto N, Demitsu T, Kakurai M, et al. Two cases of cutaneous phaeohyphomycosis due to exophiala jeanselmei: diagnostic significance of direct microscopic examination of the purpulent discharge. Clin Exp Dermatol. 2009;34(7):e351–3.

137. Singh N, Chang FY, Gayowski T, Marino IR. Infections due to dematiaceous fungi in organ transplant recipients: case report and review. Clin Infect Dis. 1997;24(3):369–74.

138. Saint-Jean M, St-Germain G, Laferrière C, Tapiero B. Hospital-acquired phaeohyphomycosis due to Exserohilum rostratum in a child with leukemia. Can J Infect Dis Med Microbiol. 2007;18(3):200–2.

139. Sutton DA, Rinaldi MG, Kielhofner M. First U.S. report of subcutaneous phaeohyphomycosis caused by Veronaea botryosa in a heart transplant recipient and review of the literature. J Clin Microbiol. 2004;42:2843–6.

140. Gerdsen R, Uerlich M, De Hoog GS, Bieber T, Horré R. Sporotrichoid phaeohyphomycosis due to Alternaria infectoria. Br J Dermatol. 2001;154:484–6.

141. Calabrò G, Nino M, Gallo L, Scalvenzi M. Cutaneous alternariosis in a kidney transplantation recipient: report of a case. J Dermatolog Treat. 2008;19:246–8.

142. Lin SC, Sun PL, Ju YM, Chan YJ. Cutaneous phaeohyphomycosis caused by Exserohilum rostratum in a patient with cutaneous T cell lymphoma. Int J Dermatol. 2009;48:295–8.

143. Segner S, Jouret F, Durant JF, Marot L, Kanaan N. Cutaneous infection by Alternaria infectoria in a renal transplant patient. Transpl Infect Dis. 2009;11:330–2.

144. Martínez-González MC, Verea MM, Velasco D, et al. Three cases of cutaneous phaeohyphomycosis by Exophiala jeanselmei. Eur J Dermatol. 2008;18(3):313–6.

145. Brasch J, Busch JO, de Hoog GS. Cutaneous phaeohyphomycosis caused by Alternaria infectoria. Acta Derm Venereol. 2008;88:160–1.

146. Romano C, Bilenchi R, Alessandrini C, Miracco C. Case report. Cutaneous phaeohyphomycosis caused by Cladosporium oxysporum. Mycoses. 1999;42:111–5.

147. Gené J, Azón-Masoliver A, Guarro J, et al. Cutaneous phaeohyphomycosis caused by Alternaria longipes in an immunosuppressed patient. J Clin Microbiol. 1995;33:2774–6.

148. Harris JE, Sutton DA, Rubin A, et al. Exophiala spinifera as a cause of cutaneous phaeohyphomycosis: case study and review of the literature. Med Mycol. 2009;47(1):87–93.

149. Dubois D, Pihet M, Clec'h CL, et al. Cutaneous phaeohyphomycosis due to Alternaria infectoria. Mycopathologica. 2005;160:117–23.

150. Yehia M, Thomas M, Pilmore H, Van Der Merwe W, Dittmer I. Subcutaneous black fungus (phaeohyphomycosis) infection in renal transplant recipients: three cases. Transplantation. 2004;77:140–2.

151. McCown HF, Sahn EE. Subcutaneous phaeohyphomycosis and nocardiosis in a kidney transplant patient. J Am Acad Dermatol. 1997;36(5 Pt 2):863–6.

152. Arnoldo BD, Purdue GF, Tchorz K, Hunt JL. A case report of phaeohyphomycosis caused by Cladophialophora bantiana treated in a burn unit. J Burn Care Rehabil. 2005;26:285–7.

153. O'Quinn RP, Hoffmann JL, Boyd AS. Colletotrichum species as emerging opportunistic fungal pathogens: a report of 3 cases of phaeohyphomycosis and review. J Am Acad Dermatol. 2001;45(1):56–61.

154. Pereiro Jr M, Pereiro Ferreirós MM, De Hoog GS, Toribio J. Cutaneous infection caused by Alternaria in patients receiving tacrolimus. Med Mycol. 2004;42(3):277–82.

155. Mayser P, Nilles M, de Hoog GS. Case report. Cutaneous phaeohyphomycosis due to Alternaria alternata. Mycoses. 2002;45(8):338–40.

156. Al-Attar A, Williams CG, Redett RJ. Rare lower extremity invasive fungal infection of an immunosuppressed patient: Exserohilum longirostratum. Plast Reconstr Surg. 2006;117(3):44e–7e.

157. Chen YT, Lin HC, Huang CC, Lo YH. Cutaneous phaeohyphomycosis caused by an Itraconazole and Amphotericin B resistant strain of Veronaeae botryose. Int J Dermatol. 2006;45:429–32.

158. Revankar SG, Patterson JE, Sutton DA, Pullen R, Rinaldi MG. Disseminated phaeohyphomycosis: review of an emerging mycosis. Clin Infect Dis. 2002;34:467–76.

159. Ohira S, Isoda K, Hamanaka H, et al. Case report. Phaeohyphomycosis caused by Philaphora verrucosa developed in a patient with non-HIV acquired immunodeficiency syndrome. Mycoses. 2002;45(1–2):50–4.

160. Keyser A, Schmid FX, Linde HJ, Merk J, Birnbaum DE. Disseminated Cladophialophora bantiana infection in a heart transplant recipient. J Heart Lung Transplant. 2002;21:503–5.

161. Levy I, Stein J, Ashkenazi S, et al. Ecthyma gangrenosum caused by disseminated Exserohilum in a child with leukemia: case report and review of the literature. Pediatr Dermatol. 2003;20:495–7.

Scedosporium and Pseudallescheria

162. Cortez KJ, Roilides E, Quiroz-Telles F, et al. Infections caused by Scedosporium spp. Clin Microbiol Rev. 2008;21(1):157–97.

163. Husain S, Muñoz P, Forrest G, et al. Infections due to Scedosporium apiospermum and Scedosporium prolificans in transplant recipients: clinical characteristics and impact of antifungal agent therapy on outcome. Clin Infect Dis. 2005;40(1):89–99.

164. Ginter G, de Hoog GS, Pschaid A, et al. Arthritis without grains caused by Pseudallescheria boydii. Mycoses. 1995;38(9–10):369–71.

165. Bower CP, Oxley JD, Campbell CK, Archer CB. Cutaneous Scedosporium apiospermum infection in an immunocompromised patient. J Clin Pathol. 1999;52(11):846–8.

166. Lavigne C, Maillot F, de Muret A, et al. Cutaneous infection with Scedosporium apiospermum in a patient treated with corticosteroids. Acta Derm Venereol. 1999;79(5):402–3.

167. Talbot TR, Hatcher J, Davis SF, et al. Scedosporium apiospermum pneumonia and sternal wound infection in a heart transplant recipient. Transplantation. 2002;74(11):1645–7.

168. Lainscak M, Hocevar A, Logar D, et al. Subcutaneous infection with Pseudallescheria boydii in an immunocompromised patient. Clin Rheumatol. 2007;26:1023–4.

169. Uenotsuchi T, Moroi Y, Urabe K, et al. Cutaneous Scedosporium apiospermum infection in an immunocompromised patient and a review of the literature. Acta Derm Venereol. 2005;85(2):156–9.

170. Castiglioni B, Sutton DA, Rinaldi MG, Fung J, Kusne S. Pseudallescheria boydii (Anamorph Scedosporium apiospermum). Infection in solid organ transplant recipients in a tertiary medical center and review of the literature. Medicine (Baltimore). 2002;81(5):333–48.

171. Chaveiro MA, Vieira R, Cardoso J, Afonso A. Cutaneous infection due to *Scedosporium apiospermum* in an immunosuppressed patient. J Eur Acad Dermatol Venereol. 2003;17(1):47–9.

172. Shinohara MM, George E. *Scedosporium apiospermum* an emerging opportunistic pathogen that must be distinguished from *Aspergillus* and other hyalohyphomycetes. J Cutan Pathol. 2009;36 Suppl 1:39–41.

173. Kusuhara M, Hachisuka H. Lymphocutaneous infection due to *Scedosporium apiospermum*. Int J Dermatol. 1997;36(9):684–8.

174. Ruxin TA, Steck WD, Helm TN, Bergfeld WF, Bolwell BJ. *Pseudallescheria boydii* in an immunocompromised host. Successful treatment with debridement and itraconazole. Arch Dermatol. 1996;132(4):382–4.

175. Hagari Y, Ishioka S, Ohyama F, Mihara M. Cutaneous infection showing sporotrichoid spread caused by *Pseudallescheria boydii* (*Scedosporium apiospermum*): successful detection of fungal DNA in formalin-fixed, paraffin-embedded sections by seminested PCR. Arch Dermatol. 2002;138(2):271–2.

176. Török L, Simon G, Csornai A, Tápai M, Török I. *Scedosporium apiospermum* infection imitating lymphocutaneous sporotrichosis in a patient with myeloblastic-monocytic leukaemia. Br J Dermatol. 1995;133(5):805–9.

177. Bernstein EF, Schuster MG, Stieritz DD, Heuman PC, Uitto J. Disseminated cutaneous *Pseudallescheria boydii*. Br J Dermato. 1995;132(3):456–60.

178. Barbaric D, Shaw PJ. Scedosporium infection in immunocompromised patients: successful use of liposomal amphotericin B and itraconazole. Med Pediatr Oncol. 2001;37(2):122–5.

179. Elm MK, Ahmed A, Gokselo D, Heming JS. Cutaneous and systemic infection with *Scedosporium apiospermum*. Cutis. 2009; 84:275–8.

180. Berenguer J, Rodríguez-Tudela JL, Richard C, et al. Deep infections caused by *Scedosporium prolificans*. A report on 16 cases in Spain and a review of the literature. *Scedosporium prolificans* Spanish Study Group. Medicine (Baltimore). 1997;76(4):256–65.

181. Rodriguez-Tudela JL, Berenguer J, Guarro J, et al. Epidemiology and outcome of *Scedosporium prolificans* infection, a review of 162 cases. Med Mycol. 2009;47(4):359–70.

Sporotrichosis

182. Dong JA, Chren MM, Elewski BE. Bonsai tree: risk factor for disseminated sporotrichosis. J Am Acad Dermatol. 1995;33:839–40.

183. Cohen PR, Grossman ME, Silvers DN. Mucocutaneous manifestations of systemic fungal infections in the HIV-seropositive patient. AIDS Read. 1993;3:47–60.

184. Yang DJ, Krishnan RS, Guillen DR, et al. Disseminated sporotrichosis mimicking sarcoidosis. Int J Dermatol. 2006;45:450–3.

185. Ramos-e-Silva M, Vasconcelos C, Carneiro S, Cestari T. Sporotrichosis. Clin Dermatol. 2007;25(2):181–7.

186. al-Tawfiq JA, Wools KK. Disseminated sporotrichosis and Sporothrix schenckii fungemia as the initial presentation of human immunodeficiency virus infection. Clin Infect Dis. 1998;26(6):1403–6.

187. Bonifaz A, Peniche A, Mercadillo P, Saúl A. Successful treatment of AIDS-related disseminated cutaneous sporotrichosis with itraconazole. AIDS Patient Care STDS. 2001;15(12):603–6.

188. Carvalho MT, de Castro AP, Baby C, et al. Disseminated cutaneous sporotrichosis in a patient with AIDS: report of a case. Rev Soc Bras Med Trop. 2002;35(6):655–9.

189. Sharma NL, Mehta KI, Mahajan VK, et al. Cutaneous sporotrichosis of face: polymorphism and reactivation after intralesional triamcinolone. Indian J Dermatol Venereol Leprol. 2007;73(3): 188–90.

190. Donabedian H, O'Donnell E, Olszewski C, MacArthur RD, Budd N. Disseminated cutaneous and meningeal sporotrichosis in an AIDS patient. Diagn Microbiol Infect Dis. 1994;18(2):111–5.

191. Yelverton CB, Stetson CL, Bang RH, Clark JW, Butler DF. Fatal sporotrichosis. Cutis. 2006;78(4):253–6.

192. Kim S, Rusk MH, James WD. Erysipeloid sporotrichosis in a woman with Cushing's disease. J Am Acad Dermatol. 1999;40: 272–4.

193. Rocha MM, Dassin T, Lira R, et al. Sporotrichosis in patient with AIDS: report of a case and review. Rev Iberoam Micol. 2001;18(3): 133–6.

194. Fontes PC, Kitakawa D, Carvalho YR, et al. Sporotrichosis in an HIV-positive man with oral lesions: a case report. Acta Cytol. 2007;51(4):648–50.

195. Aarestrup FM, Guerra RO, Vieira BJ, Cunha RM. Oral manifestation of sporotrichosis in AIDS patients. Oral Dis. 2001;7(2): 134–6.

196. Johnson RA. HIV disease: mucocutaneous fungal infections in HIV disease. Clin Dermatol. 2000;18(4):411–22.

197. Silva-Vergara ML, Maneira FR, De Oliveira RM, et al. Multifocal sporotrichosis with meningeal involvement in a patient with AIDS. Med Mycol. 2005;43(2):187–90.

198. Severo LC, Festugato M, Bernardi C, Londero AT. Widespread cutaneous lesions due to *Sporothrix schenckii* in a patient under a long-term steroids therapy. Rev Inst Med Trop Sao Paulo. 1999;41(1):59–62.

199. Hardman S, Stephenson I, Jenkins DR, Wiselka MJ, Johnson EM. Disseminated *Sporothix schenckii* in a patient with AIDS. J Infect. 2005;51(3):e73–7.

200. Vilela R, Souza GF, Fernandes Cota G, Mendoza L. Cutaneous and meningeal sporotrichosis in a HIV patient. Rev Iberoam Micol. 2007;24(2):161–3.

201. Bickley LK, Berman IJ, Hood AF. Fixed cutaneous sporotrichosis: unusual histopathology following intralesional corticosteroid administration. J Am Acad Dermatol. 1985;12(6):1007–12.

202. Ware AJ, Cockerell CJ, Skiest DJ, Kussman HM. Disseminated sporotrichosis with extensive cutaneous involvement in a patient with AIDS. J Am Acad Dermatol. 1999;40(2 Pt 2):350–5.

Zygomycosis/Mucormycosis

203. Moraru RA, Grossman ME. Palatal necrosis in an AIDS patient: a case of mucormycosis. Cutis. 2000;66(1):15–8.

204. Sanchez MR, Ponge-Wilson I, Moy JA, Rosenthal S. Zygomycosis and HIV infection. J Am Acad Dermatol. 1994;30(5 Pt 2):904–8.

205. Samant JS, Namgoong SH, Parveen T, Katner HP. Cytomegalovirus vasculitis and mucormycosis coinfection in late-stage HIV/AIDS. Am J Med Sci. 2007;333(2):122–4.

206. Mitchell SJ, Gray J, Morgan ME, Hocking MD, Durbin GM. Nosocomial infection with *Rhizopus microsporus* in preterm infants: association with wooden tongue depressors. Lancet. 1996;348(9025):441–3.

207. Barnes PD, Marr KA. Risks, diagnosis and outcomes of invasive fungal infections in haematopoietic stem cell transplant recipients. Br J Haematol. 2007;139(4):519–31.

208. Ramos A, Cuervas-Mons V, Noblejas A, et al. Breakthrough rhinocerebral mucormycosis in a liver transplant patient receiving caspofungin. Transplant Proc. 2009;41(5):1972–5.

209. Fujimoto A, Nagao K, Tanaka K, et al. The first case of cutaneous mucormycosis caused by *Rhizopus azygosporus*. Br J Dermatol. 2005;153(2):428–30.

210. Mantadakis E, Samonis G. Clinical presentation of zygomycosis. Clin Microbiol Infect. 2009;15 Suppl 5:15–20.

211. Takabayashi M, Sakai R, Sakamoto H, et al. Cutaneous mucormycosis during induction chemotherapy for acute lymphocytic leukemia. Leuk Lymphoma. 2004;45(1):199–200.

212. Wirth F, Perry R, Eskenazi A, Schwalbe R, Kao G. Cutaneous mucormycosis with subsequent visceral dissemination in a child with neutropenia: a case report and review of the pediatric literature. J Am Acad Dermatol. 1997;36(2 Pt 2):336–41.

213. Roden MM, Zaoutis TE, Buchanan WL, et al. Epidemiology and outcome of zygomycosis: a review of 929 reported cases. Clin Infect Dis. 2005;41(5):634–53.

214. Rubin AI, Grossman ME. Bull's-eye cutaneous infarct of zygomycosis: a bedside diagnosis confirmed by touch preparation. J Am Acad Dermatol. 2004;51:996–1001.

215. Alsuwaida K. Primary cutaneous mucormycosis complicating the use of adhesive tape to secure the endotracheal tube. Can J Anaesth. 2002;49(8):880–2.

216. Woods SG, Elewski BE. Zosteriform zygomycosis. J Am Acad Dermatol. 1995;32(2 Pt 2):357–61.

217. Skiada A, Petrikkos G. Cutaneous zygomycosis. Clin Microbiol Infect. 2009;15 Suppl 5:41–5.

2

Hyalohyphomycosis

Hyalohyphomycosis (hyaline septate molds) is a term used to encompass a variety of less common yet medically opportunistic mycotic pathogens.[1] They are non-dematiaceous molds or yeasts in which the tissue form is a colorless (hyaline) septate fungal hyphae with no pigment within the walls. This term is the counterpart to phaeohyphomycosis in which pathogens develop septate brown-walled hyphae in tissue. Hyalohyphomycosis does not represent a recognizable clinical syndrome, but in histologic tissue sections they can be misidentified as *Aspergillus*. Hyaline septate molds are identified by their macroscopic and microscopic morphology in culture. However, greater than 50% of hyaline molds indentified in tissue cannot be cultivated for definitive identification. The members of this group are extremely heterogeneous and include *Fusarium*, *Penicillium*, *Paecilomyces*, *Acremonium*, *Scopulariopsis*, and *Trichoderma*.

FUSARIUM

Fusarium species are common contaminants, ubiquitous soil saprophytes, important plant pathogens and are present in water worldwide.[2,3] *Fusarium* species can be pathogens in immunocompromised patients and have rarely been reported to cause disease in immunocompetent individuals. The two major risk factors for systemic *Fusarium* infection are neutropenia and corticosteroid therapy, usually occurring in hematologic malignancies (especially acute leukemia) and hematopoietic stem cell transplant (HSCT) recipients. Most fusarial infections occur in patients with prolonged (greater than 14 days) and severe neutropenia (less than 100 cells/mm³) that occurs mainly in acute leukemia. In the bone marrow transplant population the infection may occur in the early posttransplant period during neutropenia, at a median of 70 days after transplant among patients with acute graft versus host disease

(GVHD) receiving corticosteroids and greater than 1 year posttransplant during treatment of chronic extensive GVHD. Severe T-cell immunodeficiency is the major risk factor for fusariosis in these patients. Breakthrough fusarial infections in neutropenic patients receiving empiric therapy or anti-fungal prophylaxis (with itraconazole, voriconazole, or fluconazole) is rare.[4] Fusarial infections that occur after solid organ transplantation tend to be localized and the outcome is better than in neutropenic patients. Infection is acquired by inhalation of spores, through traumatized skin of burn patients, following finger or toe cellulitis[5-7] with or without onychomycosis or secondary to indwelling catheters.

Fusarium causes locally invasive infection in the immunocompromised host which may disseminate. The clinical scenarios for the portals of entry include: (1) localized cellulitis at an injection site or insect bite, (2) great toe cellulitis, (3) *Fusarium* paronychia especially in the setting of onychomycosis, (4) traumatic digital ulcer or eschar, (5) painful toe web sloughing with toe/foot cellulitis[8] and (6) facial/periorbital cellulitis from fusarial sinusitis (rhinocerebral infection). Disseminated infection by *Fusarium* species occurs almost exclusively in granulocytopenic cancer patients and recipients of bone marrow transplants who have indwelling central lines causing breaks in the skin barrier, disruptions in mucosal barriers from cytotoxic therapy and are receiving broad-spectrum antibiotics empirically or therapeutically.

The typical clinical presentations of *Fusarium* infection include persistent refractory neutropenic fever, pulmonary infiltrates (a wide spectrum of pulmonary involvement may be present from non-specific alveolar and interstitial infiltrates to nodules and cavities), sinusitis and painful skin lesions both primary and metastatic. The skin lesions evolve from painful disseminated red papules or nodules to violaceous purpuric necrotic or centrally ulcerated papules or nodules with concurrent severe

M.E. Grossman et al., *Cutaneous Manifestations of Infection in the Immunocompromised Host*,
DOI 10.1007/978-1-4419-1578-8_2, © Springer Science+Business Media, LLC 2012

myalgias and fevers. The characteristic lesion of *Fusarium* infection is a red or grey macule with a central ulceration or black eschar, which appears as a target lesion with necrosis within a rim of erythema.[9] Skin lesions due to *Fusarium* are typically numerous and widespread and lesions at different stages of evolution may be present simultaneously in the same patient.[10] Cutaneous lesions develop rapidly over days. The evolution of a skin lesion that later becomes necrotic in the center is a helpful clue to the diagnosis of *Fusarium* infection. Similar lesions can be produced by other angioinvasive opportunistic fungi including *Aspergillus* and *Mucor* species.

The clinical characteristics of disseminated *Fusarium* infection are similar to disseminated *Aspergillus*: (1) evolution of skin lesions from erythema to necrosis; (2) frequent sinopulmonary involvement (both sinus infections cause nasal and periorbital erythema often associated with black eschars on the bridge of the nose, nasal septum or palate); (3) propensity for vascular invasion and thrombosis leading to tissue infarction; (4) the spores of both can be cultured from routine air samples as well as from soil, plants and other environmental sources; and (5) appearance in tissues as acute branching (at 45° angles) broad septate hyaline hyphae. It is not possible to distinguish between *Fusarium* species and *Aspergillus* species simply by histopathologic examination of tissues. Diagnosis depends on confirmation by culture.

Important differences between *Fusarium* and Aspergillosis infections are that: (1) *Fusarium* species are frequently associated with widespread skin lesions which is uncommon in disseminated aspergillosis; (2) there is a high rate of isolation of *Fusarium* species from the blood (approximately 70%) in contrast to the rare detection of *Aspergillus* species in the blood; (3) skin lesions are common in disseminated *Fusarium* infections (75–90%) but are uncommon in disseminated aspergillosis; (4) mature skin lesions caused by *Aspergillus* species are characteristically few in number, large (2–3 cm in diameter), generally consist of a black eschar and adjacent lesions may coalesce; (5) *Fusarium* skin lesions are usually numerous, often widespread, smaller (1 cm in diameter), and demonstrate various stages of evolution simultaneously in the same patient; and (6) disseminated *Fusarium* infection has been almost uniformly fatal.

Clinical manifestations of disseminated *Fusarium* infection in the immunocompromised host diagnosed with histology and culture include: acral bullae in a 15-year-old with aplastic anemia and paranasal cellulitis[8]; non-palpable purpura with a central flaccid pustule and multiple facial pustules with umbilicated centers and some with central necrosis in relapsed or refractory leukemia[11]; painful, well-circumscribed round ulcers of the lower leg in a diabetic with non-Hodgkin's lymphoma[12]; sporotrichoid nodules on the arm of a 41-year-old with relapsed acute lymphocytic leukemia (ALL) and neutropenic fever[13]; disseminated vesicles mimicking varicella or disseminated varicella-zoster virus (VZV) as the presentation of *Fusarium solani* sepsis on the day of stem cell transplant for leukemia with zero neutrophils[14]; panniculitis-like tender red nodules on the legs of a neutropenic 11-year-old with ALL[15]; the combination of vesicular and necrotic lesions in a 32-year-old with relapsing ALL, who was febrile, on broad-spectrum antibiotics, and neutropenic from chemotherapy[16]; the combination of tender flaccid pustules, necrotic pustules, and tense hemorrhagic bullae of *F. proliferatum* sepsis in a 59-year-old with ALL and neutropenic fever post chemotherapy[17]; and flaccid pustules on the scalp, tender intramuscular nodules, and a fluctuant subcutaneous nodule on the forehead of a 69-year-old with acute myelogenous leukemia (AML) who was febrile, neutropenic post chemotherapy, and on antibiotics with muscle tenderness in his extremities due to *F. solani*.[18] *F. falciforme* produced numerous vesicular and pustular targetoid lesions which evolved into central necrotic nodules on the legs of a 58-year-old neutropenic woman following failed induction chemotherapy for AML.[19]

Localized cutaneous *Fusarium* infections have been reported as a subcutaneous foot abscess, necrotic ulcers in the lower extremities and focally necrotic violaceous plaques on the lower leg in a renal transplant recipient.[20] A similar forearm ulceration with a central black eschar due to *F. solani* was reported in a 43-year-old man with a stem cell transplant for Hodgkin's disease.[21]

Most systemic infections involve *Fusarium solani* (the most virulent and most commonly isolated species) followed by *Fusarium oxysporum*, *F. moniliforme* / *F. verticillioides*, and rarely *F. falciforme*.

The clinical course of *Fusarium* infection is either resolution associated with reconstitution of the white blood cell count or death secondary to overwhelming infection.[22] Relapse was observed exclusively among patients who received additional myeloablative therapy after apparent resolution of the initial fusarial infection.

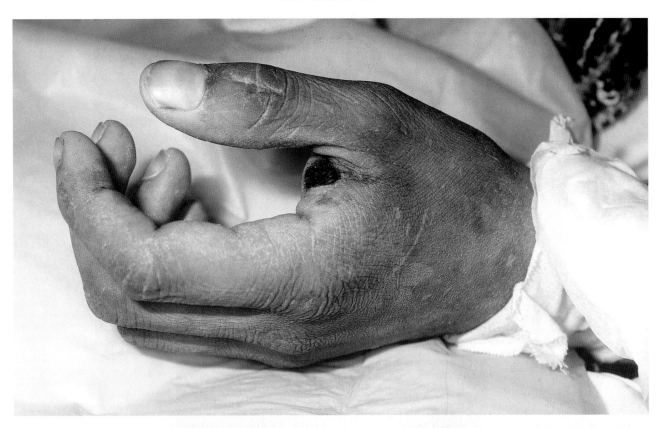

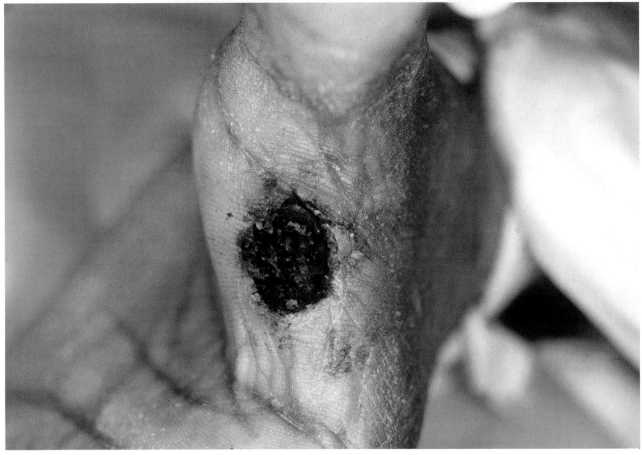

Figure 2.1. and 2.2. A necrotic subcutaneous nodule in the web space between the thumb and index finger developed in a febrile, neutropenic patient with end stage Hodgkin's disease. Skin biopsy and culture demonstrated *Fusarium* species

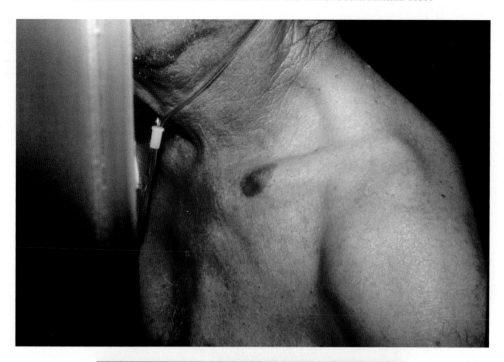

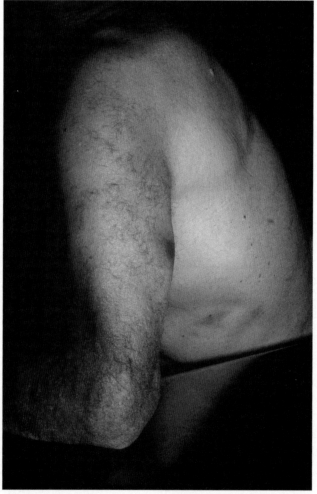

Figure 2.3. and 2.4. A 75-year-old man with refractory anemia developed acute myelogenous leukemia (AML). During chemotherapy, he developed multiple erythematous to violaceous nodules on his thumb, arms, chest, and abdomen. Skin biopsy and culture confirmed a diagnosis of *Fusarium* (Courtesy of Phillip Cohen, M.D.)

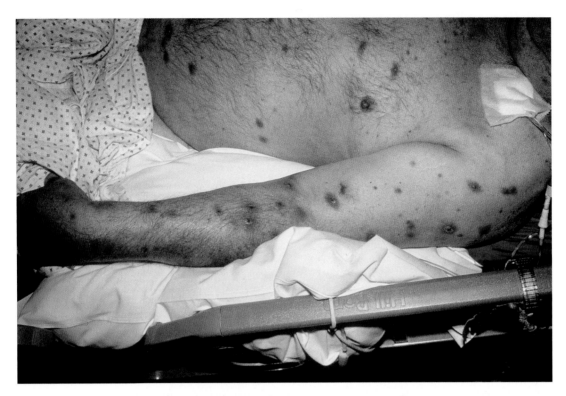

Figure 2.5. A 59-year-old diabetic with acute lymphocytic leukemia, on broad-spectrum antibiotics for *Klebsiella* and *Staphylococcus epidermidis* sepsis after chemotherapy-induced neutropenia, developed generalized erythematous macules and nonpalpable and palpable purpura with flaccid pustules. Potassium hydroxide (KOH) examination revealed septate hyphae. Skin biopsy demonstrated fungal vasculitis, and cultures grew *Fusarium proliferatum* (From Helm et al.[17])

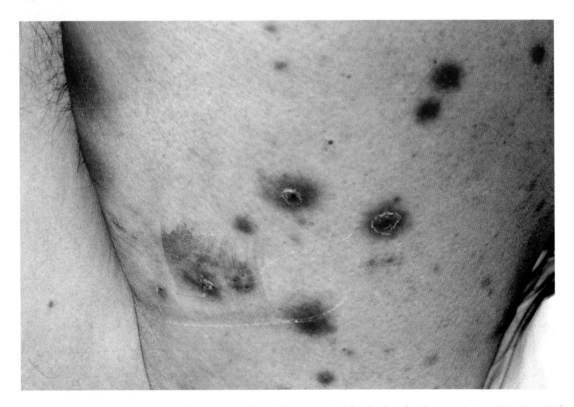

Figure 2.6. Erythematous macules, purpura, and necrotic pustules with concentric scales developed with worsening myalgias (From Helm et al.[17])

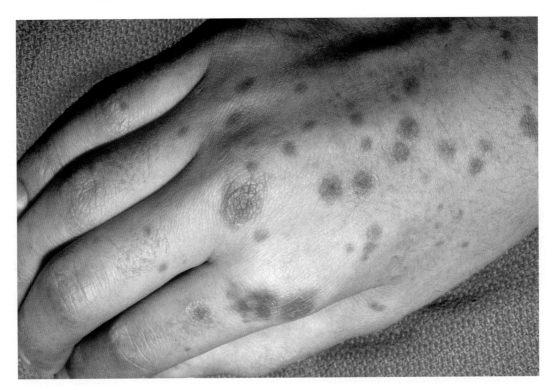

Figure 2.7. Erythematous macules and papules, many with central necrosis, on the hand of a febrile, neutropenic 18-year-old with acute lymphocytic leukemia and severe myalgias (Courtesy of Amy S. Paller, M.D. From Alvarez-Franco M, Reyes-Mugica M, Paller AS. Cutaneous *Fusarium* infection in an adolescent with leukemia. Pediatr Dermatol 1992;9:62. Reprinted by permission of Blackwell Scientific Publications, Inc.)

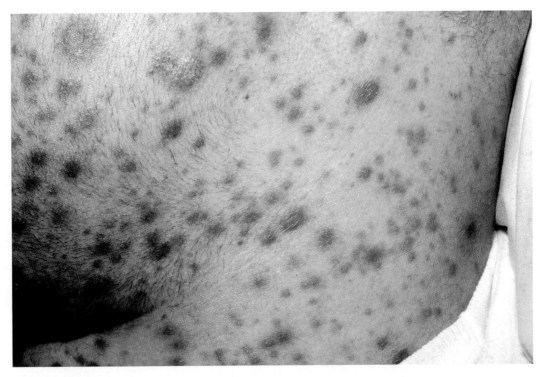

Figure 2.8. Painful erythematous papules with vesicles and central erosions on the trunk. Skin biopsy demonstrated hyphal vascular invasion, a minimal inflammatory reaction, and cultured *Fusarium* (Courtesy of Amy S. Paller, M.D. From Alvarez-Franco M, Reyes-Mugica M, Paller AS. Cutaneous *Fusarium* infection in an adolescent with leukemia. Pediatr Dermatol 1992;9:62. Reprinted by permission of Blackwell Scientific Publications, Inc.)

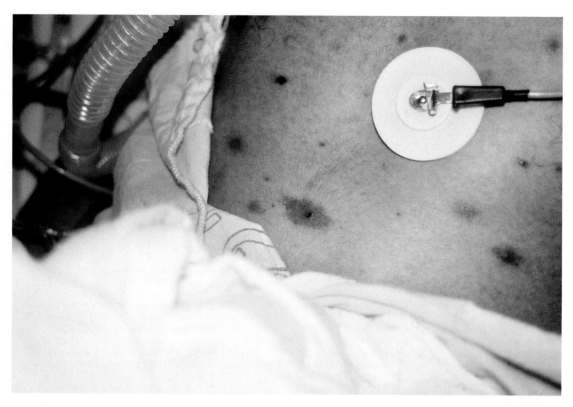

Figure 2.9. Scattered erythematous and purpuric papules with central necrosis due to *Fusarium* in a febrile, neutropenic 19-year-old patient with acute myelogenous leukemia (Courtesy of Geetinder Chattha, M.D.)

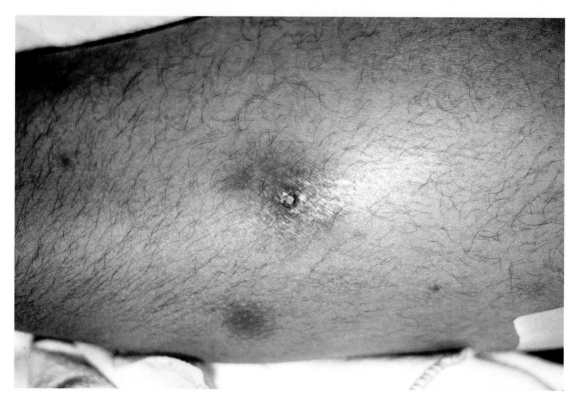

Figure 2.10. Papulonecrotic skin lesion of *Fusarium* on the extremity of the patient depicted in Figure 2.9 (Courtesy of Geetinder Chattha, M.D.)

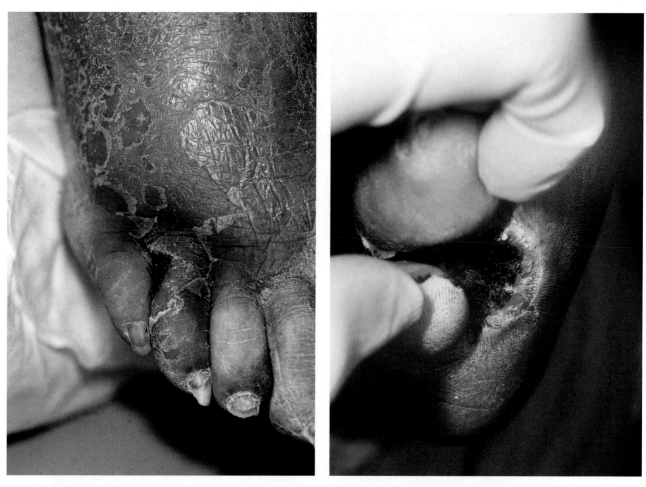

Figure 2.11. and 2.12.   A 66-year-old with relapsed refractory acute monoblastic leukemia and pancytopenia developed redness and swelling of the fourth and fifth toes with a necrotic toe web due to *Fusarium*. He developed enlarging bilateral pulmonary nodules and died a few days later

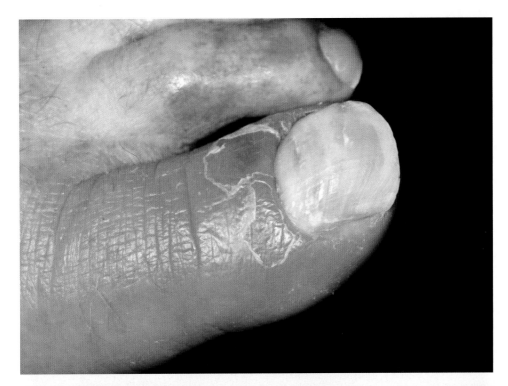

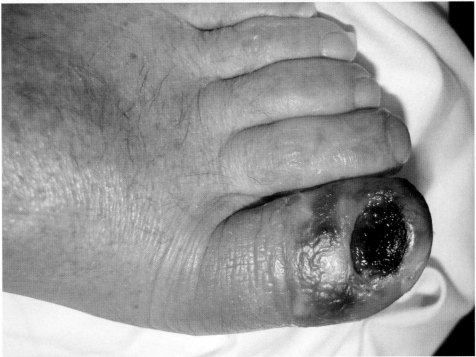

Figure 2.13.–2.16. A 57-year-old man with a history of myelofibrosis status post matched unrelated donor allogeneic stem cell transplant with newly diagnosed AML presented with "toe cellulitis" (Fig. 2.13). The patient had completed idarubicin and cytarabine chemotherapy 7 days prior to dermatology consultation. He was neutropenic and febrile on broad-spectrum antimicrobials. Twelve days later the patient's toenail demonstrated necrosis (Fig. 2.14), and he had numerous scattered erythematous papules on his head, abdomen, and lower extremities accompanied by myalgias. Magnetic resonance imaging (MRI) of his leg revealed intramuscular enhancing lesions (Fig. 2.15). KOH of his toe (Fig. 2.16) and skin biopsy of a forehead papule revealed the presence of *Fusarium* (Reprinted from Journal of the American Academy of Dermatology, Vol 65, King BA, Seropian S, Fox LP, Disseminated fusarium infection with muscle involvement, p. 235–237, 2011, with permission from Elsevier)

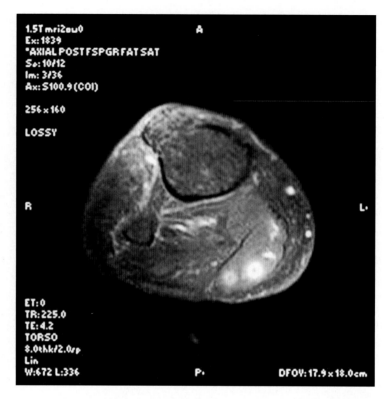

Figure 2.15.

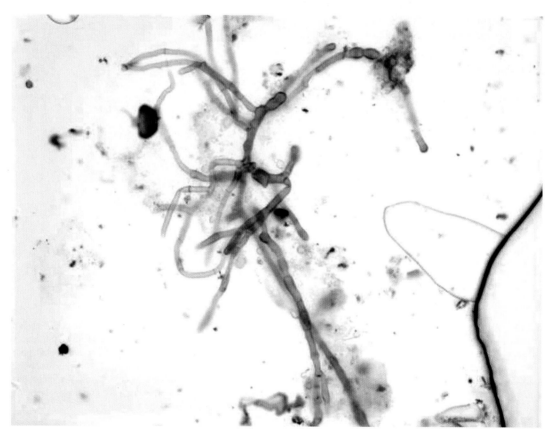

Figure 2.16.

PENICILLIUM MARNEFFEI (PM)

Penicillium marneffei (PM) is a thermally dimorphic fungus endemic to Southeast Asia (particularly in Vietnam and Thailand) and the southern part of China (Guangxi Province). Humans and bamboo rats are infected with PM from a common source, most likely the soil especially during the rainy season from May to October.[23] The incidence of penicilliosis has risen markedly since the first natural infection in a minister with Hodgkin's disease reported in 1973. The increased incidence runs parallel to that of human immunodeficiency virus (HIV) infection and acquired immune deficiency syndrome (AIDS). Penicilliosis in HIV-infected patients has been classified as an AIDS-defining illness for those who live in or visit regions to which this fungus is endemic. In HIV-infected patients *Penicillium marneffei* usually occurs in the advanced stage when the CD4 count falls below 100 cells/mm^3.[24] A significant increase in world travel and tourism across Southeast Asia has contributed to an increase in the number of cases of PM in other countries and demonstrated that penicilliosis is no longer confined to a specific region in Southeast Asia. The skin lesions are often the first indicator of PM dissemination as well as an HIV infection.

Reactivation of *Penicillium marneffei* occurs from a latent pulmonary focus in an immunocompromised host and spreads hematogenously. Visceral dissemination at the time of clinical presentation is common. *Penicillium marneffei* produces a clinical picture most commonly in HIV-infected males consisting of fever, weight loss, hepatosplenomegaly, generalized lymphadenopathy, pulmonary infiltrates, cough, symptomatic anemia, markedly elevated lactic acid dehydrogenase level, and skin lesions. Cutaneous involvement with numerous umbilicated papules with or without central necrosis, resembling molluscum contagiosum is characteristic but not diagnostic. The lesions occurred more frequently above the waist up, on the face, pinnae, upper trunk, and arms. Less often vesicular, necrotic, pustular, and acneiform lesions, subcutaneous nodules, and ulcerated papules are observed. Occasionally patients have papules on the palate, chronic genital or pharyngeal ulcers, soft tissue abscesses, or nodules.[25]

Abnormal chest x-rays were commonly encountered in patients with respiratory symptoms showing reticulonodular patterns, interstitial or localized infiltrates, pleural effusions, and rarely single or multiple cavitary lesions.[26]

Clinically and histopathologically PM mimics disseminated histoplasmosis.[27] Both proliferate within histiocytes and are similar in size (2–5 mm). PM differ by the presence of transverse septae, the absence of buds since the yeast form multiplies by fission and not by budding, and sausage shaped and tubular forms present outside of histiocytes. Histopathologic examination of skin biopsy specimens, touch smears of lymph node aspirates or bone marrow aspirates readily demonstrate the intracellular organisms of PM. Culture will provide the definitive diagnosis if microbiologists recognize *Penicillium* as a pathogen and not discard it as a saprophyte and common laboratory contaminant or simply report it as *Penicillium* species.[28] Cultures from bone marrow, lymph node aspiration, skin biopsy, or blood are simple diagnostic tools. An enzyme-linked immunosorbent assay (ELISA) based antibody test with Mp1p, an antigenic cell wall mannoprotein of *Penicillium marneffei*, may be useful for the diagnosis.

Rapid diagnosis can be made in the AIDS patient with sepsis by carefully examining the peripheral blood smear for the presence of yeast cells within neutrophils.[29] Demonstrating the organism in smears or scrapings of skin lesions can also result in prompt diagnosis and initiation of appropriate life saving therapy.

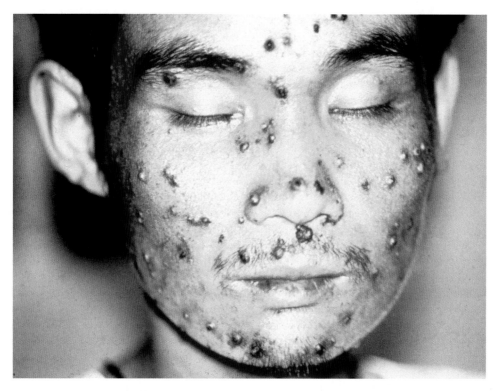

Figure 2.17.   Numerous molluscum-like papules of disseminated *Penicillium marneffei* infection on the face of a human immunodeficiency virus (HIV)-positive man from Southeast Asia (Courtesy of Konrad E. Nelson, M.D., and Thira Sirisanthana, M.D.)

Figure 2.18.   *Penicillium marneffei* infection on the face of an HIV-positive man from China (Courtesy of Toby Maurer, M.D.)

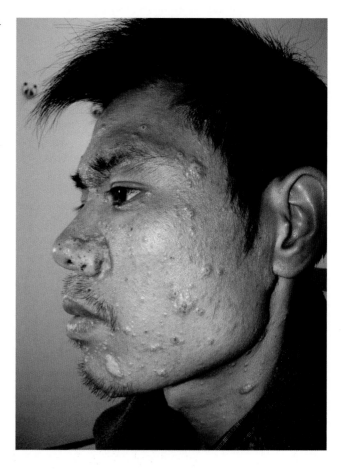

Paecilomyces

Paecilomyces is a rare emerging opportunistic saprophytic fungus found in soil, saunas, and contaminated medical materials. It can be an airborne laboratory contaminant or a contaminant in sterile solutions or moisturizing body lotions.[30,31] *Paecilomyces* has been labeled the "bottle imp" because of its resistance to standard sterilization techniques and its propensity to contaminate sterile solutions.[32] This explains why infections with this organism are often associated with surgical procedures.

Paecilomyces infections in immunocompetent hosts occur iatrogenically (with surgery or medical implants) or following minor injuries or previous trauma. Most reports of *Paecilomyces* have involved the eye after cataract extraction or intraocular lens implantation. The source of infection was the neutralizing solution used to bathe the lens prior to implantation which was contaminated with *Paecilomyces*. The majority of case reports on *Paecilomyces* infections are in the immunocompromised host with solid organ or bone marrow transplant, lymphoma, chronic granulomatous disease or immunosuppression secondary to chronic systemic corticosteroid use. The portal of entry for *Paecilomyces* usually involves breakdown of the skin barrier (onychomycosis or interdigital tinea pedis)[33] or indwelling catheters.[34] The fingernail or toenail may serve as the reservoir of *Paecilomyces* infection with contiguous spread of the infection, which explains the frequent involvement of the lower extremities, greater than upper extremities. *Paecilomyces* may cause extensive cutaneous infection of the arm or leg with a wide range of clinical features: erythematous macules, vesicles, pustules, or painful red nodules.[35,36] It mimics bacterial infections, looking like cellulitis[37,38] or furuncles.[39,40] Wolfson et al. reported two renal transplant patients who developed an ulcerating cellulitis following lacerating trauma to the anterior tibial region virtually identical to a previously reported case.[41] Satellite lesions or sporotrichoid nodules have been described in a renal transplant patient with *P. lilacinus*.[42] *Paecilomyces* produced a sternal wound infection in a lung transplant recipient.[43] Long-term cure was achieved by complying with the important surgical procedure of vigorous and adequate surgical debridement in addition to antifungal therapy. This is the same treatment principle in fungal infections associated with foreign body implants which includes removal of the device for a successful outcome.

Diagnosis of *Paecilomyces* infection is based on culture of the fungus and histology of the lesions. A peculiar characteristic of *P. lilacinus* is its ability to produce reproductive structures similar to those observed in vitro, including phialides and conidia in infected tissues. This type of sporulation in infected tissue, called adventitious sporulation, is a helpful diagnostic finding but also seen with *Fusarium* and *Acremonium*.[44] Identification of *Paecilomyces* as a pathogen should be followed by species identification because antifungal susceptibilities vary. *P. lilacinus* and *P. variotii* are the two species most frequently reported as causes of infection. Other species reported to infect humans occasionally are *P. marquandii* and *P. javanicus* and *P. viridis*. Correct diagnosis of *P. lilacinus* is important because of its

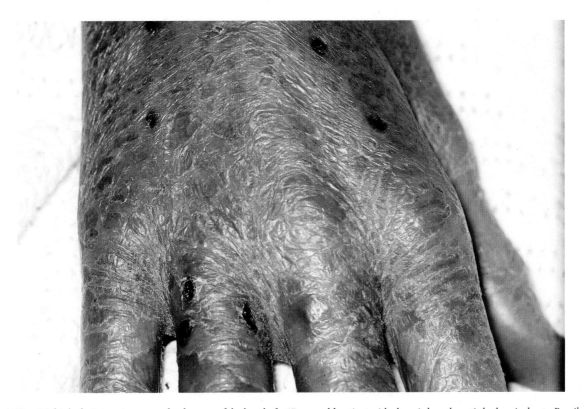

Figure 2.19. Multiple draining sinuses on the dorsum of the hand of a 47-year-old patient with chronic lymphocytic leukemia due to *Paecilomyces lilacinus* and not a bacterial cellulitis as initially diagnosed (Courtesy of Michael F. Lyons II, M.D. From Jade et al.[38])

intrinsic resistance to conventional antifungal drugs including amphotericin, flucytosine, and fluconazole. Most cases of *Paecilomyces* in immunocompromised patients were localized cutaneous infections and were cured with treatment.

Acremonium

Acremonium (*Cephalosporium*) species are extremely common environmental fungal contaminants and soil saprophytes but are infrequent pathogens in humans. Since *Acremonium* rarely causes invasive disease in man, they are often considered as contaminants when isolated in the medical laboratory. The majority of infections have been mycetomas or corneal infections (mycotic keratitis) following penetrating cutaneous or ocular injuries in immunocompetent individuals. *Acremonium* species are being increasingly recognized as opportunist fungal pathogens that cause a variety of infections in immunocompromised patients. These are organ transplant recipients, those with multiple myeloma, leukemia, or chronic granulomatous disease and those receiving chronic systemic corticosteroids.

Numerous species have been implicated in infections including *A. falciforme*, *A. kiliense*, *A. recifei*, *A. strictum*, *A. murorum*, and *A. roseogriseum*. More than 80% of human infections are caused by the first three species. *Acremonium* species grow slowly and cultures must be kept for at least 2 weeks to ensure detection of a positive sample. The high frequency of positive blood cultures (similar to *Fusarium*, unlike *Aspergillus*) during *Acremonium* infections is explained by angioinvasion and adventitious spo-rulation with sustained release of fungal spores into the bloodstream.[45]

The number and diversity of invasive infections caused by *Acremonium* species have increased in recent years. A two centimeter dark nodule developed on the index finger of a 62-year-old during induction chemotherapy for acute lymphoblastic leukemia.[46] Multiple cutaneous nodules and muscle abscesses of both legs developed during induction chemotherapy induced neutropenia in a 15-year-old with acute myelogenous leukemia.[47] A 34-year-old with myelodysplastic syndrome and neutropenia on high dose systemic steroids for severe GVHD following unrelated donor cord blood transplantation developed *Acremonium* pneumonia and multiple painful erythematous papules on her extremities and back.[48] A similar case of painful, violaceous papules generalized over the extremities and body (about 30) with severe myalgias due to *Acremonium strictum* was reported in a febrile neutropenic leukemic.[49] *Acremonium* or *Fusarium* should be considered if the clinical picture includes refractory fever, myalgias, and disseminated nodules or papules with necrotic centers in patients with profound neutropenia.[50] A case reported as mycetoma due to *Acremonium falciforme* in a renal transplant manifested as multiple large subcutaneous nodules and abscesses of the hands, forearms, and elbows. He continued to get new draining and ulcerated nodules on antifungal medications, with repeatedly positive *Acremonium* cultures for 16 months until he suffered a fatal cardiac arrest.[51] A mycetoma of the foot due to *Acremonium murorum/roseogriseum* in a heart transplant recipient was neither aggressive nor distinctive despite immunosuppressive medications. It was locally invasive without systemic symptoms and did not disseminate. The *Acremonium mycetoma* responded to standard surgical and medical treatment.[52]

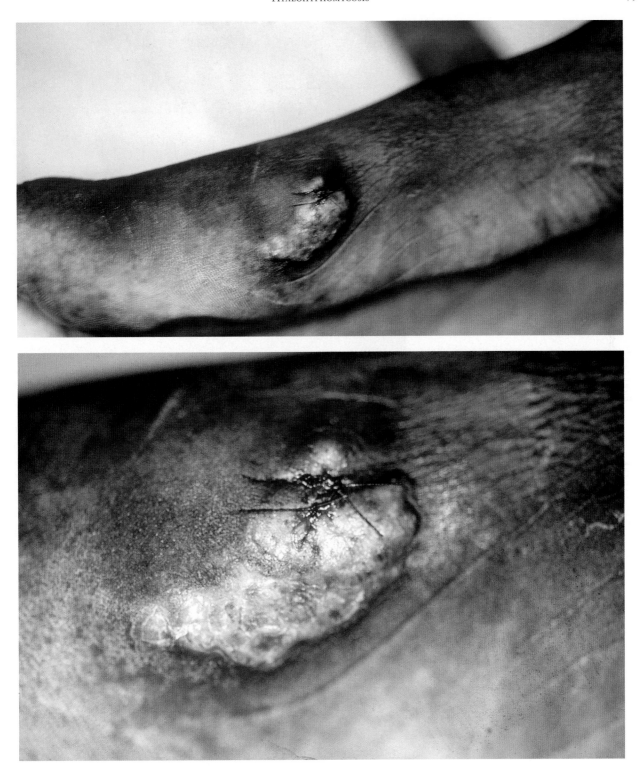

Figure 2.20. and 2.21. *Acremonium mycetoma* developed 6 years after a heart transplant in a 46-year-old from Gambia

Figure 2.22. *Acremonium* infection in a barefoot gardener with aggressive chronic lymphocytic leukemia (CLL) on chemotherapy

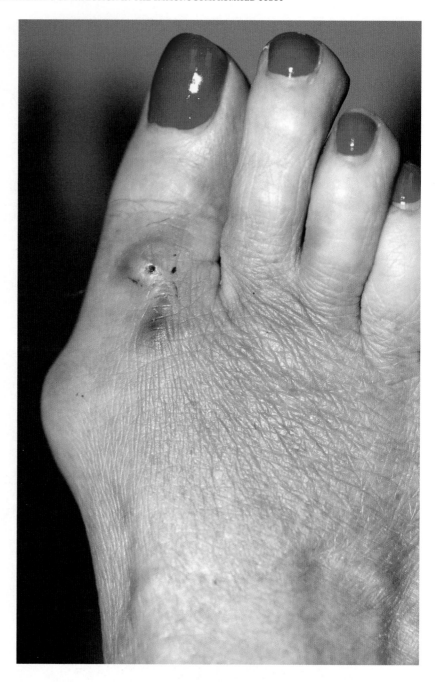

SCOPULARIOPSIS

Scopulariopsis is a ubiquitous soil saprophyte also isolated from food, paper, California beaches, caves in Mexico, and sauna baths in the German Democratic Republic.[53] Eight species of *Scopulariopsis* have been reported as causing infection in humans (*S. acremonium*, *S. asperula*, *S. flava*, *S. fusca*, *S. koningii*, *S. brevicaulis*, *S. brumptii*, and *S. candida*). Some species of *Scopulariopsis* have either *Microascus* or *Kernia* teleomorphs (sexual states, perfect form) and have been reported under these names as human pathogens. The majority of cases of *Scopulariopsis* species infections have been due to *S. brevicaulis*. *Scopulariopsis* species are keratinophilic and are most commonly associated with onychomycosis particularly involving the large toenails. A clinical clue to *S. brevicaulis* infection of the toenail (rather than the usual dermatophyte) is the absence of tinea pedis (a dermatophyte) or other toenails being affected.[54]

Clinical manifestations of *Scopulariopsis* infection in the immunocompromised patient can vary. *Scopulariopsis* has presented as recurrent red-wine colored exophytic ulcerative subcutaneous nodules on the extremities of a liver transplant recipient.[55] A case of locally invasive otomycosis and a case of paresthesias of the tip of the nose with fever and recurrent epistaxis both in leukemic patients have been described. Both were presumed to have aspergillosis until *Scopulariopsis* species

was identified by culture.[56] *Scopulariopsis* produced a black eschar or necrotic ulcer under an adhesive bandage for an intravascular catheter in a 10-year-old with graft versus host disease following stem cell transplant for acute myelogenous leukemia. This clinical picture has been also described for *Rhizopus* and *Aspergillus*.[57] Several reports of inflammatory nodules of the extremities, histologically and mycologically positive for *Scopulariopsis*, have occurred in immunocompromised patients.[58-60] The multifocal nature of the cutaneous infection suggested the possibility of either inoculation or hematogenous dissemination. The poor sensitivity of blood cultures for detection and identification of *Scopulariopsis* make it difficult to know the true mechanism. A 40-year-old with aplastic anemia on amphotericin for Candida esophagitis developed pain and periungual erythema of the big toe. The cellulitis developed a black necrotic lesion adjacent to the toenail which demonstrated angioinvasive *S. brevicaulis* histologically and by culture. Despite amphotericin the toe lesion progressed and required amputation. Histopathology revealed *Scopulariopsis* invading bone.[61] This case illustrates how an immunocompromised host receiving antifungal prophylaxis can develop a rare relatively drug resistant opportunistic fungal infection. Most strains of *Scopulariopsis* are resistant to amphotericin, itraconazole, or 5-fluorocytosine. Successful eradication of invasive *Scopulariopsis* infection requires aggressive surgical débridement in addition to newer antifungal drugs.

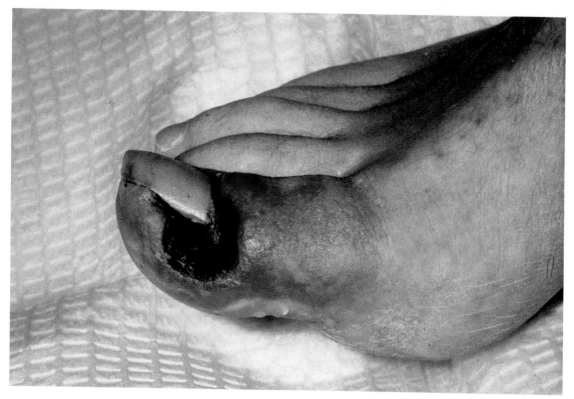

Figure 2.23. Paronychial and lateral nail fold necrotic ulcer surrounded by erythema due to biopsy and culture-proven *Scopulariopsis brevicaulis*. *Scopulariopsis* invaded into the bone requiring amputation of the great toe of this 40-year-old man with aplastic anemia who received a bone marrow transplant (Reprinted by permission of the publisher from Phillips et al.[61] Copyright 1989 by Elsevier Science Inc.)

TRICHOSPORON

Trichosporonosis is an uncommon but frequently fatal emerging opportunistic fungal infection in immunocompromised patients. The taxonomy of the genus *Trichosporon* (175 species) has been revised and the previously named single species *T. beigelii* (formerly *T. cutaneum*) in the most recent classification corresponds to six different species: *T. asahii, T. asteroides, T. cutaneum, T. inkin, T. mucoides,* and *T. ovoides.*[62] All are recognized as potential human pathogens (as well as *T. pullulans* and *T. loubieri*) and each are associated with different types of infection: *T. cutaneum* and *T. asteroides,* superficial infections; *T. ovoides,* white piedra of the scalp; *T. inkin,* white piedra of the pubic area; *T. asahii* and *T. mucoides,* white piedra and deep seated infections. All species have been implicated in invasive infections in patients with hematologic malignancies, most frequently neutropenic acute leukemics. *T. asahii* is thought to be the most common cause of disseminated trichosporonosis.[63] Invasive trichosporonosis also occurs in the setting of cytotoxic chemotherapy induced neutropenia, corticosteroids, underlying malignancy, hemochromatosis, and AIDS. *T. inkin* is a rare infection encountered almost exclusively in chronic granulomatous disease.[64,65]

Trichosporon is a natural inhabitant of the soil and occasionally part of the normal flora of human skin. It colonizes the throat and lower gastrointestinal tract. The majority of patients with disseminated Trichosporon infection have acute leukemia and are neutropenic. Some granulocytopenic patients were receiving amphotericin B empirically for fever unresponsive to broad-spectrum antibacterial agents when they developed breakthrough trichosporonosis. Patients may present with a syndrome suggestive of disseminated candidiasis with fever, severe myalgias, endophthalmitis with multiple round white spots on fundus examination and multiple purpuric nodules that progress to centrally necrotic lesions.[66,67] Compared to Candida, trichosporonosis is associated with higher positive blood culture yield, more frequent visceral involvement and a poorer prognosis. Cutaneous involvement occurs in 30–43% of patients with disseminated trichosporonosis.[68] The most frequently documented skin lesions are purpuric papules and nodules with central necrosis and ulceration. The trunk, arms and face were most commonly involved. Other morphologies have been reported in immunocompromised hosts including: pink nodules on the face and scalp of a patient with AIDS[68]; tender hemorrhagic bullous cellulitis in a pancytopenic man,[69] sporotrichoid purple nodules in a renal transplant patient,[70] black necrotic lesions of the buccal mucosa in an acute leukemia patient,[71] purpuric papules with pale centers in a bone marrow transplant recipient,[72] erythematous papulopustules in a pancytopenic man with carcinoma of the lung,[73] and multiple linear ulcerative hemorrhagic nodules due to *T. inkin* on the forearm of a steroid dependent woman with rheumatoid arthritis.[74]

Skin biopsy and culture, like blood culture, is a high yield source of diagnosis. Although the microscopic appearance can be confused with Candida or *Aspergillus,* close observation of biopsy specimens containing *T. beigelii* by a skilled dermatopathologist reveals pseudohyphae, the presence of numerous rectangular arthroconidia and a few blastoconidia permitting an accurate diagnosis. *Trichosporon* shares cross-reactive antigenicity with the capsular polysaccharide of cryptococcus that results in a positive cryptococcal antigen test, as would be expected in cases of disseminated infection with either of these two pathogens. During the course of invasive Trichosporon infection, antigen positivity to *Aspergillus* galactomannan may also be positive potentially leading to misdiagnosis and inadequate treatment.[75] Fungal cultures of cutaneous lesions are positive in greater than 90% of cases and can minimize the possibility of mistaken histologic identification.

Disseminated Trichosporon infections are often fatal despite antifungal treatment. The death rate approaches 80%. In neutropenic patients the success of treatment was associated with resolution of neutropenia.

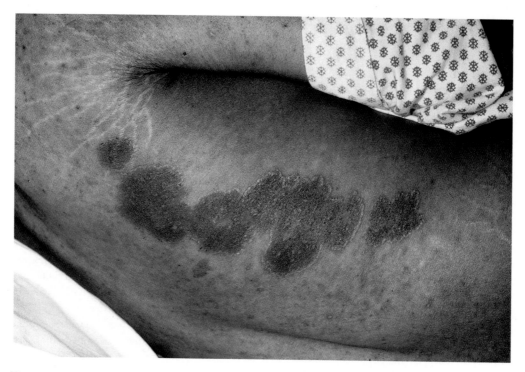

Figure 2.24. Tinea corporis, an unusual morphology for KOH and culture-positive *Trichosporon beigelii* in a patient with acquired immune deficiency syndrome (AIDS)

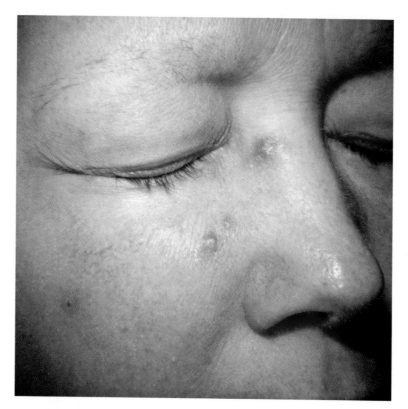

Figure 2.25. Erythematous papules and papulopustules caused by *T. beigelii* on the face of a patient with acute lymphocytic leukemia (From Dreizen et al. Unusual mucocutaneous infections in immuno-suppressed patients with leukemia – expansion of an earlier study. Postgrad Med 1986;79(4):287–294)

Trichoderma

Trichoderma infections in humans are rare but they are increasingly being reported in the immunocompromised patient. *Trichoderma* are ubiquitous saprophytic fungi with a worldwide distribution. They occur in soil, especially water-logged soil, wood, decaying vegetation, cellulose containing substances and moisture damaged building materials. Six species have been identified as etiologic agents of infections in immunocompromised hosts: *T. harzianum*, *T. koningii*, *T. longibrachiatum*, *T. pseudokoningii*, *T. citrinoviride*, and *T. viride*. Risk factors for invasive *Trichoderma* include prolonged and severe neutropenia, prolonged treatment with broad-spectrum antimicrobial agents, steroid therapy, mucosal barrier damage, and transplantation.[76] *Trichoderma* infection can be misdiagnosed as aspergillosis and other hyalohyphomycoses because the hyphae are morphologically similar on direct examination.[77] Culture of biopsy material is needed for definitive diagnosis. *Trichosporum* is characterized by very fast growth. Blood culture does not appear to be a valuable diagnostic tool.

Three similar necrotic ulcerated plaques due to *Trichoderma* that developed on the extremities at the insertion site of intravenous cannulas have been reported. A 45-year-old bone marrow transplant recipient on amphotericin and fluconazole developed fatal disseminated *T. pseudokoningii* from an ulcero-necrotic skin lesion (histologic and mycologic positive skin, brain and lungs)[78] at the entry point of a central venous catheter. A pediatric patient with aplastic anemia and prolonged neutropenia on fluconazole developed a painful two centimeter erythematous indurated centrally necrotic plaque at the site of a peripheral intravenous line. Skin biopsy and culture revealed *T. longibrachiatum* which was cured with a prolonged course of amphotericin.[79] Another pediatric patient with ALL developed centrally necrotic plaques/nodules with erythematous halos on the extremities, "especially in canulae entrance of the skin" during a neutropenic fever. Multiple cultures of pus from the skin lesions, sputum and throat grew *T. harzianum*.[80]

Two cases of invasive *Trichoderma* due to mucosal barrier damage, one in the oral cavity and the other in the intestinal wall were both fatal from overwhelming pulmonary infection and dissemination. A persistently neutropenic bone marrow transplant recipient (for ALL) on systemic steroids for GVHD and on amphotericin then itraconazole for *T. longibrachiatum* isolated from multiple stool surveillance cultures developed an enlarging perianal ulcer. It manifested as a necrotic lesion infiltrated with hyphae and cultured positive for *Trichoderma*. He developed multiple pulmonary nodules as the perianal ulcer continued to enlarge. *Trichoderma* was cultured from the liver, lung, brain and bowel at autopsy.[81] *Trichoderma* has been isolated from grains and food suggesting acquisition of the "non-pathogenic" fungus through the gastrointestinal tract.

A fatal case of *T. longibrachiatum* rapidly disseminated from ulcerative necrotic gingiva covered by a violaceous pseudomembrane in a neutropenic patient with non-Hodgkin's diffuse large B cell lymphoma.[82]

Blastoschizomyces Capitatus

Blastoschizomyces capitatus (previously *Geotrichium capitatum* and *Trichosporon capitatum*) is an emerging opportunistic yeast pathogen that is rarely reported. *B. capitatus* is widely distributed in soil, feces of semi-domesticated pigeons, and is part of the normal human skin flora and the respiratory and digestive tract mucosa. *B. capitatus* has been documented in immunocompetent individuals as a cause of onychomycoses. Invasive infection occurs predominantly in severely neutropenic leukemic patients and especially in those receiving intensive chemotherapy. The clinical presentation is similar to that of invasive candidiasis. Initial gastrointestinal and respiratory tract colonization is followed by hematogenous dissemination and localization in the skin and lungs.[83] The diagnosis is usually made by blood culture. The mortality rate (60% versus 24%) and percentage of patients who develop invasive organ involvement is much higher in *B. capitatus* infection compared to candidemia (60–80% versus 10–20%). The incidence of skin involvement with *B. capitatus* in acute leukemia is approximately 26%, but well documented reports of cutaneous findings are rare.

Etienne et al. reported a 59-year-old patient neutropenic from chemotherapy for acute myelocytic leukemia with *B. capitatus* in blood culture, who developed bilateral nodular pneumonia and arm papules.[84] Pérez-Sanchez described a pruritic rash, subcutaneous nodules, and gingival ulcers from which *B. capitatus* was cultured in a 44-year-old neutropenic patient with bilateral nodular pneumonia on chemotherapy for refractory anemia with excess of blasts.[85] A 1 cm erythematous nodule developed on the arm of a 47-year-old neutropenic leukemic patient with bilateral bronchopneumonia and fatal disseminated *B. capitatus* infection.[86] *B. capitatus* produced a chicken pox-like skin eruption in a febrile 6-year-old with refractory acute lymphocytic leukemia and neutropenic fever unresponsive to antibiotics. *B. capitatus* was cultured from blister fluid of skin lesions mimicking both the morphology and distribution of varicella.[87]

Hepatosplenomegaly with microabscesses, elevated alkaline phosphatase, and bull's-eye lesions with hepatic ultrasound or computerized tomography indistinguishable from hepatosplenic candidiasis is the most frequent manifestation of *B. capitatus*.[87] The other frequently involved system is the respiratory tract where *B. capitatus* can produce pulmonary infiltrates with the crescent sign (mass/nodules surrounded by a halo of low attenuation, diagnostic of pulmonary mycetoma). This finding resembles angioinvasive fungal pneumonia which differentiates *B. capitatus* from Candida pneumonia.

Paracoccidioidomycosis (South American Blastomycosis)

Paracoccidioidomycosis (Lutz' disease) is caused by the thermally dimorphic fungus *Paracoccidioides brasiliensis*, found in the soil of Latin America. It is geographically restricted and occurs mainly between the latitudes 23° north (Mexico) and 34° south (Argentina). *P. brasiliensis* is a rare infection worldwide but is an endemic deep mycosis most commonly found in Brazil followed by Columbia, Ecuador, and Venezuela. Infection with *P. brasiliensis* is acquired through inhalation of conidia, leading to pulmonary infection followed by extrapulmonary dissemination.[88]

P. brasiliensis has not been classically considered an opportunistic mycosis of the immunocompromised host.[89] *P. brasiliensis* has been described in patients receiving cancer chemotherapy, immunosuppressive medications such as azathioprine and systemic steroids, after renal transplantation, and in HIV/AIDS.[90,91] However, *P. brasiliensis* is not as common as might be expected in immunocompromised patients. The relatively small number of cases of paracoccidioidomycosis associated with AIDS when compared with histoplasmosis and cryptococcosis among HIV-infected patients is striking because the prevalence of paracoccidioidomycosis is much higher in the non-immuno-suppressed population.[92] The rarity of cases of *P. brasiliensis* in patients with HIV/ AIDS remains unexplained but it is consistent with the similarly low incidence of paracoccidioidomycosis among solid organ transplant recipients and patients with solid and hematologic malignancies.[88] The scarcity of reported cases of paracoccidioidomycosis and AIDS might be explained by the widespread use of trimethoprim-sulfamethoxazole as prophylaxis for *Pneumocystis jirovecii*. This drug combination is also very effective against *Paracoccidioides brasiliensis*. It is not known whether paracoccidioidomycosis in HIV is explained by reactivation of latent infection or whether it begins from a recent exogenously acquired infection.

Paracoccidioidomycosis most commonly occurs as a chronic form with pulmonary lesions and ulcerations of the oral, nasal, or laryngeal mucosa and occasionally with skin and other visceral lesions. The most common manifestation in patients with AIDS is disseminated disease. The acute form, rapidly progressive with HIV disease, occurs with fever, generalized lymphadenopathy, hepatosplenomegaly, skin, and bone lesions. The lungs are the most common organ infected, followed by the skin and lymph nodes, with cutaneous lesions being the most common clinical presentation at the time of diagnosis.[88] The cutaneous lesions of paracoccidioidomycosis in patients with HIV disease are multiple and widely disseminated. The skin lesions are in various stages of development including papules, nodules, nodules with central ulcerations, and ulcers.[92]

The oral involvement in paracoccidioidomycosis commonly includes painful, infiltrated ulcerations, pronounced increase in thickness of the lips, and erythematous finely granular hyperplasia of the mucosa speckled with pinpoint hemorrhages and a mulberry-like surface.[93] Although not uncommon, oral paracoccidioidomycosis can cause hard palatal perforation. Oral lesions are usually secondary to lung involvement and may be accompanied by laryngeal or esophageal involvement causing hoarseness, dysphagia, odynophagia, dysphonia, and/or cervical and submandibular lymphadenopathy.[94] Paracoccidioidomycosis can also affect other mucosal surfaces causing nasal, conjunctival, or perianal lesions.

References

Hyalohyphomycosis

1. Walsh TJ, Groll A, Hiemenz J, et al. Infections due to emerging and uncommon medically important fungal pathogens. Clin Microbiol Infect. 2004;10 Suppl 1:48–66.

Fusarium

2. Gupta Ad, Baran R, Summerbell RC. Fusarium infections of the skin. Curr Opin Infect Dis. 2000;13:121–8.
3. Nucci M, Anaissie E. Fusarium infections in immunocompromised patients. Clin Microbiol Rev. 2007;20:695–704.
4. Cooper C, MacPherson P, Angel JB. Liver toxicity resulting from syphilis and Jarish-Herxheimer reaction in cases of coinfection with HIV and hepatitis C virus. Clin Infect Dis. 2005;40(8):1211–2.
5. Polk C, Forrest G, Cross A. Cellulitis in a patient with leukemia. Clin Infect Dis. 2007;44:1240–50.
6. Child FJ, Fuller LC, Higgins EM, du Vivier AWP, Mufti GJ. Cutaneous presentation of *Fusarium solani* infection in a bone marrow transplant recipient. J R Soc Med. 1996;89:647–8.
7. Bigley VH, Duarte RF, Gosling RD, et al. *Fusarium dimerum* infection in a stem cell transplant recipient treated successfully with voriconazole. Bone Marrow Transplant. 2004;34:815–7.
8. Nucci M, Anaissie E. Cutaneous infection by *Fusarium* species in healthy and immunocompromised hostes: implications for diagnosis and management. Clin Infect Dis. 2002;35:909–19.
9. Bordeaux JS, O'Brien M, Mahalingam M, Wiss K. Clinicopathologic challenge. Int J Dermatol. 2008;47:13–4.
10. Bodey GP, Boktour M, Mays S, et al. Skin lesions associated with *Fusarium* infection. J Am Acad Dermatol. 2002;437:659–66.
11. Musa MO, Al Eisa A, Halim M, et al. The spectrum of *Fusarium* infection in immunocompromised patients with haematological malignancies and in non-immunocompromised patients: a single institution experience over 10 years. Br J Haematol. 2000;108:544–8.
12. Pérez-Pérez L, Pereiro Jr M, Sánchez-Aguilar D, Toribio J. Ulcerous lesions disclosing cutaneous infection with *Fusarium solani*. Acta Derm Venereol. 2007;87:422–4.
13. Watsky KL. Sporotrichoid nodules in an immunocompromised host. Arch Dermatol. 1995;131:1329–30.
14. Hamaki T, Kami M, Kishi A, et al. Vesicles as initial skin manifestations of disseminated fusariosis after non-myeloablative stem cell transplantation. Leuk Lymphoma. 2004;45:631–3.
15. Zhang CZ, Fung MA, Eiser DB. Disseminated fusariosis presenting as panniculitis-like lesions on the legs of a neutropenic gril with acute lymphoblastic leukemia. Dermatol Online J. 2009;15:5.
16. Durand-Joly I, Alfandari S, Benchikh Z, et al. Successful outcome of disseminated *Fusarium* infection with skin localization treated with voriconazoleand amphotericin B-lipid complex in a patient with acute leukemia. J Clin Microbiol. 2003;41:4898–900.
17. Helm TN, Longworth DL, Hall GS, et al. Case report and review of resolved fusariosis. J Am Acad Dermatol. 1990;23:393–8.
18. Matsuda T, Matsumoto T. Disseminated hyalohyphomycosis in a leukemic patient. Arch Dermatol. 1986;123:1171–5.
19. Yun SJ, Shin MG, Choi C, et al. Fatal disseminated angioinvasive Fusarium falciforme infection in a patient with acute myeloid leukemia. Br J Dermatol. 2007;157:407–9.
20. Cocuroccia B, Gaido J, Gubinelli E, Annessi G, Girolomoni G. Localized cutaneous hyalohyphomycosis caused by *Fusarium* species infection in a renal transplant patient. J Clin Microbiol. 2003;41:905–7.
21. Gardner JM, Nelson MM, Heffernan MP. Chronic cutaneous fusariosis. Arch Dermatol. 2005;141:794–5.
22. Nucci M, Anaissie EJ, Queiroz-Telles F, et al. Outcome predictors of 84 patients with hematologic malignancies and *Fusarium* infection. Cancer. 2003;98:315–9.

Penicillium marneffei (PM)

23. Ungpakorn P. Cutaneous manifestations of *Penicillium morneffei* infection. J Infect Dis. 2000;13:129–34.
24. Carey J, Hofflich H, Amre R, Protic J, Perlman DC. *Penicillium marneffei* infection in an immunocompromised traveler: a case report and literature review. J Travel Med. 2005;12:291–4.
25. Supparatpinyo K, Chiewchanvit S, Hirunsri P, et al. *Penicillium marneffei* infection in patients infected with human immunodeficiency virus. Clin Infect Dis. 1992;14:871–4.
26. Wu TC, Chan JW, Ng CK, et al. Clinical presentations and outcomes of *Penicillium marneffei* infections: a series from 1994 to 2004. Hong Kong Med J. 2008;12:103–9.
27. Duong TA. Infection due to *Penicillium marneffei*, an emerging pathogen: review of 155 reported cases. Clin Infect Dis. 1996;23:125–30.
28. Walsh TJ, Groll AH. Emerging fungal pathogens: evolving challenges to immunocompromised patients for the twenty-first century. Transpl Infect Dis. 1999;1:247–61.
29. Supparatpinyo K, Sirisanthana T. Disseminated *Penicillium marneffei* infection diagnosed on examination of a peripheral blood smear of a patient with human immunodeficiency virus infection. Clin Infect Dis. 1994;18:246–7.

Paecilomyces

30. Itin PH, Frei R, Lautenschlager S, et al. Cutaneous manifestations of *Paecilomyces lilacinus* infection induced by a contaminated skin lotion in patients who are severely immunosuppressed. J Am Acad Dermatol. 1998;39:401–9.
31. Orth B, Frei R, Itin PH, et al. Outbreak of invasive mycoses caused by *Paecilomyces lilacinus* from a contaminated skin lotion. Ann Intern Med. 1996;125:799–806.
32. Hall VC, Goyal S, Davis MD, Walsh JS. Cutaneous hyalohyphomycosis caused by *Paecilomyces lilacinus*: report of three cases and review of the literature. Int J Dermatol. 2004;43:648–53.
33. Hilmarsdóttir I, Thorsteinsson SB, Asmundsson P, Bödvarsson M, Arnadóttir M. Cutaneous infection caused by *Paecilomyces lilacinus* in a renal transplant patient: treatment with voriconazole. Scand J Infect Dis. 2000;32:331–2.
34. Lin WL, Lin WC, Chiu CS. *Paecilomyces lilacinus* cutaneous infection associated with peripherally inserted central catheter insertion. J Eur Acad Dermatol Venereol. 2008;22:1267–78.
35. Safdar A. Progresssive cutaneous hyalohyphomycosis due to *Paecilomyces lilacinus*: rapid response to treatment with saspofungin and itraconzole. Clin Infect Dis. 2002;43:1415–7.
36. Hecker MS, Weinberg JM, Bagheri B, et al. Cutaneous *Paecilomyces lilacinus* infection: report of two novel cases. J Am Acad Dermatol. 1997;37:270–1.
37. Harris LF, Dan BM, Lefkowitz Jr LB, Alford RH. *Paecilomyces* cellulitis in a renal transplant patient: successful treatment with intravenous miconazole. South Med J. 1979;72:987.
38. Jade KB, Lyons MF, Gnann Jr JW. *Paecilomyces lilacinus* cellulitis in an immunocompromised patient. Arch Dermatol. 1986;122:1169.
39. Castro LGM, Salebian A, Sotto MN. Hyalohyphomycosis by *Paecilomyces lilacinus* in a renal transplant patient and a review of human *Paecilomyces* species infection. J Med Vet Mycol. 1990;28:15.
40. Silliman CC, Lawellin DW, Lohr JA, Rodgers BM, Donowitz LG. *Paecilomyces lilacinus* infection in a child with chronic granulamatous disease. J Infect. 1992;24:191.
41. Wolfson JS, Sober AJ, Rubin RN. Dermatologic manifestations of infections in immunocompromised patients. Medicine (Baltimore). 1985;64:115–33.
42. Lott ME, Sheehan DJ, Davis LS. *Paecilomyces lilacinus* with a sporotrichoid pattern in a renal transplant patient. J Drugs Dermatol. 2007;6:436–9.

43. Lee J, Yew WW, Chiu CS, et al. Delayed sternotomy wound infection due to *Paecilomyces variotii* in a lung transplant recipient. J Heart Lung Transplant. 2002;21:1131–4.

44. Pastor FJ, Guarro J. Clinical manifestations, treatment and outcome of *Paecilomyces lilacinus*. Clin Microbiol Infect. 2006;12:948–60.

Acremonium

45. Schell WA, Perfect JR. Fatal, disseminated Acremonium strictum infection in a neutropenic host. J Clin Microbiol. 1996;34:1333–6.

46. Fincher RM, Fisher JF, Lovell RD, et al. Infection due to the fungus *Acremonium (Cephalosporium)*. Medicine (Baltimore). 1991;70:398–409.

47. Chang YH, Huang LM, Hsueh PR, et al. *Acremonium* pyomyositis in a pediatric patient with acute leukemia. Pediatr Blood Cancer. 2005;44:521–4.

48. Yamazaki R, Mori T, Aisa Y, et al. Systemic infection due to *Acremonium* after allogeneic peripheral blood stem cell transplantation. Intern Med. 2006;45:989–90.

49. Foell JL, Fischer M, Seibold M, et al. Lethal double infection with *Acremonium strictum* and *Aspergillus fumigates* during induction chemotherapy in a child with all. Pediatr Blood Cancer. 2007;49(6):858–61.

50. Mattei D, Mordini N, Lo Nigro C, et al. Successful treatment of *Acrenomium*-Fungämien mit voriconazol. Mycoses. 2003;46:511–4.

51. Van Etta LL, Peterson LR, Gerding DN. *Acremonium falciforme (Cephalosporium falciforme)* mycetoma in a renal transplant patient. Arch Dermatol. 1983;119:707–8.

52. Geyer AS, Fox LP, Husain S, Della-Latta P, Grossman ME. *Acremonium* mycetoma in a heart transplant recipient. J Am Acad Dermatol. 2006;55:1095–100.

Scopulariopsis

53. Ragge NK, Dean Hart JC, Easty DL, Tyers AG. A case of fungal keratitis caused by *Scopulariopsis brevicaulis*: treatment with antifungal agents and penetrating heratoplasty. Br J Ophthalmol. 1990;74:561–2.

54. Gupta AK, Elewski BE. Nondermatophyte causes of onychomycosis and superficial mycoses. Curr Top Med Mycol. 1996;7:87–97.

55. Sellier P, Monsuez JJ, Lacroix C, et al. Recurrent subcutaneous infection due to *Scopulariopsis brevicaulis* in a liver transplant recipient. Clin Infect Dis. 2000;30:820–3.

56. Neglia JP, Hurd DD, Ferrieri P, Snover DC. Invasive *Scopulariopsis* in the immunocompromised host. Am J Med. 1987;83:1163–6.

57. Steinbach WJ, Schell WA, Miller JL, Perfect JR, Martin PL. Fatal *Scopulariopsis brevicaulis* infection in a paediatruc stem-cell transplant pateine treated with voriconazole and caspofungin and a review of *Scopulariopsis* infections in immunocompromised patients. J Infect. 2004;48:112–6.

58. Patel R, Gustaferro CA, Krom RA, et al. Phaeohyphomycosis due to *Scopulariopsis brumptii* in a liver transplant recipient. Clin Infect Dis. 1994;19:198–200.

59. Karam A, Hery G, Eveillard JR, et al. Subcutaneous mycosis due to *Scopulariopsis brevicaulis* in an aplastic patient. Ann Dermatol Venereol. 2003;130:783–6.

60. Martel J, Faisant M, Lebeau B, et al. Subcutaneous mycosis due to *Scopulariopsis brevicaulis* in an immunocompromised patient. Ann Dermatol Venereol. 2001;128:130–3.

61. Phillips P, Wood WS, Phillips G, Rinaldi MG. Invasive hyalohyphomycosis caused by *Scopulariopsis brevicaulis* in a patient undergoing allogeneic bone marrow transplant. Diagn Microbiol Infect Dis. 1989;12:429–32.

Trichosporon

62. Girmenia C, Pagano L, Martino B, et al. Invasive infections caused by *Trichosporon* species and *Geotrichum capitatum* in patients with hematological malignancies: a retrospective multicenter study from Italy and review of the literature. J Clin Microbiol. 2005;43:1818–28.

63. Takamura S, Oono T, Kanzaki H, Arata J. Disseminated trichosporonosis with *Trichosponon asahii*. Eur J Dermatol. 1999;9:577–9.

64. Wynne SM, Kwon-Chung KJ, Shea YR, et al. Invasive infection with *Trichosporon inkin* in 2 siblings with chronic granulomatous disease. J Allergy Clin Immunol. 2004;114:1418–24.

65. Reichenbach J, Lopatin U, Mahlaoui N. Actinomyces in chronic granulomatous disease: an emerging and unanticipated pathogen. Clin Infect Dis. 2009;49:1703–9.

66. Hoy J, Hsu KC, Rolston K, Luna M, Bodey GP. *Trichosporon beigelii* infection: a review. Rev Infect Dis. 1986;8:959–67.

67. Fournier S, Pavageau W, Feuillhade M, et al. Use of voriconazole to successfully treat disseminated *Trichosporon asahii* infection in a patient with acute myeloid leukaemia. Eur J Clin Microbiol Infect Dis. 2002;21:892–6.

68. Nahass GT, Rosenberg SP, Leonardi CL, Penneys NS. Disseminated infection with *Trichosporon beigelii*. Arch Dermatol. 1993;129:1020–3.

69. Libertin CR, Davies NJ, Halper J, Edson RS, Roberts GD. Invasive disease caused by *Trichosporon beigelii*. Mayo Clin Proc. 1983;58:684–6.

70. Hughes CE, Serstock D, Wilson BD, Payne W. Infection with *Trichosporon pullulans*. Ann Intern Med. 1988;108:772–3.

71. Gold JW, Poston W, Mertelsmann R, et al. Systemic infection with *Trichosporon cutaneum* in a patient with acute leukemia. Cancer. 1981;48:2163–7.

72. Winston DJ, Blasley GE, Rhodes J, Linne SR. Disseminated *Trichosporon capitatum* infection in an immunosuppressed host. Arch Intern Med. 1977;137:1192–5.

73. Walsh TJ, Newman KR, Moody M, Wharton RC, Wade JC. Trichosporonosis in patients with neoplastic disease. Medicine. 1986;65:268–79.

74. Song HJ, Chung SL, Lee KS. Trichosporon in skin subcutaneous infection in a rheumatoid arthritis patient. Int J Dermatol. 2007;46:282–3.

75. Fekkar A, Brun S, D'Ussel M, et al. Serum cross-reactivity with *Aspergillus* galactonmannan and cryptococcal antigen during fatal disseminated *Trichonsporon dermatis* infection. Clin Infect Dis. 2009;49:1457–8.

Trichoderma

76. De Miguel D, Gómez P, González R, et al. Nonfatal pulmonary *Trichoderma viride* infection in an adult patient with acute myeloid leukemia: report of one case and review of the literature. Diagn Microbiol Infect Dis. 2005;53:33–7.

77. Chouaki T, Lavarde V, Lachaud L, Raccurt CP, Hennequin C. Invasive infections due to *Trichoderma* species: report of 2 cases, findins of in vitro susceptibility testing, and review of the literature. Clin Infect Dis. 2002;35:1360–7.

78. Gautheret A, Dromer F, Bourhis JH, Andremont A. *Trichoderma pseudokoningii* as a cause of fatal infection in bone marrow transplant recipient. Clin Infect Dis. 1995;20:1060–3.

79. Munoz FM, Demmler GJ, Travis WR, et al. *Trichoderma longibrachiatum* infection in a pediatric patient with aplastic anemia. J Clin Microbiol. 1997;35:499–503.

80. Kantarcioğlu AS, Celkan T, Yücel A, et al. Fatal *Trichoderma harzianum* infection in a leukemic pediatric patient. Med Mycol. 2009;47:207–15.

81. Richter S, Cormican MG, Pfaller MA, et al. Fatal disseminated *Trichoderma longibrachiatum* infection in an adult bone marrow transplant patient: species identification and review of the literature. J Clin Microbiol. 1999;37:1154–60.

82. Myoken Y, Sugata T, Fujita Y, et al. Fatal necrotizing stomatitis due to *Trichoderma longibrachiatum* in a neutropenic patient with malignant lymphoma: a case report. Int J Oral Maxillofac Surg. 2002;31:688–91.

Blastoschizomyces capitatum

83. Martino R, Salavert M, Parody R, et al. *Blastoschizomyces capitatus* infection in patients with leukemia: report of 26 cases. Clin Infect Dis. 2004;38:335–41.

84. Etienne A, Datry A, Gaspar N, et al. Successful treatment of disseminated *Geotrichum capitatum* infection with a combination of caspofungin and voriconazole in an immunocompromised patient. Mycoses. 2008;54:270–2.

85. Pérez-Sanchez I, Anguita J, Martín-Rabadan P, et al. *Blastoschizomyces capitatus* infection in acute leukemia patients. Leuk Lymphoma. 2000;39:209–12.

86. Kassamali H, Anaissie E, Ro J, et al. Disseminated *Geotrichum candidum* infection. J Clin Microbiol. 1987;25:1782–3.

87. Huang CL, Lu MY, Lin KH, Huang LM. *Geotrichum candidum* fungemia with skin lesions similar to varicella in a patient with acute lymphocytic leukemia. Acta Paediatr Taiwan. 2004;45:38–40.

Paracoccidioidomycosis (South American Blastomycosis)

88. Goldani LZ, Sugar AM. Paracoccidioidomycosis and AIDS: an overview. Clin Infect Dis. 1995;21(5):1275–81.

89. Silva-Vergara ML, Teixeira AC, Curi VG, et al. Paracoccidioidomycosis associated with human immunodeficiency virus infection. Report of 10 cases. Med Mycol. 2003;41(3):259–63.

90. Zavascki AP, Bienardt JC, Severo LC. Paracoccidioidomycosis in organ transplant recipient: case report. Rev Inst Med Trop Sao Paulo. 2004;46(5):279–81.

91. Paniago AM, de Freitas AC, Aguiar ES, et al. Paracoccidioidomycosis in patients with human immunodeficiency virus: review of 12 cases observed in an endemic region in Brazil. J Infect. 2005;51(3):248–52.

92. Morejón KM, Machado AA, Martinez R. Paracoccidioidomycosis in patients infected with and not infected with human immunodeficiency virus: a case-control study. Am J Trop Med Hyg. 2009;80(3):359–66.

93. Almeida OP, Jacks Jr J, Scully C. Paracoccidioidomycosis of the mouth: an emerging deep mycosis. Crit Rev Oral Biol Med. 2003;14(5):377–83. Review.

94. Brunaldi MO, Rezende RE, Zucoloto S, et al. Co-infection with paracoccidioidomycosis and human immunodeficiency virus: report of a case with esophageal involvement. Am J Trop Med Hyg. 2010;82(6):1099–101.

3

Superficial Mycoses

DERMATOPHYTOSES

Dermatophyte infections are superficial fungal infections of the hair, nails, and typically the stratum corneum of the skin. Causative organisms include fungi in the *Trichophyton*, *Microsporum*, or *Epidermophyton* groups. The dermatophytes typically do not invade living tissue. Subcutaneous and systemic involvements are rare. However, in immunosuppressed patients, such as transplant patients, patients on chemotherapy or other immunosuppressive medications, or patients with compromised immunity due to human immunodeficiency virus (HIV) infection, these fungi can become invasive. *Trichophyton rubrum* is the most common dermatophyte isolated.

Invasion into the dermis through a ruptured hair follicle has been reported as Majocchi's granuloma. However, direct invasion into the dermis without evidence of follicular rupture has also been described.[1] The presence of deep dermal or subcutaneous involvement without any evidence of follicular location, absence of keratin or hair elements in the dermis, and scarcity of foreign body giant cells are all suggestive of invasive dermatophyte.[2] Few cases of widespread invasive dermatophytosis have been described in immunosuppressed patients, and they may initially present with violaceous, erythematous, or hemorrhagic nodules in an area of chronic dermatophyte infection, such as the feet, lower legs, or buttocks.[3,4] Invasive dermatophyte nodules can also occur on the face, scalp, or trunk. Deep cutaneous infections with dermatophyte can present as a dermatophyte abscess, a cold abscess, chronic draining nodules,[5] a fluctuant nodule, or chronic ulceration. Most patients have only a few nodules, but up to 100 nodules have been reported. Although the lesions are usually 1 cm to several centimeters in diameter, some have been reported as large as 10 cm. Most patients with invasive tinea have onychomycosis[6] or chronic superficial dermatophyte infection. Dermatophyte abscesses

can appear and progress even in the immunocompromised patient receiving intravenous amphotericin. Despite an excellent in vitro profile against dermatophytes, systemic amphotericin is not generally effective against dermatophytes because it is not secreted in sweat or sebum and low tissue levels are achieved in the outer layers of skin only by passive diffusion.[7]

Dermatophyte infections can be readily misdiagnosed because they mimic other cutaneous diseases.[8,9] Tinea infection of the face has been described as simulating dermatomyositis, seborrheic dermatitis, acne rosacea, photosensitivity rashes, and discoid and systemic lupus.[10] Widespread pustular eruptions due to dermatophyte infection may mimic bacterial folliculitis, pustular psoriasis, subcorneal pustular dermatitis, or a pustular drug eruption.[11] Widespread vesicular or bullous dermatophyte infection may mimic herpes or varicella zoster virus infection, as well as autoimmune blistering diseases.[11] Invasive dermatophyte infection can produce numerous red-blue nodules on the feet mimicking Kaposi sarcoma.[12-14] Deep dermatophyte infection can produce subcutaneous swelling with multiple draining sinuses without grains, known as a pseudomycetoma.[15,16]

In the immunocompromised host, one can see extensive and widespread involvement of the skin with a dermatophyte infection, which usually produces only a localized or trivial infection in the immunocompetent host. Dermatophyte infection often extends from long-standing onychomycosis and moccasin-type tinea pedis across the dorsa of the toes and feet to the ankles. Annular erythematous plaques can also be found anywhere on the body. A severe widespread dermatophytosis may be seen with unusual morphologies, with multiple lesions, in unusual locations and may be difficult to control. Dermatophyte infection may also resemble palmoplantar keratoderma with diffuse thickening of the palms and soles or keratoderma blennorrhagica. Disseminated tinea corporis appeared in a profoundly immunosuppressed HIV-positive man after initiation of highly active antiretroviral therapy

M.E. Grossman et al., *Cutaneous Manifestations of Infection in the Immunocompromised Host*, DOI 10.1007/978-1-4419-1578-8_3, © Springer Science+Business Media, LLC 2012

(HAART); immune restoration occurred accompanied by an inflammatory reaction in the form of a generalized rash (immune restoration inflammatory syndrome or IRIS).[17]

Tinea capitis, rarely seen in adults, may present in HIV infected patients with alopecia or seborrhea like scaling patches. Favus classically[18] affects the scalp and is usually due to *Trichophyton schoenleinii*. Favus like lesions of the scrotal skin or scutular tinea rarely reported in HIV infection may be due to *Microsporum gypseum*, a geophilic dermatophyte.[19]

Local immunosuppression because of the application of topical corticosteroids or immunomodulators, such as tacrolimus or pimecrolimus, given erroneously to an undiagnosed dermatophyte infection can produce tinea incognito.[20] The features are similar to those seen in patients with tinea infections receiving systemic corticosteroids. The inflammatory response is suppressed so that scaling becomes absent and the margins become indistinct. The fungus is allowed to grow unchecked and the area involved may become very extensive. At times, multiple annular rings are seen with little or no erythema in the intervening areas resembling tinea imbricata. Tinea incognito may mimic entities such as granuloma annulare, discoid lupus erythematosus, seborrheic dermatitis, or erythema migrans.[20] Follicular papules and pustules are common. With continued use of the topical corticosteroid creams, their adverse effects on the skin become evident: atrophy, telangiectasias, and purpura because of skin fragility.

Diagnosis may be difficult in tinea incognito because of the absence of scale for scraping for a potassium hydroxide (KOH) preparation. However, if an adequate specimen is obtained, it is loaded with hyphae that can be readily identified and cultured. Skin biopsy may be useful to identify fungal organisms and to differentiate the dermatophytosis from the skin diseases that it may mimic. When *Trichophyton rubrum* grows in the dermis, as in Majocchi's granuloma, the hyphae may assume unusual morphologic forms and may be absent from the stratum corneum, its usual habitat.

Onychomycosis is frequent in the immunocompromised host, but paronychial involvement and proximal white subungual onychomycoses are distinctive clinical appearances seen with immunosuppression, most often with HIV infection. Proximal white subungual onychomycosis is characterized by white patches on the proximal portion of the nail, initially limited to the lunula but may involve the entire nail. The surface of the nail is usually smooth and normal. *Trichophyton rubrum* is the fungus most commonly isolated from the nail. Proximal white onychomycosis has been described in renal transplant patients and patients with connective tissue disease on systemic steroid therapy.[21-23]

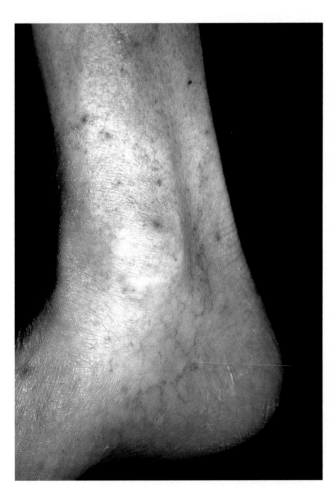

Figure 3.1. Routine tinea pedis in a 60-year-old with Hodgkin's disease before chemotherapy. *T. rubrum* was cultured

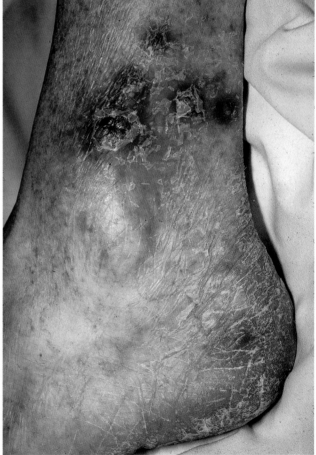

Figure 3.2. Neutropenic during chemotherapy, the same patient shown in Fig. 3.1 6 weeks later developed multiple hemorrhagic nodules in the areas of the superficial dermatophyte infection

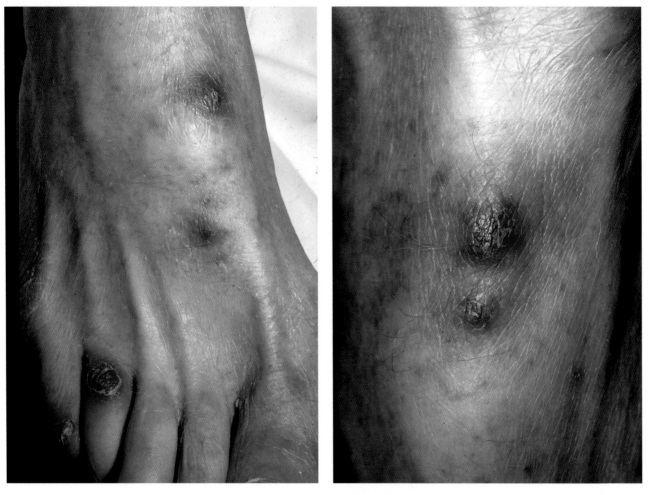

Figure 3.3. and 3.4. Purple nodules on the foot and knee of a neutropenic patient with Hodgkin's disease during chemotherapy. Skin biopsy and culture confirmed *T. rubrum* invasion into the dermis and subcutis

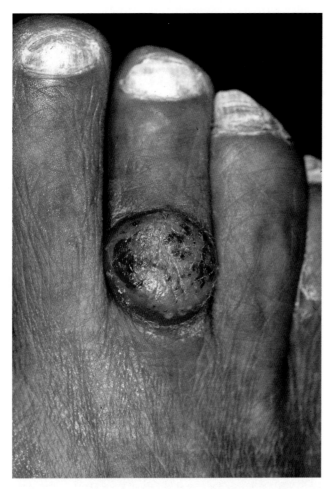

Figure 3.5. Chronic onychomycoses and a dome-shaped erythematous nodule with minute pustules due to invasive *Trichophyton rubrum* on the toe of a renal transplant recipient. Histopathology suggested the microform of *Blastomyces dermatitidis*

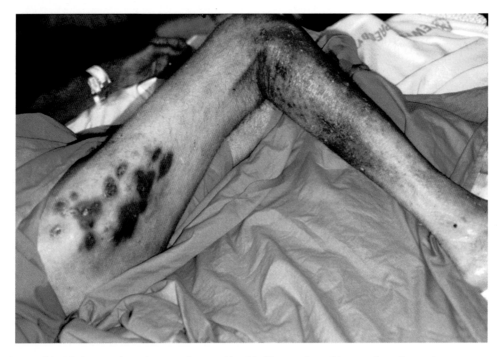

Figure 3.6. A 50-year-old with dermatophyte abscesses diagnosed by skin biopsy prior to his second renal transplant

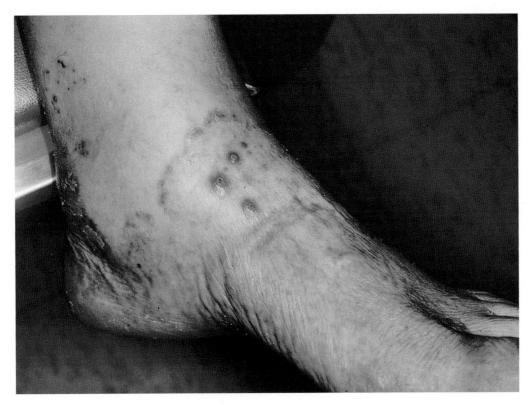

Figure 3.7. Hemorrhagic nodules of invasive dermatophyte surrounded by extensive moccasin-type tinea pedis on the ankle of a renal transplant recipient

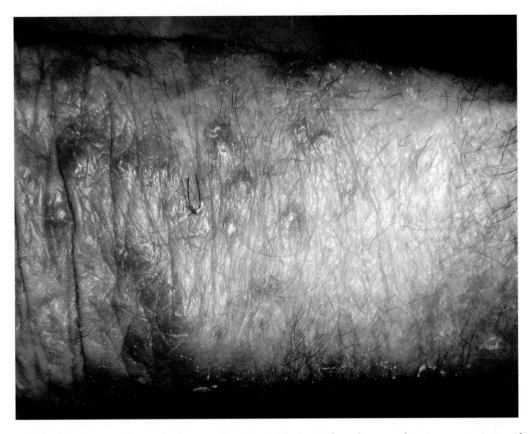

Figure 3.8. Dusky erythematous papules on the forearm of a patient with chronic lung disease on long-term systemic steroids. Skin biopsy confirmed the presence of dermatophytes in the dermis and epidermis

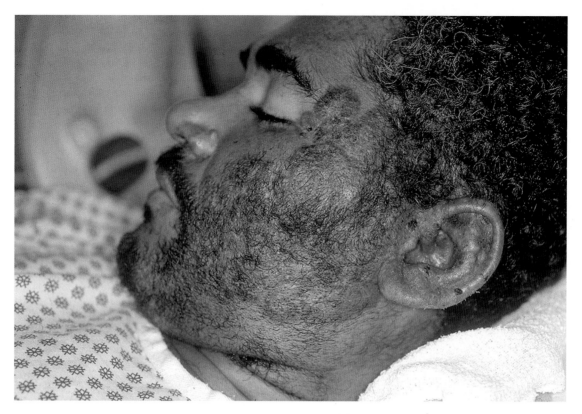

Figure 3.9. Coalescent purple plaques of the face due to widespread *T. rubrum* infection in adult T-cell leukemia associated with human T-cell lymphotrophic virus type I (HTLV-I)

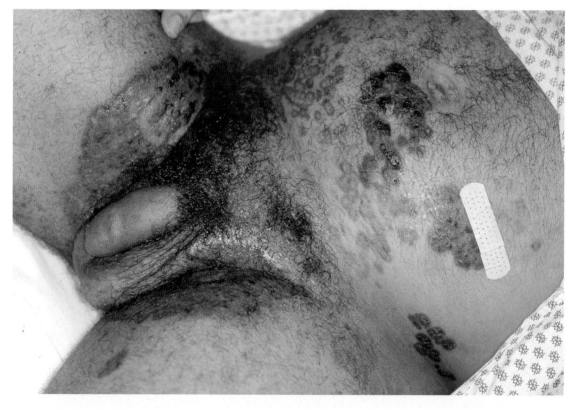

Figure 3.10. Purple truncal nodules due to invasive *T. rubrum*, along with annular and bicrural tinea in HTLV-I leukemia

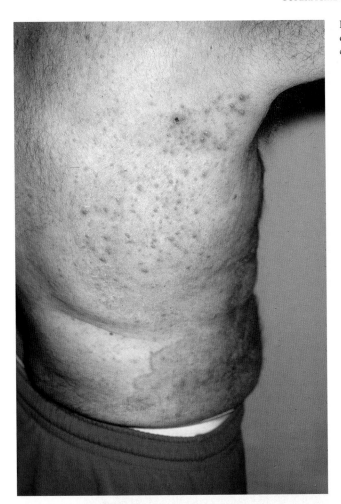

Figure 3.11. Papulonodules of invasive *T. rubrum* infection developed within the extensive chronic dermatophyte infection in a cardiac transplant patient undergoing an episode of rejection

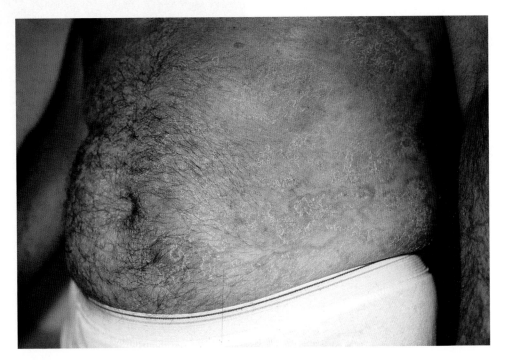

Figure 3.12. Extensive *T. rubrum* infection in a heart transplant patient. Annular scaling plaques were present over the abdomen, chest, groin, buttocks, legs, and feet

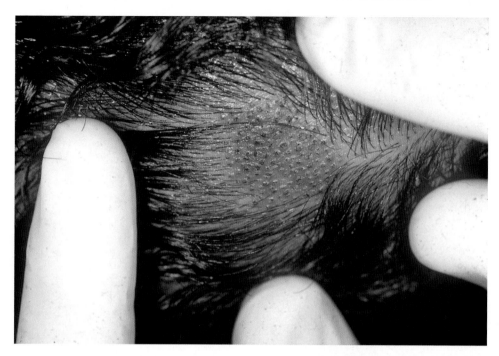

Figure 3.13. Tinea capitis due to *Microsporum canis* in a human immunodeficiency virus (HIV)-positive adult. Generally a disease of prepubertal children, tinea capitis occurs in the immunocompromised adult. The black dot ringworm seen here with *M. canis* is most often caused by *Trichophyton tonsurans* or *Trichophyton violaceum*

Figure 3.14. A 19-year-old with systemic lupus erythematosus on high-dose immunosuppressives presented with worsening skin rash and persistent headaches. The clinical impression was flaring lupus with lupus cerebritis and cutaneous disease. Erythematous scaling papules and plaques on the face, chest, and arms were present in a photodistribution

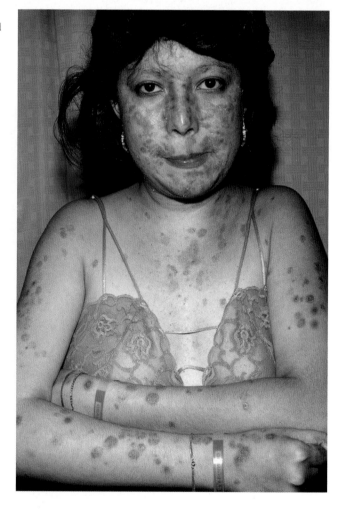

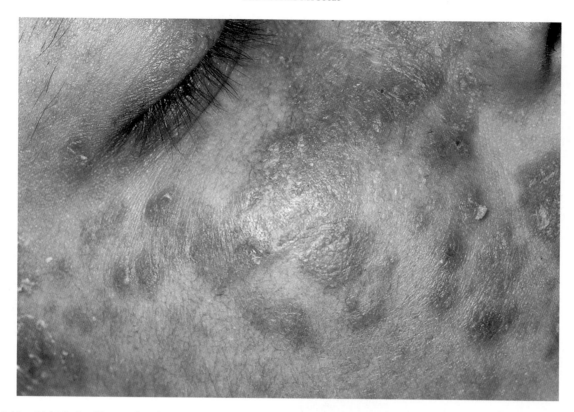

Figure 3.15. Multiple facial lesions thought to be discoid lupus with scalp involvement causing alopecia

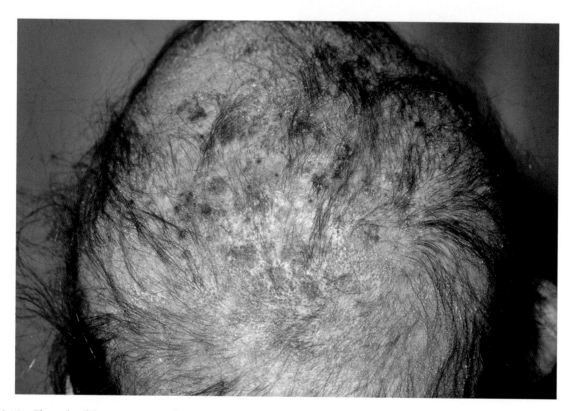

Figure 3.16. The scalp of the patient in Figs. 3.14 and 3.15 (after the wig was removed) was boggy, minimally erythematous with scattered crusts and a few pustules. Potassium hydroxide preparations demonstrated numerous hyphae which were *M. canis* on culture. All the skin lesions cleared and the hair regrew with ketoconazole

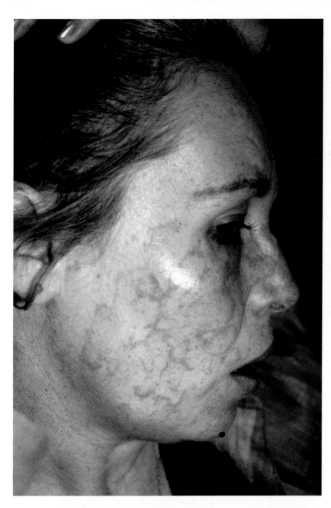

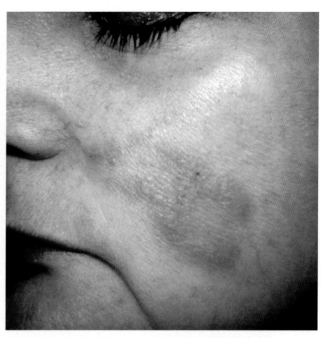

Figure 3.18. A nonscaling erythematous plaque with indistinct margins treated with a corticosteroid cream until the diagnosis of tinea faciei was made

Figure 3.17. An extensive dermatophyte infection extending from the cheek to the nose and chin. Shiny skin and multiple annular rings are due to the frequent use of a fluorinated corticosteroid cream

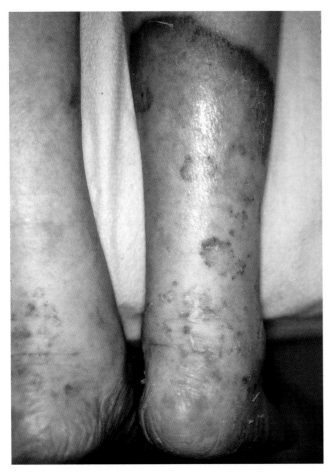

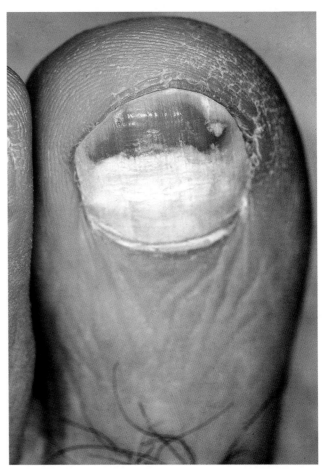

Figure 3.19.   An annular hemorrhagic border of tinea that spread up the leg because of the inappropriate use of a fluorinated corticosteroid cream. Onychomycoses and tinea pedis were long-standing

Figure 3.20.   Proximal white subungual onychomycosis in a patient with HIV infection. The area of white discoloration sometimes extends to involve the entire nail plate

MALASSEZIA SPECIES

Malassezia (previously known as *Pityrosporum ovale* and *Pityrosporum orbiculare*) is a ubiquitous fungus of low pathogenicity that colonizes normal skin. *Malassezia furfur* is a dimorphic fungus that requires an exogenous source of medium- and long-chain fatty acids for growth. The yeast forms are round to oval, thick-walled cells measuring 2–5 μm in diameter. In humans, *M. furfur* is considered normal resident flora of the pilosebaceous units (hair follicles and their associated sebaceous glands). The skin of the human chest, back, and scalp are sebaceous regions rich in fatty acids, providing an exogenous source of lipids for the growth of *M. furfur.* Culture of *Malassezia* requires supplementation of the medium with a source of fatty acids such as sterile olive oil.

Malassezia is thought to play a role, or to be the causative factor, in the development of several skin diseases, such as seborrheic dermatitis, tinea versicolor, *Pityrosporum* folliculitis, and possibly atopic dermatitis, particularly in adults.[24] Overgrowth of *Pityrosporum* yeasts has been implicated in the high incidence of seborrheic dermatitis in patients with HIV/AIDS (acquired immune deficiency syndrome).

Impaired host immunity or suppression of normal bacterial skin flora by antibiotics may permit *Pityrosporum* overgrowth within the hair follicle. *Pityrosporum* folliculitis may be seen in patients immunocompromised as a result of organ transplantation, malignancy, pregnancy, AIDS, prolonged antibiotic treatment, or chronic renal failure. Neutropenia and the use of broad spectrum antimicrobials do not appear to be significant risk factors for *Malassezia* infections unlike more common opportunistic fungal infections in immunocompromised patients.[25] The lesions of *Pityrosporum* folliculitis are predictable, distributed over the chest, shoulders, and upper back, where pilosebaceous units are most abundant. The erythematous follicular papules and pustules are minimally pruritic and may number from fewer than ten to hundreds. The pustular lesions of *Pityrosporum* folliculitis may mimic disseminated candidiasis, bacterial folliculitis, or severe acne.[26-29]

In recent years, yeast has been implicated in causing invasive disease (albeit without specific skin manifestations) in premature infants receiving lipid rich intravenous infusions and in severely immunocompromised patients with central venous access devices (CVAD).[30] The fungus colonizes the skin and gains access to the CVAD causing fever and fungemia. Resolution of the infection follows removal of the CVAD, discontinuation of parenteral nutrition including intralipids, and may or may not require parenteral antifungal therapy.

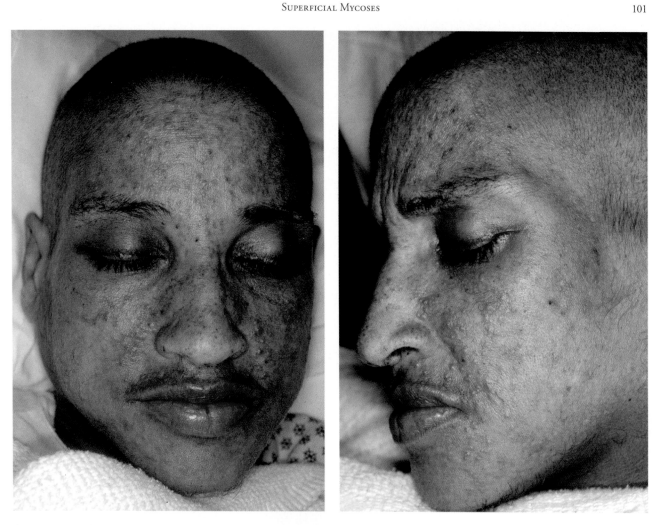

Figures 3.21. and 3.22.   Erythematous papules and rare papulopustules on the face of an HIV-positive patient with *Pityrosporum* folliculitis (Fig. 3.22 courtesy of Paul Schneiderman, M.D.)

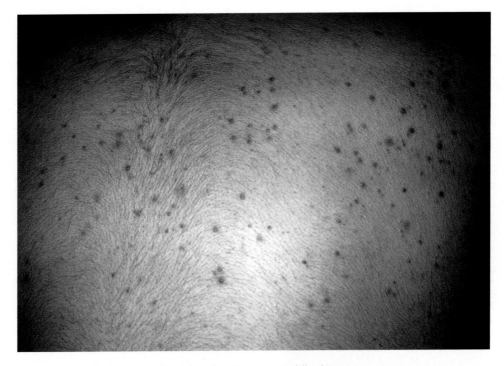

Figure 3.23.   Erythematous follicular papulopustules and crusts of *Pityrosporum* folliculitis

Figure 3.24.   Coalescent patches of widespread tinea versicolor in a renal transplant patient

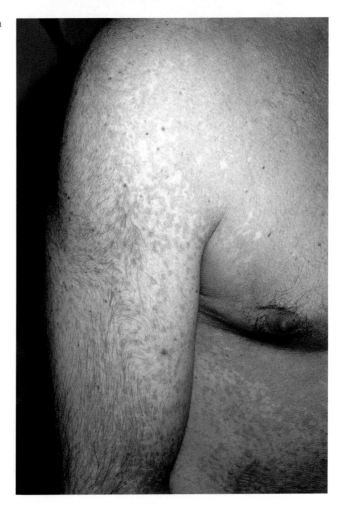

REFERENCES

Dermatophytoses

1. Smith KJ, Welsh M, Skelton H. Trichophyton rubrum showing deep dermal invasion directly from the epidermis in immunosuppressed patients. Br J Dermatol. 2001;145(2):344–8.
2. Erbaği Z. Deep dermatophytoses in association with atopy and diabetes mellitus: Majocchi's granuloma tricophyticum or dermatophytic pseudomycetoma? Mycopathologia. 2002;154(4):163–9.
3. Squeo RF, Beer R, Silvers D, Weitzman I, Grossman M. Invasive *Trichophyton rubrum* resembling blastomycosis infection in the immunocompromised host. J Am Acad Dermatol. 1998;39(2 Pt 2):379–80.
4. Baker RL, Para MF. Successful use of ketoconazole for invasive cutaneous *Trichophyton rubrum* infection. Arch Intern Med. 1984; 144(3):615–7.
5. Demidovich CW, Kornfeld BW, Gentry RH, Fitzpatrick JE. Deep dermatophyte infection with chronic draining nodules in an immunocompromised patient. Cutis. 1995;55(4):237–40.
6. Novick NL, Tapia L, Bottone EJ. Invasive *Trichophyton rubrum* infection in an immunocompromised host. Am J Med. 1987;82(2):321–5.
7. Elewski BE, Sullivan J. Dermatophytes as opportunistic pathogens. J Am Acad Dermatol. 1994;30(6):1021–2.
8. Shapiro L, Cohen HJ. Tinea faciei simulating other dermatoses. JAMA. 1971;215:2106–7.
9. Rist TE, Abele DC, Caves JM. Tinea faciale: an often misdiagnosed clinical entity. South Med J. 1974;67:331–4.
10. Almeida L, Grossman ME. Widespread dermatophyte infections that mimic collagen vascular disease. J Am Acad Dermatol. 1990;23: 855–7.
11. Ziemer M, Seyfarth F, Elsner P, Hipler UC. Atypical manifestations of tinea corporis. Mycoses. 2007;50 Suppl 2:31–5.
12. Brod C, Benedix F, Röcken M, Schaller M. Trichophytic Majocchi granuloma mimicking Kaposi sarcoma. J Dtsch Dermatol Ges. 2007;5(7):591–3.
13. Crosby DL, Berger TG, Woosley JT, Resnick SD. Dermatophytosis mimicking Kaposi's sarcoma in human immunodeficiency virus disease. Dermatologica. 1991;182(2):135–7.
14. Kwon KS, Jang HS, Son HS, et al. Widespread and invasive *Trichophyton rubrum* infection mimicking Kaposi's sarcoma in a patient with AIDS. J Dermatol. 2004;31(10):839–43.
15. Petrov I, Kempf W, Stoilova D, et al. Disseminated dermatophytic pseudomycetomas arising in an immunocompromised patient. Br J Dermatol. 2006;155(3):628–30.
16. Franco RC. Deep dermatophytosis in a post transplant recipient. Int J Dermatol. 2001;40(5):363–4.
17. van Hal SJ, Kotsiou G. An HIV-positive man with generalized rash. Clin Infect Dis. 2005;40(1):113, 182–183.
18. Bournerias I, De Chauvin MF, Datry A, et al. Unusual *Microsporum canis* infections in adult HIV patients. J Am Acad Dermatol. 1996;35 (5 Pt 2):808–10.
19. Prochnau A, de Almeida HL, Jr SPR, Souza PR, et al. Scutular tinea of the scrotum: report of two cases. Mycoses. 2005;48(3):162–4.
20. Rallis E, Koumantaki-Mathioudaki E. Pimecrolimus induced tinea incognito masquerading as intertriginous psoriasis. Mycoses. 2008; 51(1):71–3.
21. Rongioletti F, Persi A, Tripodi S, Rebora A. Proximal white subungual onychomycosis: a sign of immunodeficiency. J Am Acad Dermatol. 1994;30:129–30.
22. Sentamil Selvi G, Kamalam A, Ajithados K, Janaki C, Thambiah AS. Clinical and mycological features of dermatophytosis in renal transplant recipients. Mycoses. 1999;42(1–2):75–8.
23. Tlacuilo-Parra A, Guevara-Gutiérrez E, Mayorga J, Salazar-Páramo M. Proximal white subungual onychomycosis caused by *Microsporum canis* in systemic lupus erythematosus. Rheumatol Int. 2002;21(6): 250–2.

Malassezia Species

24. Gupta AK, Batra R, Bluhm R, Boekhout T, Dawson Jr TL. Skin diseases associated with *Malassezia* species. J Am Acad Dermatol. 2004;51(5):785–98.
25. Morrison VA, Weisdorf DJ. The spectrum of Malassezia infections in the bone marrow transplant population. Bone Marrow Transplant. 2000;26(6):645–8.
26. Klotz SA, Drutz DJ, Huppert M, Johnson JE. *Pityrosporum* folliculitis: its potential for confusion with skin lesions of systemic candidiasis. Arch Intern Med. 1982;142:2126–9.
27. Bufill JA et al. *Pityrosporum* folliculitis after bone marrow transplantation. Ann Intern Med. 1988;108:560–3.
28. Yohn JJ, Lucus J, Camisa C. *Malassezia* folliculitis in immunocompromised patients. Cutis. 1985;35:536–8.
29. Rhie S, Turcios R, Buckley H, Suh B. Clinical features and treatment of Malassezia folliculitis with fluconazole in orthotopic heart transplant recipients. J Heart Lung Transplant. 2000;19(2):215–9.
30. Devlin RK. Invasive fungal infections caused by *Candida* and *Malassezia* species in the neonatal intensive care unit. Adv Neonatal Care. 2006;6(2):68–77.

4

Algae

PROTOTHECOSIS

Prototheca species are ubiquitous but rare pathogens. They are achlorophillic aerobic unicellular algae, which have been isolated from salt and fresh water (including sea water, marshes, ponds, streams, and lakes), sewage, soil, tree sap, potato peels, and bananas. *Prototheca* is closely related to the green algae *Chlorella*. They may colonize human skin, fingernails, the respiratory tract, and the gastrointestinal tract. *Prototheca* are spherical, 5–14 mm in diameter, and reproduce asexually by internal septation and cleavage with the formation of a sporangium containing up to 20 endospores. There have been three species (*P. wickerhamii, P. zopfi, P. stagnora*) described, but only *Prototheca wickerhamii* has been associated with human disease in the compromised host. These include organ transplant recipients, patients receiving immunosuppressive medications or chemotherapy for malignancies, diabetics,[1] human immunodeficiency virus (HIV) infection, and prolonged use of topical corticosteroids. *Prototheca* infections have a worldwide distribution and are often initiated by local trauma or surgery.

In normal hosts, *Prototheca* infections present as olecranon bursitis and a single lesion of the skin or subcutaneous tissue. The typical lesion is a painless slowly progressive plaque or papulonodular lesion that becomes eczematous or ulcerated. Lesions typically enlarge over weeks to months. The papules, plaques, or eczematous dermatitis are usually limited to the exposed portions of the body, especially the extremities and/or face. Most patients reported trauma with contamination of wounds with water. An immunocompromised 74-year-old with rheumatoid arthritis receiving infliximab was reported with olcecranon bursitis and a 3-cm nodule on the third metacarpal phalangeal joint.[2]

Cutaneous lesions of protothecosis in patients on immunosuppressive medications for transplantation or other medical conditions have been variously described: vesicles that ruptured leaving superficial ulcers with seropurulent drainage mimicking a bacterial pyoderma in a renal transplant patient[3]; painful papules and nodules that developed pustules and necrotic crusts on the shins of a women with systemic lupus erythematosus on immunosuppressive medications[4]; ulcerating cellulitis of the fingers of a diabetic renal transplant patient after extensive immersion of his hands in water[5]; cellulitis in a renal transplant patient[6]; nontender fluctuant papulonodules on the forearm and a draining abscess at the site of an old arteriovenous shunt in a renal transplant patient[7]; a large well-demarcated erythematous plaque on the forearm with papules at the margin in a farmer with a long history of steroid use[8]; and a thick scaly erythematous confluent plaque with multiple erosions and pustules over the right forearm in a woman with a history of intermittent steroid injections for arthritis.[9]

Numerous patients with diabetes mellitus have been reported with protothecosis: boggy erythematous plaques with several small ulcerations and prominent scarring on the lower leg of a diabetic woman on hemodialysis[10]; an 11 × 11 cm eczematous patch with multiple subcutaneous satellite nodules on the arm of a man with diabetes and steroid-dependent asthma after a verrucous nodule of chromoblastomycosis (*Philophora gougerotti*) was excised[11]; and a large erythematous plaque on the lower leg with pustules and purulent ulcers in a farmer with untreated diabetes.[8]

Other manifestations of protothecosis include: tender papulopustules on the leg of a woman with metastatic breast cancer[12]; painful grouped vesicles on an erythematous base resembling herpes simplex in a woman with myasthenia gravis[13]; yellowish vesiculobullous lesions on the hand and elbow of a

M.E. Grossman et al., *Cutaneous Manifestations of Infection in the Immunocompromised Host,*
DOI 10.1007/978-1-4419-1578-8_4, © Springer Science+Business Media, LLC 2012

woman on systemic steroids for severe chronic obstructive pulmonary disease (COPD)[14]; a verrucous plaque on the dorsum of the hand of an HIV-positive woman[15]; and mildly pruritic erythematous papules that gradually enlarged to form a large (4 × 9 cm) plaque on the back of a man with acquired immune deficiency syndrome (AIDS).[16]

The course of cutaneous protothecosis is chronic with low grade inflammation and indolence. These lesions seem less acute and tender clinically so non-bacterial infections are often suspected. Disseminated protothecosis from primary cutaneous inoculation has rarely been described and are most often reported in patients with neutrophil dysfunction. A woman with refractory acute myelocytic leukemia (AML) presented with an abscess on the thigh, which progressed to generalized tender subcutaneous nodules on the extremities, and subsequent development of

multiple lung abscesses.[17] Another woman with AML presented with a necrotic, ulcerated, and hemorrhagic plaque on the chest after the traumatic removal of a Hickman catheter.[18]

Clinically, the diagnosis of cutaneous protothecosis may be difficult because of its rarity and variable presentation. In contrast, the microscopic appearance is very specific. Prothecal organisms are readily identified in tissues with periodic acid-Shiff (PAS) and silver stains, although they are visible with routine hematoxylin and eosin staining. If endosporulation with a characteristic morula (mulberry) is not seen, the organism may be difficult to differentiate from several deep mycoses. Both microabscesses and granulomas with multinucleated giant cells may be seen. *Prototheca* can be cultured on Sabouraud's dextrose agar as long as cycloheximide is not added to the medium.

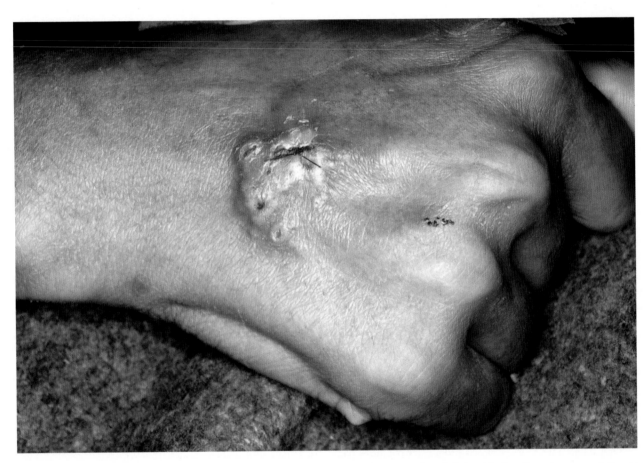

Figure 4.1. An erythematous to yellowish 2 × 3-cm verrucous plaque on the dorsum of the hand of a 33-year-old human immunodeficiency virus (HIV)-positive woman. Skin biopsy, culture, and biochemical assimilation tests identified *P. wickerhamii* as the cause of the skin infection (Courtesy of Andrew Woolrich, M.D.)

References

Protototothecosis

1. Torres HA, Bodey GP, Tarrand JJ, Kontoyiannis DP. Prototothecosis in patients with cancer: case series and literature review. Clin Microbiol Infect. 2003;9:786–92.
2. Curbelo A, Pankey GA. A man presenting with nodules on hands and elbows. Clin Infect Dis. 2009;48(8):1114–5, 1160–1.
3. Wolfe ID, Sacks HG, Samorodin CS, Robinson HM. Cutaneous protothecosis in a patient receiving immunosuppressive therapy. Arch Dermatol. 1976;112(6):829–32.
4. Thianprasit M, Youngchaiyud V, Suthipinittharm P. Protothecosis: a report of two cases. Mykosen. 1983;26(9):455–61.
5. Wolfson JS, Sober AJ, Rubin RH. Dermatologic manifestations of infections in immunocompromised patients. Medicine (Baltimore). 1985;64(2):115–33.
6. Mezger E, Eisses JF, Smith MJ. Prothecal cellulitis in a renal transplant patient. Lab Invest. 1981;44:81A.
7. Dagher FJ, Smith AG, Pankoski D, Ollodart RM. Skin protothecosis in a patient with renal allograft. South Med J. 1978;71(2):222–4.
8. Chao SC, Hsu MM, Lee JY. Cutaneous protothecosis: report of five cases. Br J Dermatol. 2002;146(4):688–93.
9. Cho BK, Ham SH, Lee JY, Choi JH. Cutaneous protothecosis. Int J Dermatol. 2002;41(5):304–6.
10. Schumann K, Hollandsworth K, Ormsby A. Nonhealing leg ulceration. Arch Dermatol. 2000;136:1263–8.
11. McAnally T, Parry EL. Cutaneous protothecosis presenting as recurrent chromomycosis. Arch Dermatol. 1985;121(8):1066–99.
12. Klintworth GK, Fetter BF, Nielsen Jr HS. Protothecosis, an algal infection: report of a case in man. J Med Microbiol. 1968;1(2):211–6.
13. Goldstein GD, Bhatia P, Kalivas J. Herpetiform protothecosis. Int J Dermatol. 1986;25(1):54–5.
14. Heitzman HB, Books TJ, Phillips BJ. Protothecosis. South Med J. 1984;77(11):1477–8.
15. Woolrich A, Koestenblatt E, Don P, Szaniawski W. Cutaneous protothecosis and AIDS: a case report and review of the literature. J Am Acad Dermatol. 1994;31:920–4.
16. Piyophirapong S, Linpiyawan R, Mahaisavariya P, et al. Cutaneous protothecosis in an AIDS patient. Br J Dermatol. 2002;146(4):713–5.
17. Wirth FA, Passalacqua J-A, Kao G. Disseminated cutaneous protothecosis in an immunocompromised host: a case report and literature review. Cutis. 1999;63(3):185–8.
18. Gaur S, Marrin C, Barnes RA. Disseminated protothecosis following traumatic Hickman line removal in a patient with leukaemia. Med Mycol. 2010;48(2):410–2.a

5

Mycobacteria

MYCOBACTERIUM TUBERCULOSIS

M. tuberculosis infection of the skin occurs as a result of direct inoculation from an exogenous source, autoinoculation, or through contiguous or hematogenous spread. Cutaneous tuberculosis shows a spectrum of morphological presentations that include lupus vulgaris, scrofuloderma, tuberculosis verrucosa cutis, primary cutaneous tuberculosis (tuberculous chancre or primary inoculation), tuberculosis cutis orificialis, and miliary cutaneous tuberculosis. Tuberculids are *Mycobacterium tuberculosis*-induced skin diseases due to the host's immunologic response to the organism. These include erythema induratum, papulonecrotic tuberculid, lichen scrofulosorum, or nodular tuberculid.[1]

Acute fulminating dissemination to the skin (tuberculosis cutis miliaris disseminata, miliary cutaneous tuberculosis) once a rare form of tuberculosis, has re-emerged among patients infected with human immunodeficiency virus (HIV) as 1–4 mm erythematous-to-brown papules, some of which become papulovesicules or papulopustules. At this stage the lesions may be mistaken for folliculitis and may be ignored. The tiny vesicles or pustules rupture and form a central crust on the papule. Removal of the crust leaves a minute but sharply defined umbilication or dell. These lesions occur predominantly on the trunk, thighs, buttocks, genitalia, and extremities, particularly the extensor surfaces.[2,3] The face is generally spared. The lesions are generally asymmetric and number several dozen in total.[4] Cutaneous miliary tuberculosis has also presented in HIV-positive patients as hyperpigmented macules,[5] a diffuse maculopapular eruption,[6] and diffuse pustules or acneiform lesions on the trunk and extremities.[7] Small follicular papules with central crusting have also been described.[8] Skin biopsy of miliary cutaneous tuberculosis shows a dermal microabscess with a scant to dense polymorphonuclear leukocyte and mononuclear cell infiltrate. Cutaneous miliary tuberculosis in HIV disease and other immunocompromised patients is typically characterized by absence of a granulomatous response, giant cells, and true caseating granulomas.[4] An acid-fast stain (if the diagnosis is considered and the stain requested) usually shows numerous acid-fast bacilli (AFB) seen quite easily. A miliary pattern on chest x-ray does not have to be present to see hematogeneous dissemination of the bacilli to the skin.[8] The finding of typical choroidal tubercles on ophthalmologic examination would support the diagnosis of cutaneous miliary tuberculosis before the results of histological examination of a skin biopsy specimen are available.[6]

Patients with HIV disease have presented with several other manifestations of cutaneous tuberculosis, including reports of multiple reddish plaques on the cheek, consistent with lupus vulgaris,[9] ulcers,[10,11] and subcutaneous abscesses.[12] Tuberculids reported in HIV-infected patients include focal minute follicular-based lichenoid papules of lichen scrofulosorum,[13] widespread papulonecrotic tuberculid lesions,[14] and a nodular tuberculid reaction manifesting as multiple, nontender, mobile, firm, subcutaneous nodules with slight hyperpigmentation or erythema on the lower extremities.[1]

Tuberculosis in solid organ transplant patients is one of the most serious opportunistic infections encountered. *M. tuberculosis* may be either primary infection, reactivation of latent disease, or acquired through the transplanted organ. A widespread eruption of discrete erythematous pinhead-sized papules and macules covering the entire trunk and both upper and lower extremities, which evolved into vesiculopustules, was described in a 62-year-old renal transplant recipient on azathioprine and prednisone. After she developed acute respiratory failure and her sputum was noted to contain numerous acid-fast bacilli, then a review of her skin biopsy was undertaken. It showed numerous AFB.[15] A case of miliary *M. tuberculosis*

M.E. Grossman et al., *Cutaneous Manifestations of Infection in the Immunocompromised Host*,
DOI 10.1007/978-1-4419-1578-8_5, © Springer Science+Business Media, LLC 2012

presenting with both erythema and edema mimicking cellulitis and erythematous, violaceous nodules on the leg of a 37-year-old renal transplant patient maintained on azathioprine and methylprednisolone has been reported.[16] Subcutaneous nodules were the first sign of fatal disseminated *M. tuberculosis* in two renal transplant recipients.[17] Isolated cutaneous tuberculosis has also presented as a chest nodule in a 68-year-old patient following living-donor renal transplant.[18] *M. tuberculosis* was cultured from multiple ulcerating nodules on the bilateral lower extremities in 27-year-old a renal allograft recipient taking prednisolone, azathioprine, and cyclosporine.[19] Necrotizing tuberculous fasciitis of the gluteus muscle was an unusual presentation of miliary tuberculosis in a woman with rheumatoid arthritis on prednisolone and methotrexate.[20]

Figure 5.1. Tuberculosis cutis miliaris disseminata in a human immunodeficiency virus (HIV)-positive patient

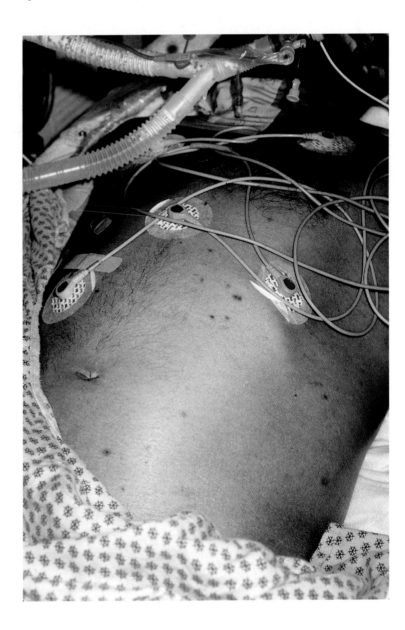

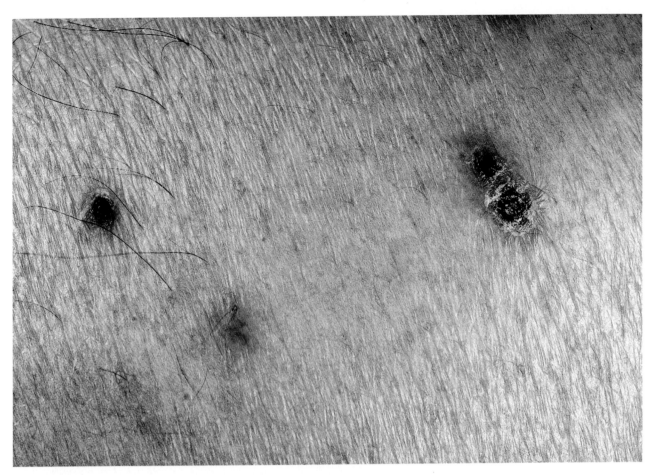

Figure 5.2. Groups of centrally necrotic papules and dell-shaped crusted papules on the trunk. Skin biopsy was floridly positive on acid-fast bacilli (AFB) stain and cultured *M. tuberculosis*

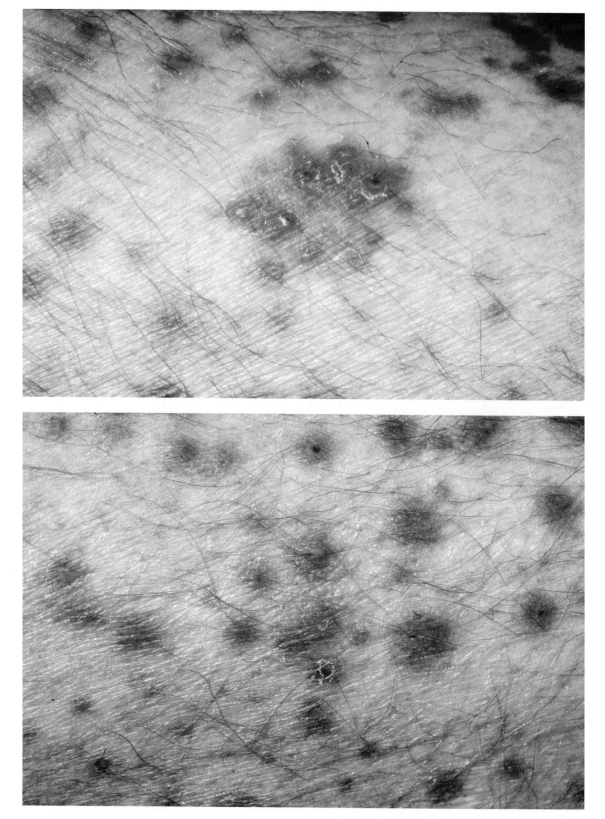

Figure 5.3. and 5.4.   Miliary tuberculosis involving the skin in a patient with acquired immune deficiency syndrome (AIDS). Disseminated erythematous papules with some papulopustules and papules with central necrosis and crusts were seen. *M. tuberculosis* was confirmed by skin biopsy and culture (Courtesy of Mary Ruth Buchness, M.D.)

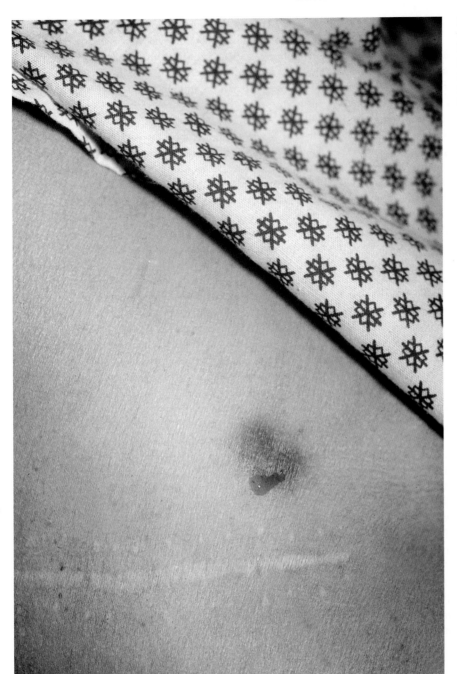

Figure 5.5.   A 32-year-old HIV-positive woman presented with a several-month history of a "boil" in the right axillary region 2 years after a right lobectomy for pulmonary tuberculosis. Culture of the chest wall abscess grew multi-drug-resistant *M. tuberculosis*

NONTUBERCULOUS MYCOBACTERIA

Atypical or nontuberculous mycobacteria are ubiquitous in the environment, present in soil, environmental water sources, drinking water, and in certain animal reservoirs.[21] Runyon organized these pathogens into a classification system in 1954 based on growth and morphological characteristics: Runyon group I, photochromogens, are slow-growing mycobacteria whose colonies produce pigment upon exposure to light; Runyon group II, scotochromogens, are slow growers that produce pigment in the dark; Runyon group III, nonphotochromogens, are nonpigmented slow growers; and Runyon group IV are the rapid growers. While this classification system at one time served to organize the nontuberculous mycobacteria, rapid advances in laboratory technology have allowed for the identification of more than 100 species of nontuberculous mycobacteria, making Runyon's classification system largely of historical significance.

Cutaneous disease with nontuberculous mycobacteria follows two general patterns. In the immunocompetent host, traumatic or surgical injury, usually to an extremity (frequently the upper arm or fingers), is followed 4–6 weeks later by the development of localized cellulitis or abscess formation with or without lymphatic spread.[22] The classic example is the "swimming pool" or "fish tank" granuloma of *Mycobacterium marinum*, which usually presents as a papule or nodule on an extremity after minor trauma. The nodule may ulcerate and spread via regional lymphatics in a "sporotrichoid" pattern. In the immunocompromised individual, a history of trauma is usually absent and the patient presents with either multiple localized erythematous or violaceous subcutaneous nodules or widespread disease with variable morphology that ranges from single or multiple nodules similar to those in otherwise healthy hosts, to sinus tracts, non-healing ulcers, subcutaneous abscesses, fluctuant nodules, or broad erythema and ulcers.[23] The most common presentations of nontuberculous mycobacterial infection following solid organ transplantation are cutaneous lesions of the extremities, tenosynovitis, and arthritis.[24] In transplant recipients, chronic indwelling central venous catheter-related infection is one of the most common presentations of a nontuberculous mycobacterial infection.[25] It is essential to maintain a high index of suspicion for atypical mycobacterial infection, as acid-fast organisms may be difficult to identify on histologic sections, and many of these fastidious pathogens are challenging to grow in culture, often requiring weeks for the culture to turn positive, and in some cases requiring specific media. Polymerase chain reaction (PCR) is an emerging technique which may aid in the diagnosis of mycobacterial infections. Speciation of the offending organism is crucial, as the antibiotic susceptibility profiles differ among the organisms and are essential to achieving therapeutic success.

GROUP 1

M. marinum presents as an erythematous or violaceous nodule or pustule which may develop a verrucous crust or ulcerate, typically over a bony prominence and almost always on an extremity. These lesions usually develop 2 to 3 weeks after minor trauma to the skin in combination with exposure to a marine environment, such as stagnant water, swimming pools, or fish tanks. While the disease is frequently limited to a single lesion in immunocompetent hosts, immunosuppressed patients may demonstrate "sporotrichoid" spread with multiple nodules present following lymphatic drainage patterns. Dissemination of *M. marinum* to multiple cutaneous sites has been described in lymphoma and in a patient following combined simultaneous kidney and pancreas transplantation who was on cyclosporine, azathioprine, and prednisone at the time of presentation.[26,27] Widespread skin nodules with cellulitis progressing to ulceration and osteomyelitis was reported in a 41-year-old marine biologist renal transplant patient on long-term corticosteroids.[28] Multiple ulcerative nodules and upper limb swelling was noted in a 50-year-old female on tacrolimus, prednisolone, and mycophenolate mofetil for renal transplant immunosuppression.[29] Cellulitis, synovitis, and lower extremity ulceration was reported in a 35-year-old Thai woman with lupus nephritis on high-dose corticosteroids.[30] The more classic presentation of multiple tender erythematous nodules in a linear sporotrichoid pattern on the exposed extremities has been described in a number of solid organ transplant recipients on a variety of immunosuppressive regimens[27,31] as well. Very rarely does the infection disseminate systemically and this could be due to its optimal growth requirement of lower temperatures between 28°C and 32°C. The higher core body temperature may inhibit systemic dissemination.[27] Multiple lesions in a sporotrichoid pattern have also been reported following infliximab therapy for ankylosing spondylitis in a 45-year-old man,[32] and multiple papules and subcutaneous nodules with an associated digital tenosynovitis occurred in a 49-year-old woman with rheumatoid arthritis on combination infliximab and methotrexate.[33] A presentation of multiple nodules that ulcerated was reported in 63-year-old man with rheumatoid arthritis on corticosteroids and methotrexate.[34] A 66-year-old man who lived on a saltwater lagoon was treated for presumed rheumatoid arthritis of the right hand and wrist with oral prednisone and methotrexate, later followed by infliximab for worsening arthritis of the hands and inability to walk. When he developed exudative, ulcerating nodules on the face, extremities, and penis, cultures of the skin lesions revealed *M. marinum* to be the cause of the skin lesions, likely disseminating from the initial rheumatoid arthritis-like joint presentation 5 years prior.[35]

Rare examples of disseminated *M. marinum* in the normal and the immunocompromised host illustrate the diagnostic missteps and potential serious course of swimming pool granuloma. Several clues to suspect *M. marinum* include: (1) the appearance of a common cutaneous infection that fails to completely respond to standard antibiotics, progresses during therapy, or recurs shortly after finishing the course of treatment; (2) a skin biopsy with granulomatous or chronic inflammation and negative stains and cultures; (3) any history of water exposure including swimming pool, spa, fresh or salt water beaches, aquariums, or hobbies such as tropical fish, fishing, swimming, or boating; (4) worsening skin lesions after intralesional steroid injections, or worsening joint symptoms after intra-articular steroid treatment;

and (5) synovitis or arthritis that does not respond to conventional therapy should be re-evaluated, even if synovial biopsies show granulomatous inflammation consistent with rheumatoid arthritis. The cascade of immunosuppressive therapies for "unresponsive arthritis" can cause disseminated or invasive *M. marinum* infection with a delay of accurate diagnosis up to 1 year.

Cutaneous infection due to *M. kansasii* in the immunocompromised patient may produce an acute, febrile, rapidly progressive course, or may present as an indolent, slowly growing skin lesion. *M. kansasii* may mimic the pyogenic reaction of bacterial infections of the soft tissues and resemble bacterial cellulitis,[36] papulopustules,[37] fluctuant abscesses,[38] palatal ulcers,[39] or scattered erythematous subcutaneous nodules in the renal transplant patient.[24] A 38-year-old male renal transplant recipient maintained on high dose prednisone for episodes of rejection developed an erythematous, warm, swollen knee with an overlying ragged ulcer.[40] Infection mimicking cellulitis following minor trauma and swimming exposure was also noted in a 38-year-old woman with lupus on combination therapy including prednisolone and azathioprine.[41] One patient with systemic lupus erythematosus maintained on prednisone and hydroxychloroquine presented with fever and recurrent widespread tender nodules resembling lupus profunda involving the wrists, hands, arm, thighs, and back which spontaneously drained a beige fluid, AFB stain and culture positive.[42] A 47-year-old male renal transplant recipient presented with an annular, granulomatous plaque with central clearing over the heel while on prednisone and azathioprine.[40] An erythematous plaque studded with papules and associated discrete papules distributed in an ascending, sporotrichoid pattern on the forearm of a heart transplant patient was an asymptomatic infection.[43]

In patients with acquired immune deficiency syndrome (AIDS), *M. kansasii* has presented with sporotrichoid lesions on the hand and arms, some of which ulcerated,[44] and with an intracutaneous abscess with painful regional lymph node enlargement.[45]

Chronic *M. kansasii* cutaneous lesions described include a slowly growing nasolabial crusted ulceration in a 51-year-old with leukopenia and impaired cell-mediated immunity,[46] and a scaly erythematous plaque on the elbow in a 43-year-old on prednisone and azathioprine for kidney transplant.[40]

M. simiae, first isolated from *Macacus rhesus* monkeys in 1965 and later from environmental sources, rarely causes cutaneous disease. There is one report of disseminated *M. simiae* infection in a 29-year-old man with advanced AIDS where the organism was isolated from the ear with no further clinical description.[47] There is another report of disseminated *M. simiae* presenting as crusted or ulcerated subcutaneous nodules on the buttocks and legs in a 44-year-old patient with AIDS.[48]

described in a 32-year-old man with AIDS.[49] A 59-year-old woman status post bone marrow transplant for breast cancer developed a red nontender nodule on the volar surface of the right index joint due to *M. scrofulaceum* following a paper cut and handling of thorny roses from slimy water.[50]

M. malmoense infection presented in a 48-year-old woman with chronic myelogenous leukemia as widespread multiple pea-sized, red, tender, indurated nodules.[51] A scanty, disseminated papular exanthem on the extremities and abdomen followed by the development of ulceronodular lesions on the lower legs was reported in a patient with hairy cell leukemia.[52] Ulcerated nodules and papulokeratotic lesions in a sporotrichoid distribution on the arm of a patient with myelodysplastic syndrome has been described.[53]

M. szulgai infection has been described in a patient on chronic corticosteroids for sarcoidosis who developed bilateral foot and leg cellulitis, a 6 × 7-cm nontender thigh mass with multiple draining sinuses, and discrete cutaneous nodules on the elbow, knee, and abdomen. Cultures from all these different types of skin lesions grew *M. szulgai*.[54] *M. szulgai* produced a similar clinical picture in a 51-year-old patient with desquamative interstitial pneumonitis maintained on chronic steroids who presented with boggy red nodules on the elbow, knee, and back and osteomyelitis of the distal fibula with overlying cellulitis.[55] A 4-year-old boy with T-cell leukemia treated with allogeneic bone marrow transplantation developed a paronychia of the great toe, which became diffusely indurated and erythematous, progressing to develop vesicles and pustules over the sole and dorsal foot. Two nontender fluctuant masses with overlying red-blue discoloration developed in the right groin. Cultures from both the foot and the lymph node grew *M. szulgai*.[56] *M. szulgai* has also presented as an isolated subcutaneous nodule in a patient with systemic lupus erythematosus on daily high dose prednisolone[57] and as painful erythematous nodules with central induration progressing to ulceration and associated multifocal osteomyelitis in a 66-year-old patient with chronic lymphocytic leukemia.[58]

M. gordonae infection in a steroid-dependent asthmatic a few months following a rat bite while collecting frogs in a pond produced small ulcerated red or bluish nodules on the dorsum of the affected hand.[59] The first case of cutaneous disease due to *M. gordonae* in an HIV-infected patient manifested as 4–5 cm subcutaneous nodules of the extensor arms and legs with fever and polyarthritis. *M. gordonae* was isolated from cloudy fluid in the skin lesions, blood, bone marrow, and joint aspirate.[60] A patient with HIV infection developed widespread pruritic nodules on her face and arms while on multidrug therapy for *M. tuberculosis*. Culture of these lesions revealed a resistant strain of *M. gordonae*.[61]

GROUP 2

M. scrofulaceum usually presents with a localized lymphadenitis, particularly in children. Disseminated disease presenting with chronic ulcerative and nodular lesions has been

GROUP 3

M. avium-intracellulare complex (MAC), a common opportunistic pathogen in patients with AIDS and disseminated disease, is common even in the era of highly active antiretroviral therapy (HAART). Disseminated MAC is characterized by fever, weight loss, diarrhea, anemia, lymphadenitis, pulmonary symptoms, and signs of liver involvement. Despite the frequency of disseminated MAC in AIDS, cutaneous manifestations are uncommon, but may occur as cellulitis,[62] a chronic skin ulcer at an injection site, perianal erosions and abscesses,[10] necrotizing oral ulcers,[63] an isolated red, tender, non-fluctuant nodule,[64] or sporotrichosis-like nodules.[65,66]

Cutaneous MAC has been reported as part of the immune reconstitution inflammatory syndrome (IRIS) in patients receiving HAART. Reported presentations include an erythematous, indurated, 3.5 × 3.5 cm round plaque with central nodules,[67] multiple painful subcutaneous nodules with areas of necrosis on the legs and abdomen,[68] and a 4-cm painful subcutaneous nodule on the lateral thigh which ulcerated and drained *M. avium*.[69] The immune restoration syndrome may reveal latent or occult mycobacterial infection by increased inflammation and unmasking clinical disease.

MAC has caused skin lesions in other immunocompromised hosts including a yellow-orange scaly papule on the forearm of a steroid-treated asthmatic,[70] widespread panniculitis,[71] multiple abscess-like nodular skin lesions in a renal allograft recipient,[72] subcutaneous nodules on the hand and arms of a heart transplant recipient,[73] indurated erythematous plaques on the legs of a bone marrow transplantation recipient,[74] and ulcerated arm abscesses in a patient with sarcoidosis on prednisolone and azathioprine.[75]

M. ulcerans is the third most common mycobacterial disease worldwide (after tuberculosis and leprosy),[76] endemic in parts of Africa, Asia, and South America. Inoculation may occur directly through minor skin injuries, or secondarily with the organism colonizing existing lesions. The vast majority of cases occur on the extremities. The organism then slowly grows, producing the characteristic painless ulcer. While there does not appear to be an increased risk of infection in immunocompromised hosts, *M. ulcerans* has been reported in patients with AIDS.[77] The clinical manifestations in HIV-positive patients appear similar to infections in immunocompetent hosts, with infection presenting as a large painless ulcer.[78] Nontender subcutaneous nodules that ulcerated and caused destructive scarring of the soft tissues with osteomyelitis in an HIV-positive patient have also been described.[78,79] Some authors have suggested that immune compromise may facilitate multifocal aggressive forms of *M. ulcerans* disease.[79]

Group 4

Mycobacterium fortuitum, *Mycobacterium abscessus*, and *Mycobacterium chelonae* are collectively referred to as "rapid growers." These rapidly growing environmental pathogens can cause posttraumatic skin infection, as well as nosocomial infection, following surgical procedures and injections, or through use of contaminated dialysis equipment. Injections of illicit drugs and acupuncture have also been associated with spread of these pathogens.[80] *M. fortuitum* infection is more common in immunocompetent patients, while *M. chelonae* and *M abscessus* more often infect immunocompromised patients.[81] Infection with rapidly growing mycobacterium (RGM) is rare in HIV-infected patients. In HIV-infected patients, the major RGM is *M. fortuitum*.[82]

M. fortuitum infection develops weeks after injury. In immunocompetent hosts lesions may present as tender nodules, abscesses, ulcers, draining tracts, or cellulitis.[83] Lower extremity furunculosis has been reported following an outbreak in nail salons.[84] Two women with systemic lupus erythematosus on systemic steroids were reported with a large buttock abscess and leg nodules[85] and multiple purple-red nodules on the trunk and extremities which ulcerated and drained AFB-smear and *M. fortuitum* culture positive material.[86] Ulcerated erythematous sporotrichoid nodules on the arm were described in a patient following bone marrow transplantation for acute lymphoblastic leukemia.[87] Nodules and pustules in an HIV-positive man,[88] a maculopapular eruption in a woman with chronic myelocytic leukemia,[89] and lower extremity erythema and edema with multiple nodules and ill-defined subcutaneous plaques mimicking panniculitis in a 60-year-old woman with a 14-year history of steroid-dependent asthma[90] due to *M. fortuitum* have been reported. Lymphadenopathy of the neck, including fluctuant buboes and draining masses, can be the presenting sign of *M. fortuitum* infection in HIV-positive patients.[91]

M. chelonae causes chronic cutaneous infections. Patients with disseminated or localized cutaneous disease were usually taking corticosteroids and were often renal transplant recipients. *M. chelonae* skin disease in kidney transplant recipients tends to be clinically distinctive, characterized by erythematous, cutaneous, and subcutaneous nodules with a predilection for the legs and feet. The nodules evolve into abscesses with multiple fistulas, which are typically painful only when large. Almost all lesions drain spontaneously. The drainage is cloudy, serous fluid. With pressure, thick, white, necrotic material can be expressed from nodules, which is acid-fast smear positive. A history of trauma or injury, unlike in immunocompetent hosts, is usually absent. Affected patients are afebrile, asymptomatic, and typically have an indolent clinical course.[92] Evidence of *M. chelonae* infection elsewhere is rare.

In immunosuppressed patients, the sporotrichoid pattern of *M. chelonae* infection is rare. Other clinical presentations of *M. chelonae* in the compromised host include papules, subcutaneous nodules, and vesiculopustules,[93-95] cellulitis with multiple draining fistulas,[92] and ulcerative pustulonodules with satellitosis.[96] Scaly crusts over ulcerated nodules, some displaying a sporotrichoid pattern of infection, have been described.[97,98] While rare, a pure sporotrichoid pattern of infection with multiple violaceous nodules starting distally and progressing proximally has been reported in a 52-year-old renal transplant recipient on prednisolone and azathioprine.[99] Similar lesions were reported in a 67-year-old man with chronic lymphocytic leukemia.[100] *M. chelonae* infection presented in a patient following lung transplant with thoracotomy scar associated painless subcutaneous nodules and pustules which spontaneously ruptured, transiently improving on reduced immunosuppression, and recurring as a subcutaneous plaque on the thigh.[101] A 60-year-old woman treated for a breast ulcer presumed to be pyoderma gangrenosum with systemic immunosuppression consisting of methylprednisolone, cyclosporine, and mycophenolate mofetil developed widespread subcutaneous nodules and draining ulcers due to *M. chelonae*.[102] Her original ulcer was likely to have been her initial presentation of *M. chelonae* infection. A 65-year-old renal transplant recipient with multiple purple-blue nodules on one leg suspected to be Kaposi sarcoma was AFB stain and culture positive for *M. chelonae*.[95] One report of synchronous infection with *M. chelonae* and *Paecilomyces* in a 41-year-old heart transplant recipient presented with multiple subcutaneous nodules and ulcers on the hand and lower extremities.[103]

M. abscessus infection has presented with multiple cutaneous morphologies, both localized and disseminated in solid organ transplant recipients. Cutaneous manifestations of this organism appear to be rare in patients with other causes of immunosuppression. The majority of cases occur on the lower extremities, and present as reddish papules, erythematous or violaceous nodules, or plaques that spread in a sporotrichoid fashion,[104] and frequently spontaneously ulcerate.[105-108] In some cases *M. abscessus* can mimic a severe bacterial cellulitis[109] or a wound infection. A renal transplant recipient developed nodules, induration, erythema, and purulent discharge culture positive for *M. abscessus* at the allograft incisional site.[108] Another renal transplant recipient had purulent discharge due to *M. abscessus* at the former site of a peritoneal dialysis catheter with a subcutaneous fluctuant collection.[108] *M. abscessus* infection also presented as multiple painful grouped erythematous nodules with deep pustules on the forearm of a patient self-treating arthritis symptoms with corticosteroids.[110] Another patient on systemic corticosteroids for metastatic cancer developed erythematous nodular, ulcerating skin lesions which grew *M. abscessus*.[111] Disseminated disease presented as tender red nodules and scattered erythematous, infiltrated plaques on the face, neck, and extremities in a patient with idiopathic low CD4+ T cell count[112] and as tender red nodules of the extremities with swelling of multiple joints in a multivisceral transplant recipient.[108]

M. mucogenicum is a recently characterized RGM based on 16S ribosomal RNA (rRNA) gene sequencing. It produced erythematous papules and subcutaneous lower leg nodules which drained a cloudy, yellow exudate in a 61-year-old with rheumatoid arthritis on prednisone and etanercept.[113]

M. haemophilum infections have cutaneous manifestations in 75% of cases. However, because the fastidious nature of this organism makes obtaining a positive culture difficult, the incidence of infection may be underreported. *M. haemophilum* has a predilection for infection of the skin and underlying bone and joints in patients with renal, bone marrow, and heart transplants, hematologic dyscrasias, iatrogenic immunosuppression, and HIV infection.[114-118] The skin lesions of *M. haemophilum* infection are frequently disseminated, often involving distant, acral areas overlying joints, paralleling the lower optimal growth temperature of *M. haemophilum*. When *M. haemophilum* infection is suspected, microbiology laboratories should be notified to include ferric-containing compounds (hematin, hemoglobin, ferric ammonium citrate) in plating media, which are required for growth of this pathogen. It requires a low temperature (28–30°C) for growth, as does *M. ulcerans* and *M. marinum*, as opposed to 37°C which is the optimum temperature for most other pathogenic mycobacteria.

Clinical presentations of *M. haemophilum* infections include painful erythematous or violaceous nodules on the extremities which may ulcerate or form abscesses, papules, plaques, cellulitis, and/or suppurative lymphadenitis.[115,119] Lesions presenting as cysts, scaly plaques, panniculitis,[116] erythematous nodules, and chronic nonhealing crusted ulcerations[120] have been described. Typically located on the extremities, lesions of *M. haemophilum* rarely occur on the chest, back, and face. A patient with common variable immunodeficiency and autoimmune hepatic cirrhosis on multi-agent immunosuppressive therapy with intravenous immunoglobulin, prednisone, and azathioprine presented with multiple firm, painful nodules on her hands, wrists, and anterior legs which grew slowly over a period of weeks. Biopsy and 16S ribosomal RNA gene sequencing confirmed infection with *M. haemophilum*. A patient with myasthenia gravis iatrogenically immunocompromised because of maintenance treatment with prednisone, azathioprine, and mycophenolate mofetil presented with a 1-year history of painful erythematous papules, plaques, and nodules on her arms, hands, and lower extremities due to *M. haemophilum* infection.[121] An unusual presentation of a large annular plaque on the thigh of an HIV patient with concurrent scattered reddish papulonodules on the extremities has been described.[122] The development of multiple violaceous, fluctuant, and suppurative nodules, located on the limbs in a renal transplant patient following acupuncture treatment was caused by *M. haemophilum* infection.[123]

In the immunocompromised patient with unexplained skin lesions that are smear positive for acid-fast bacilli, but culture negative, request that the microbiology laboratory add hematin or ferric ammonium citrate to the culture and incubate at lower temperatures (28–30°C) for 6–10 weeks to grow *M. haemophilum*.

Figure 5.6. A 49-year-old woman with rheumatoid arthritis treated with methotrexate, infliximab, and prednisone developed *M. marinum* infection of the soft tissue and joint of the fourth finger with sporotrichoid papules

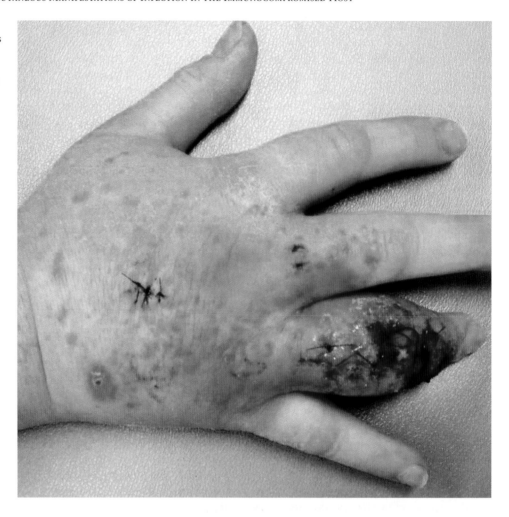

Figure 5.7.– 5.10. A 66-year-old man who lived on a lagoon, enjoyed crabbing, repairing boats, and tending to his tropical fish tank complained of swelling and tenderness of his right wrist and an erythematous painful nodule on the ring finger. He was diagnosed with sero-negative rheumatoid arthritis with a clinical course refractory to treatment which led to a cascade of immunosuppressive therapies including prednisone, methotrexate, and infliximab. When he was hospitalized for cellulitis with a 2-year history of progressive draining nodules, ulcers, and swelling of the hands, forearms, feet, and legs, *M. marinum* was cultured from the skin, blood, and joints (Courtesy of Amy Pappert, M.D., and David Najarian, M.D.)

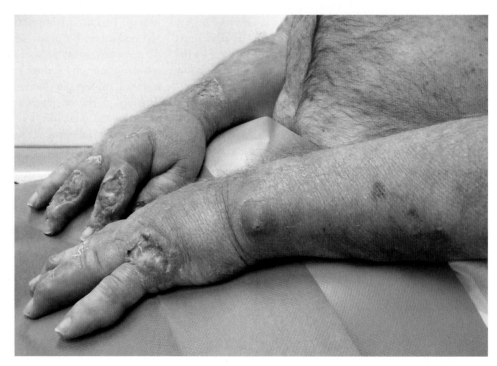

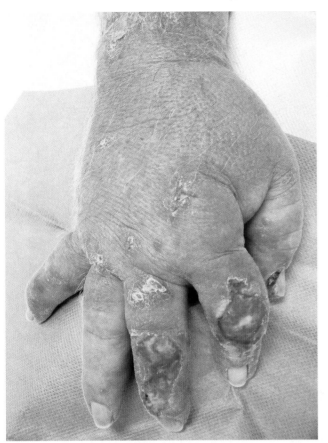

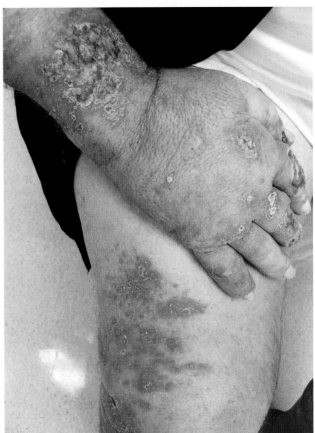

Figure 5.8.

Figure 5.9.

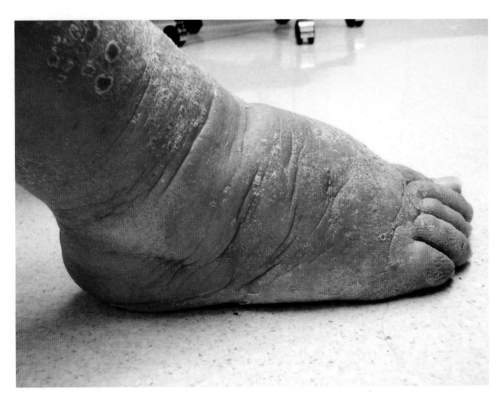

Figure 5.10.

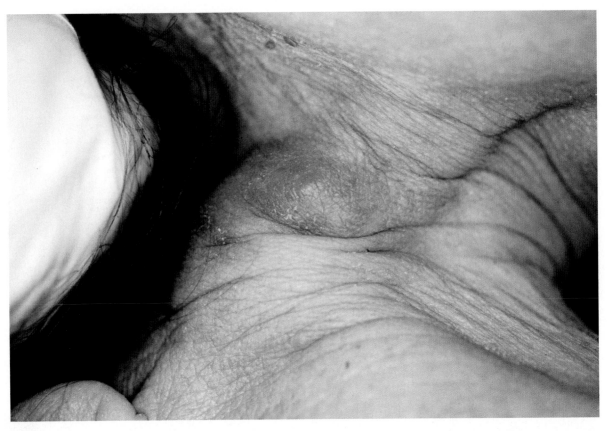

Figure 5.11. A 62-year-old woman with newly diagnosed HIV/AIDS presented with *Pneumocystis carinii* pneumonia (PCP) and *Mycobacterium avium-intracellulare* lymphadenitis. She died 2 months later of cryptococcal meningitis

Figure 5.12. An HIV-positive renal transplant patient developed multiple purple nodules, thought to be Kaposi's sarcoma, on the leg

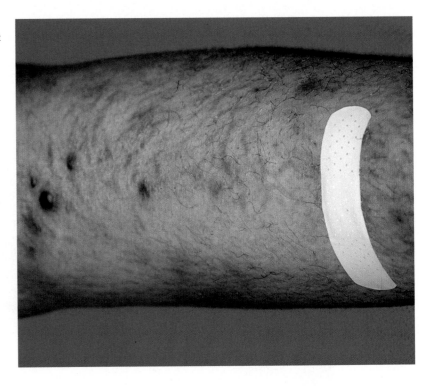

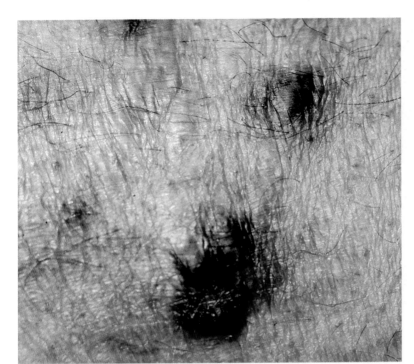

Figure 5.13. A close-up of the purple nodules of the same patient as shown in Fig. 5.12. Multiple skin biopsies and cultures demonstrated *M. avium* complex. Kaposi's sarcoma was not seen

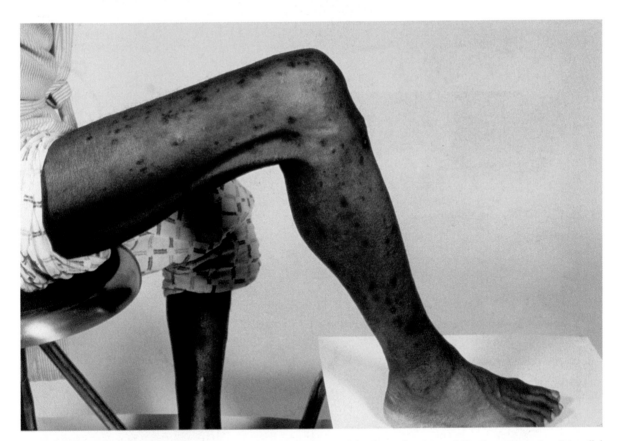

Figure 5.14. Multiple hyperpigmented to violaceous macules, papules, and nodules due to disseminated *Mycobacterium avium-intracellulare* on the legs of a patient with AIDS (Courtesy of Mary Ruth Buchness, M.D.)

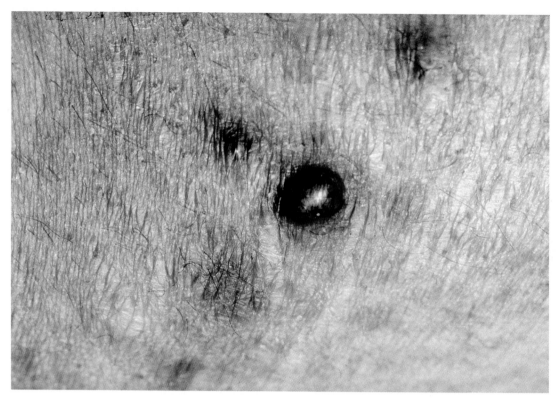

Figure 5.15. Kaposi's sarcoma-like lesion of disseminated *Mycobacterium avium-intracellulare* in an HIV-infected patient (Courtesy of Mary Ruth Buchness, M.D.)

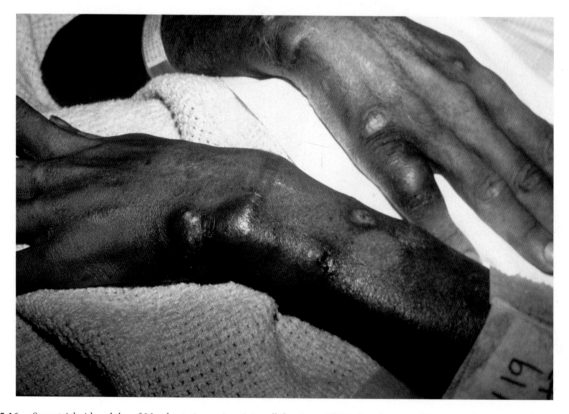

Figure 5.16. Sporotrichoid nodules of *Mycobacterium avium-intracellulare* in an HIV-infected patient (Courtesy of Robert G. Phelps, M.D.)

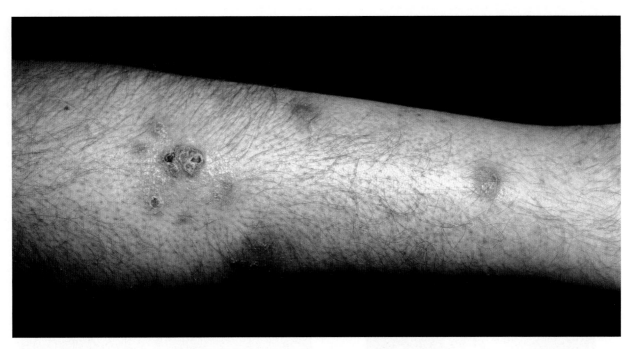

Figure 5.17. A 36-year-old renal transplant with no history of trauma presented with 4 months of skin lesions localized to one leg. Multiple subcutaneous nodules with pustules and sinus tracts were caused by *M. chelonae*

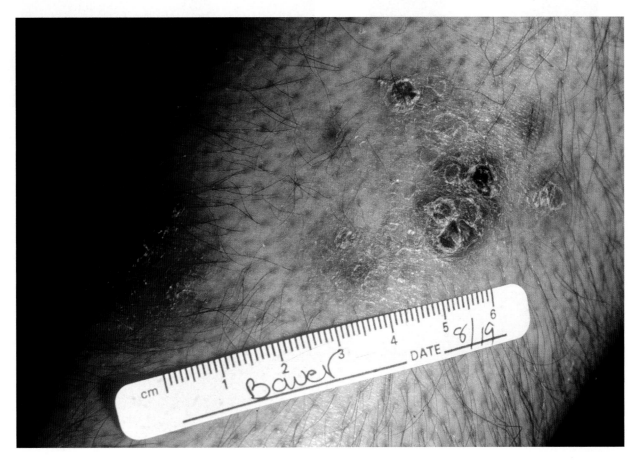

Figure 5.18. A crusted erythematous nodule was surrounded by multiple erythematous and crusted papules in a renal transplant recipient due to *M. chelonae*

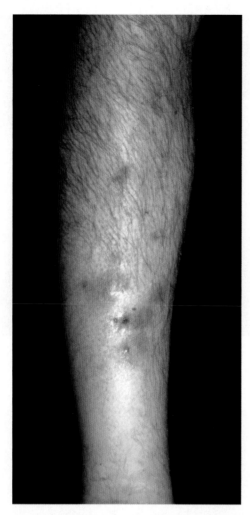

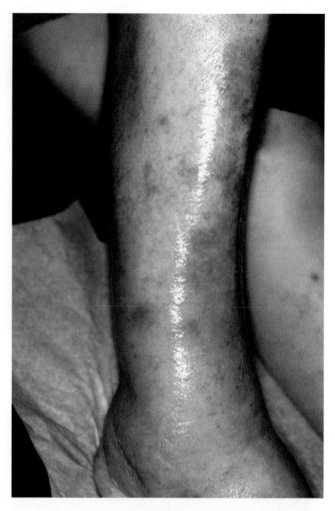

Figure 5.19. Multiple tender subcutaneous nodules were on the leg of a renal transplant patient. Skin biopsy demonstrated a suppurative panniculitis with clumps of acid-fast rods. Within 5 days, culture confirmed *M. chelonae* infection

Figure 5.20. An 83-year-old diabetic woman on systemic steroids for idiopathic thrombocytopenic purpura developed posttraumatic right lower extremity cellulitis with draining papulonodules unresponsive to ciprofloxacin. Skin biopsy was AFB positive and culture demonstrated *M. chelonae* (Courtesy of Paul Schneiderman, M.D.)

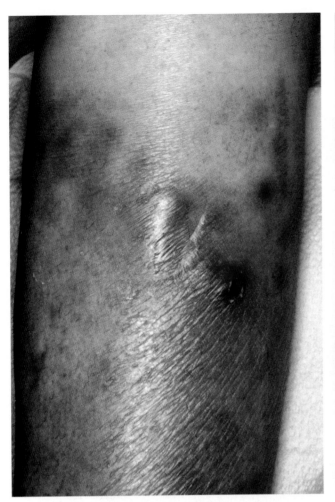

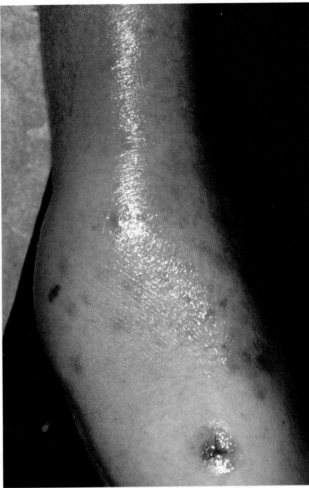

Figure 5.21. A young woman with systemic lupus erythematosus on systemic steroids developed multiple red-purple painful nodules with surrounding dull red inflammation on her leg due to *M. chelonae*

Figure 5.22. The erythema and edema extended to the ankle and foot with peripheral papulonodules. *M. chelonae* was present on skin biopsy and culture

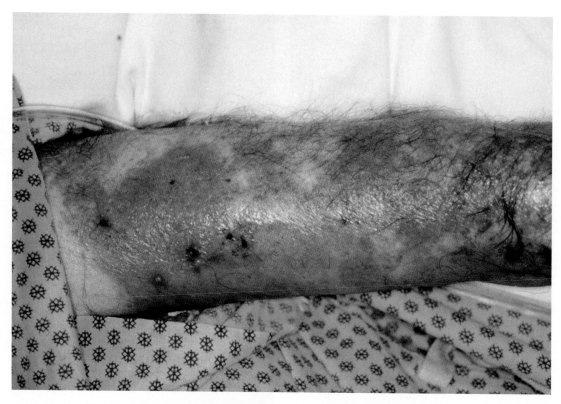

Figure 5.23. A 62-year-old HIV-negative heart transplant patient presented with a 3-month history of left arm cellulitis. A tender erythematous plaque extended from the mid-left arm distally to involve the elbow and forearm

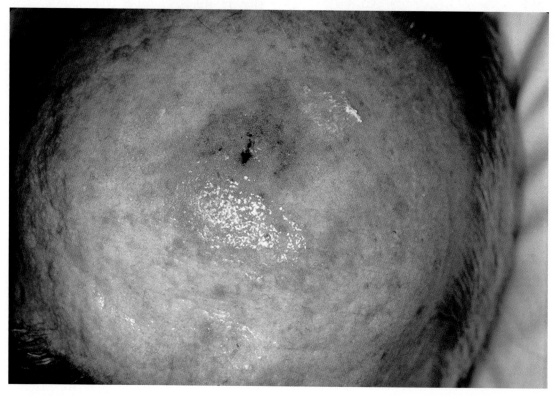

Figure 5.24. One week later, a new erythematous plaque appeared on the forehead of the same patient as shown in Fig. 5.23. Skin biopsies from both lesions demonstrated sarcoidal granulomas in the superficial and deep dermis extending into the subcutis. Numerous acid-fast bacilli were seen and cultures grew *M. haemophilum* after 90 days

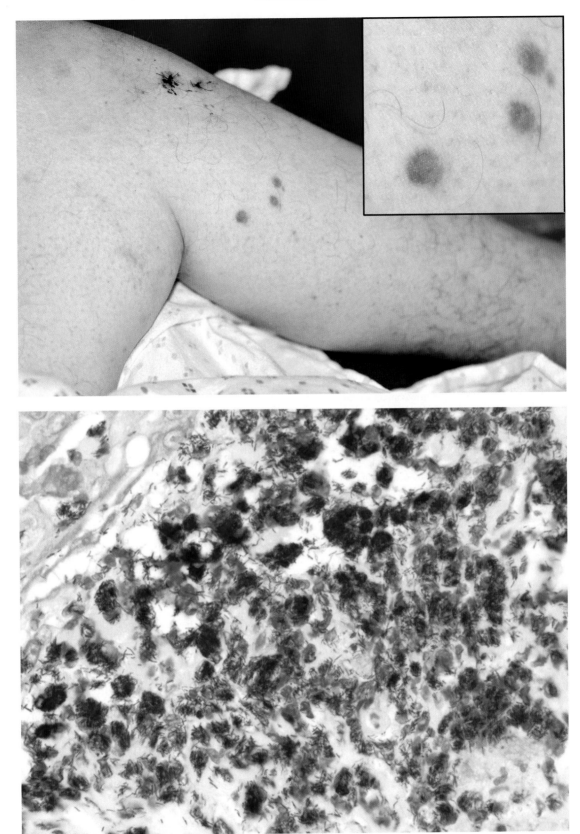

Figure 5.25. and 5.26. A 26-year-old with acute myeloid leukemia and *Mycobacterium abscessus* bacteremia with cutaneous foci (inset close-up). Skin biopsy showed globi of acid-fast positive organisms

REFERENCES

Mycobacterium tuberculosis

1. Friedman PC, Husain S, Grossman ME. Nodular tuberculid in a patient with HIV. J Am Acad Dermatol. 2005;53:S154–6.

2. Rohatgi PK, Palazzolo JV, Saini NB. Acute miliary tuberculosis of the skin in acquired immunodeficiency syndrome. J Am Acad Dermatol. 1992;26:356–9.

3. Stack RJ, Bickley LK, Coppel JG. Miliary tuberculosis presenting as skin lesions in a patient with acquired immunodeficiency syndrome. J Am Acad Dermatol. 1990;23:1031–5.

4. High WA, Evans CC, Hoang MP. Cutaneous miliary tuberculosis in two patients with HIV infection. J Am Acad Dermatol. 2004;50 (5 Suppl):S110–3.

5. Hudson CP, Wood R, O'Keefe EA. Cutaneous miliary tuberculosis in the AIDS era. Clin Infect Dis. 1997;25:1484.

6. Antinori S, Bini T, Galimberti L, et al. Cutaneous miliary tuberculosis in a patient infected with human immunodeficiency virus. Clin Infect Dis. 1997;25:1484–6.

7. Daikos GL, Uttamchandani RB, Tuda C, et al. Disseminated miliary tuberculosis of the skin in patients with AIDS: report of four cases. Clin Infect Dis. 1998;27:205–8.

8. Libraty DH, Byrd TF. Cutaneous miliary tuberculosis in the AIDS era: case report and review. Clin Infect Dis. 1996;23:706–10.

9. Hamada M, Urabe K, Moroi Y, et al. A case of multifocal lupus vulgaris that preceded pulmonary tuberculosis in an immune compromised patient. J Dermatol. 2004;31:124–8.

10. Freed JA, Pervez NF, Chen V, et al. Cutaneous mycobacteriosis: occurrence and significance in two patients with the acquired immunodeficiency syndrome. Arch Dermatol. 1987;123:1601–2.

11. Krumholz HM, Emlein G. An HIV-infected man with a neck ulcer and a fever. Hosp Pract (Off Ed). 1989;24:122–4.

12. Mellado B, Pedrol E, Casademount J, Grau JM. A tuberculotic subcutaneous abscess as the form of presentation of the acquired immunodeficiency syndrome. Rev Clin Esp. 1993;192:95–6.

13. Ariananyagam AV, Ash S, Jones RR. Lichen scrofulosorum in a patient with AIDS. Clin Exp Dermatol. 1994;19:74–6.

14. Fernandes C, Maltez F, Lourenco R, et al. Papulonecrotic tuberculid in a human immunodeficiency virus type-1 patient with multidrug-resistant tuberculosis. J Eur Acad Dermatol Venerol. 2004;18:369–70.

15. Park KW, Kim US, Shin JW, et al. Disseminated erythematous papules in a renal transplant recipient: a case of disseminated tuberculosis. Scand J Infect Dis. 2002;34:775–7.

16. Seyahi N, Apaydin S, Kahveci A, et al. Cellulitis as a manifestation of miliary tuberculosis in a renal transplant recipient. Transpl Infect Dis. 2005;7:80–5.

17. Caroti L, Zanazzi M, Rogasi P, et al. Subbcutaneous nodules and infectious complications in renal allograft recipients. Transplant Proc. 2010;42(4):1146–7.

18. Mori N, Yokoyama S, Tsutahara K, et al. Case report of skin tuberculosis after living renal transplantation. Nippon Hinyokika Gakkai Zasshi. 2006;97:60–3.

19. Ram R, Uppin S, Swarnalatha G, et al. Isolated skin ulcers due to Mycobacterium tuberculosis in a renal allograft recipient. Nephrology. 2007;3:688–92.

20. Kwon HH, Baek SH, Park SH. Miliary tuberculosis and necrotizing tuberculous fasciitis – an unusual coexistence in a rheumatoid arthritis patient. Int J Rheum Dis. 2010;13(2):171–4.

Nontuberculosis Mycobacteria

21. Falkinham JO. Nontuberculous mycobacteria in the environment. Clin Chest Med. 2002;23:529–51.

22. Dodiuk-Gad R, Dyachenko P, Ziv M, et al. Nontuberculous mycobacterial infections of the skin: a retrospective study of 25 cases. J Am Acad Dermatol. 2007;57:413–20.

23. Uslan DZ, Kowalski TJ, Wengenack NL, Virk A, Wilson JW. Skin and soft tissue infections due to rapidly growing mycobacteria. Comparison of clinical features, treatment, and susceptibility. Arch Dermatol. 2006;142:1287–92.

24. Patel R, Roberts GD, Keating MR, Paya CV. Infections due to nontuberculous mycobacteria in kidney, heart, and liver transplant recipients. Clin Inf Dis. 1993;19:263–73.

25. Doucette K, Fishman JA. Nontuberculous mycobacterial infection in hematopoietic stem cell and solid organ transplant patients. Clin Infect Dis. 2004;38:1428–39.

26. Gombert ME, Goldstein EJ, Corrado ML, Stein AJ, Butt KM. Disseminated Mycobacterium marinum infection after renal transplantation. Ann Intern Med. 1981;94(4 pt 1):486–7.

27. Pandian TK, Deziel PJ, Otley CC, et al. Mycobacterium marinum infections in transplant recipients: case report and review of the literature. Transpl Infect Dis. 2008;10:358–63.

28. Wolfson JS, Sober AJ, Rubin RH. Dermatologic manifestation of infections in immunocompromised patients. Medicine (Baltimore). 1985;64:115.

29. Lovric S, Becker JU, Kayser D, et al. Fish, flesh and a good red herring: a case of ascending upper limb infection in a renal transplant patient. Clin Nephrology. 2009;72:402–4.

30. Enzenauer RJ, McKoy J, Vincent D, Gates R. Disseminated cutaneous and synovial Mycobacterium infection in a patient with systemic lupus erythematosus. South Med J. 1990;83(4):471–4.

31. Farooqui MA, Berenson C, Lohr JW. Mycobacterium marinum infection in a renal transplant recipient. Transplantation. 1999;67: 1495–6.

32. Rallis E, Koumantaki-Mathioudaki E, Frangoulis E, et al. Severe sporotrichoid fish tank granuloma following infliximab therapy. Am J Clin Dermatol. 2007;8:385–8.

33. Hess SD, Van Voorhees AS, Chang LM, et al. Subcutaneous Mycobacterium marinum infection in a patient with chronic rheumatoid arthritis receiving immunosuppressive therapy. Int J Dermatol. 2009;48:782–3.

34. Bocher W, Galle PR, Marker-Hermann E. Skin nodules and ulcers of the limbs in a patient with rheumatoid arthritis. Dtsch Med Wochenschr. 2002;127(14):735–8.

35. Lam A, Toma W, Schlesinger N. Mycobacterium marinum arthritis mimicking rheumatoid arthritis. J Rheumatol. 2006;33(4):817–9.

36. Rosen T. Cutaneous Mycobacterium kansasii infection presenting as cellulitis. Cutis. 1983;31:87–9.

37. Bolivar R, Satterwhite TK, Floyd M. Cutaneous lesions due to Mycobacterium kansasii. Arch Dermatol. 1980;116(2):207–8.

38. Fraser DW, Buxton AE, Naji A, et al. Disseminated Mycobacterium kansasii infection presenting as cellulitis in a recipient of a renal homograft. Am Rev Respir Dis. 1975;112:125–9.

39. Lichtenstein IH, MacGregor RR. Mycobacterial infections in renal transplant recipients: report of five cases and review of the literature. Rev Infect Dis. 1983;5(2):216–26.

40. Lloveras J, Peterson PK, Simmons RL, Najarian JS. Mycobacterial infections in renal transplant recipients. Arch Intern Med. 1982;142: 888–92.

41. Hsu PY, Yang YH, Hsiao CH, et al. Mycobacterium kansasii infection presenting as cellulitis in a patient with systemic lupus erythematosus. J Formos Med Assoc. 2002;101:581–4.

42. Czelusta A, Moore AY. Cutaneous Mycobacterium kansasii infection in a patient with systemic lupus erythematosus: case report and review. J Am Acad Dermatol. 1999;40:359–63.

43. Stengem J, Grande KK, Hsu S. Localized primary cutaneous Mycobacterium kansasii infection in an immunocompromised patient. J Am Acad Dermatol. 1999;41:854–6.

44. Pennys NS. Skin manifestations of AIDS. Philadelphia: JB Lippincott; 1990. p. 43.

45. Stellbrink HJ, Koperskik AH, Greten H. Mycobacterium kansasii infection limited to skin and lymph node in a patient with AIDS. Clin Exp Dermatol. 1990;15:457–8.

46. Hirsh FS, Saffold OE. *Mycobacterium kansasii* infection with dermatologic manifestations. Arch Dermatol. 1976;112:706–8.

47. Al-Abdely HM, Revankar SG, Graybill JR. Disseminated *Mycobacterium simiae* infection in patients with AIDS. J Infect. 2000;41:143–7.

48. Vandercam B, Gala J, Vandeweghe B, et al. *Mycobacterium simiae* disseminated infection in a patient with acquired immunodeficiency syndrome. Infection. 1996;24:49–51.

49. Sanders JW, Walsh AD, Snider RL, Sahn EE. Disseminated *Mycobacterium scrofulaceum* infection: a potentially treatable complication of AIDS. Clin Infect Dis. 1995;20:549.

50. Kandyil R, Maloney D, Tarrand J, Duvic M. Red nodule on the finger of an immunosuppressed woman. Arch Dermatol. 2002;138(5):689–94.

51. Gannon M, Otridge B, Hone R, Dervan P, O'Loughlin S. Cutaneous *Mycobacterium malmoense* infection in an immunocompromised patient. Int J Dermatol. 1990;29:149–50.

52. Castor B, Juhlin I, Henriques B. Septic cutaneous lesions caused by *Mycobacterium malmoense* in a patient with hairy cell leukemia. Eur J Clin Microbiol Infect Dis. 1994;13:145–8.

53. Doutre MS, Beylot C, Mougein J, et al. Cutaneous infection caused by *Mycobacterium malmoense* in a patient with myelodysplastic syndrome. J R Soc Med. 1993;86:110–1.

54. Sybert A, Tsou E, Garagus VF. Cutaneous infection due to *Mycobacterium szulgai*. Am Rev Respir Dis. 1977;115(4):695–8.

55. Cross GM, Guill MA, Aton JK. Cutaneous *Mycobacterium szulgai* infection. Arch Dermatol. 1985;121(2):247–9.

56. Frisk P, Boman G, Pauksen K, Petrini B. Lönnerholm. Skin infection caused by *Mycobacterium szulgai* after allogeneic bone marrow transplantation. Bone Marrow Transplant. 2003;31:511–3.

57. Shimizu T, Kodama K, Kobayashi H, et al. Successful treatment using clarithromycin for a cutaneous lesion caused by *Mycobacterium szulgai*. Br J Dermatol. 2000;142:838–40.

58. Meyer JJ, Gelman SS. Multifocal osteomyelitis due to *Mycobacterium szulgai* in a patient with chronic lymphocytic leukemia. J Infect. 2008;56:151–4.

59. Gengoux P, Portaels F, Lachapelle JM, et al. Skin granulomas due to *Mycobacterium gordonae*. Int J Dermatol. 1987;26:181–4.

60. Bernard E, Michiels JF, Pinier Y, Bourdet JF, Dellamonica P. Disseminated infection as a result of *Mycobacterium gordonae* in an AIDS patient. AIDS. 1992;6(10):1217–8.

61. Rusconi S, Gori A, Vago L, et al. Cutaneous infection caused by *Mycobacterium gordonae* in a human immunodeficiency virus-infected patient receiving antimycobacterial treatment. Clin Infect Dis. 1997;25:1489–90.

62. DeCoste SD, Dover JS. Kaposi's sarcoma and MAI with cellulitis in a patient with AIDS. J Am Acad Dermatol. 1989;21:574.

63. Volpe F, Schwimmer A, Barr C. Oral manifestations of disseminated MAI in a patient with AIDS. Oral Surg Oral Med Oral Pathol. 1985;60:567–70.

64. Taylor CR, Bailey EM. Red nodule on the forearm of an HIV-positive man. Arch Dermatol. 1998;134:1279–84.

65. Piketty C, Danic DL, Weiss L, Kazatchkine MD. Sporotrichosis-like infection caused by *Mycobacterium avium* in the acquired immunodeficiency syndrome. Arch Dermatol. 1993;129:1343–4.

66. Kayal JD, McCall CO. Sporotrichoid cutaneous *Mycobacterium avium* complex infection. J Am Acad Dermatol. 2002;47:S249–50.

67. Sivanesan SP, Khera P, Buckthal-McCuin J, English JC. Cutaneous *Mycobacterium avium-intracellulare* complex associated with immune reconstitution inflammatory syndrome. J Am Acad Dermatol. 2010;62:e25–6.

68. Giudice P, Durant J, Counillon E, et al. Mycobacterial cutaneous manifestations: a new sign of immune restoration syndrome in patients with acquired immunodeficiency syndrome. Arch Dermatol. 1999;135:1129–30.

69. Pelgrom J, Bastian I, Van den Enden E, Portaels F, Colebunders R. Cutaneous ulcer caused by *Mycobacterium avium* and recurrent genital herpes after highly active antiretroviral therapy. Arch Dermatol. 2000;136:129.

70. Cole GW, Gebhard J. *Mycobacterium avium* infection of the skin resembling lepromatous leprosy. Br J Dermatol. 1979;101:71–4.

71. Sanderson TL, Moskowitz L, Hensley GT, Cleary TJ, Penneys N. Disseminated MAI infection appearing as panniculitis. Arch Pathol Lab Med. 1982;106:112–4.

72. Otaki Y, Nakanishi T, Nanami M, et al. A rare combination of sites of involvement by *Mycobacterium intracellulare* in a hemodialysis patient: multifocal synovitis, spondylitis, and multiple skin lesions. Nephron. 2002;92(3):730–4.

73. Wood C, Nickoloff BJ, Todes-Talor NR. Pseudotumor resulting from atypical mycobacterial infection: a "histoid" variety of *Mycobacterium avium-intracellulare* complex infection. Am J Clin Pathol. 1985;83(4):524–7.

74. Saruwatari H, Yoshifuku A, Kawai K, Kanekura T. Cutaneous *Mycobacterium intracellulare* infection in a bone marrow transplantation recipient. J Dermatol. 2010;37:185–7.

75. Grice K. Sarcoidosis and MAI cutaneous abscesses. Clin Exp Dermatol. 1983;8:323–7.

76. Asiedu K, Scherpbier R, Raviglione M. Buruli ulcer – *Mycobacterium ulcerans* infection. Geneve: World Health Organization Global Buruli Ulcer Initiative; 2000.

77. Allen S. Buruli ulcer and HIV infection. Int J Dermatol. 1992;31(10):744–5.

78. Johnson RC, Ifebe D, Hans-Moevi A, et al. Disseminated *Mycobacterium ulcerans* disease in an HIV-positive patient: a case study. AIDS. 2002;16:1704–5.

79. Toll A, Gallardo F, Ferran M, et al. Aggressive multifocal Buruli ulcer with associated osteomyelitis in an HIV-positive patient. Clin Exp Dermatol. 2005;30:649–51.

80. Fox LP, Geyer AS, Husain S, et al. *Mycobacterium abscessus* cellulitis and multifocal abscesses of the breasts in a transsexual from illicit intramammary injections of silicone. J Am Acad Dermatol. 2004;50:450–4.

81. Uslan DZ, Kowalski TJ, Wengenack NL, et al. Skin and soft tissue infections due to rapidly growing mycobacteria. Arch Dermatol. 2006;142:1287–91.

82. Redelman-Sidi G, Sepkowitz KA. Rapidly growing mycobacteria infection in patients with cancer. Clin Infect Dis. 2010;51(4):422–34.

83. Bhambri S, Bhambri A, Del Rosso JQ. Atypical mycobacterial cutaneous infections. Dermatol Clin. 2009;27:63–73.

84. Winthrop KL, Abrams M, Yakrus M, et al. An outbreak of mycobacterial furunculosis associated with footbaths at a nail salon. N Engl J Med. 2002;346:1366–71.

85. Hendrick SJ, Jorizzo JL, Newton RC. Giant *Mycobacterium fortuitum* abscess associated with systemic lupus erythematosus. Arch Dermatol. 1986;122(6):695–7.

86. Laborde H, Rodrigue S, Catoggio PM. *M. fortuitum* in SLE. Clin Exp Rheumatol. 1989;7:291–3.

87. Okano A, Shimazaki C, Ochiai N, et al. Subcutaneous infection with *Mycobacterium fortuitum* after allogeneic bone marrow transplantation. Bone Marrow Transplant. 2001;28:709–11.

88. Rodriguez-Barradas MC, Clarridge J, Darouiche R. Disseminated *Mycobacterium fortuitum* disease in an AIDS patient. Am J Med. 1992;93:473–4.

89. Lazo-de-la-Vega SA, Pezzarossi HE, Ponce-de-León S, Sifuentes J, Ruiz-Palacios GM. Cutaneous manifestations of disseminated infection by *Mycobacterium fortuitum* biovariant "Third Group". J Am Acad Dermatol. 1987;16:1058–60.

90. Retief CR, Tharp MD. *Mycobacterium fortuitum* panniculitis in a steroid-dependent asthmatic patient. J Am Acad Dermatol. 1998;39:650–3.

91. Smith MB, Schnadig VJ, Boyars MC, Woods GL. Clinical and pathologic features of *Mycobacterium fortuitum* infections. An emerging pathogen in patients with AIDS. Am J Surg Pathol. 2001;116:225–32.

92. Wallace RJ, Brown BA, Onyi GO. Skin, soft tissue, and bone infections due to *Mycobacterium chelonae chelonae*: importance of prior corticosteroid therapy, frequency of disseminated infections, and resistance to oral antimicrobials other than clarithromycin. J Infect Dis. 1992;166:405–12.

93. Drabick JJ, Duffy PE, Samlaska CP, Scherbenske JM. Disseminated *Mycobacterium chelonae* subspecies *chelonae* infection with cutaneous and osseous manifestations. Arch Dermatol. 1990;126:1064–7.

94. Wolfson JS, Sober AJ, Rubin RH. Dermatologic manifestations of infections in immunocompromised patients. Medicine (Baltimore). 1985;64(2):115–33.

95. Verhelst D, Goffin E, Bodarwe AD, et al. Purple-blue subcutaneous nodules after renal transplantation: not always Kaposi sarcoma. Nephrol Dial Transplant. 2001;16:1716–8.

96. Nathan DL, Singh S, Kestenbaum TM, Casparian JM. Cutaneous *Mycobacterium chelonae* in a liver transplant patient. J Am Acad Dermatol. 2000;43:333–6.

97. Kane CL, Vincent AL, Green JN, Sandin RL. Disseminated cutaneous *Mycobacterium chelonae* infection. Cancer Control. 2000;7: 181–4.

98. Ena P, Sechi LA, Molicotti P, et al. Cutaneous *Mycobacterium chelonae* infection extending in the lower extremities in a renal transplant patient. J Eur Acad Dermatol Venereol. 2005;19:504–5.

99. Jopp-McKay AG, Randell P. Sporotrichoid cutaneous infection due to *Mycobacterium chelonei* in a renal transplant patient. Australas J Dermatol. 1990;31:105–9.

100. Dungarwalla M, Field-Smith A, Jameson C, et al. Cutaneous *Mycobacterium chelonae* infection in chronic lymphocytis leukaemia. Haematologica. 2007;92:e5–6.

101. Baisi A, Nosotti M, Chella B, Santambrogio L. Relapsing cutaneous *Mycobacterium chelonae* infection in a lung transplant patient. Transpl Int. 2005;18:1117–9.

102. Hoetzenecker W, Ulmer A, Klingel K, et al. Dissemination of a localized cutaneous infection with *Mycobacterium chelonae* under immunosuppressive treatment. Arch Dermatol. 2007;143:951–2.

103. Kim JE, Sung H, Kim MN, et al. Synchronous infection with *Mycobacterium chelonae* and *Paecilomyces* in a heart transplant patient. Transpl Infect Dis. 2011;13(1):80–3.

104. Prinz BM, Michaelis S, Kettelhack N, et al. Subcutaneous infection with *Mycobacterium abscessus* in a renal transplant recipient. Dermatology. 2004;208(3):259–61.

105. Graybill JR, Silva Jr J, Fraser DW, Lordon R, Rogers E. Disseminated mycobacteriosis due to *Mycobacterium abscessus* in two recipients of renal homografts. Am Rev Respir Dis. 1974;109:4–10.

106. Endzweig CH, Strauss E, Murphy F, Rao BK. A case of cutaneous *Mycobacterium chelonae abscessus* infection in a renal transplant patient. J Cutan Med Surg. 2001;5:28–32.

107. Scholze A, Loddenkemper C, Grunbaum M, et al. Cutaneous *Mycobacterium abscessus* infection after kidney transplantation. Nephrol Dial Transplant. 2005;20:1764–5.

108. Garrison AP, Morris MI, Doblecki-Lewis S, et al. *Mycobacterium abscessus* infection in solid organ transplant recipients: report of three cases and review of the literature. Transpl Infect Dis. 2009;11:541–8.

109. Freudenberger RS, Simagranca SM. Cutaneous infection with rapidly-growing mycobacterial infection following heart transplant: a case report and review of the literature. Transplant Proc. 2006;38: 1526–9.

110. Kwon YH, Lee GY, Kim WS, Kim KJ. A case of skin and soft tissue infection caused by *Mycobacterium abscessus*. Ann Dermatol. 2009;21:84–7.

111. Vogels MT, Tjan-Heijnen VC, Alkemade JA, et al. Cutaneous infection due to *Mycobacterium abscessus*. A case report. Acta Derm Venerol. 1997;77:222–4.

112. Wang H, Jin P, Wu Q. Disseminated cutaneous infection with *Mycobacterium abscessus* in a patient with a low CD4+ T cell count. Eur J Dermatol. 2008;18:337–40.

113. Shehan JM, Sarma DP. *Mycobacterium mucogenicum*: report of a skin infection associated with etanercept. Dermatol Online J. 2008; 14(1):5.

114. Lederman C, Spitz JL, Scully B, et al. *M. haemophilum* cellulitis in a heart transplant recipient. J Am Acad Dermatol. 1994;30:804–6.

115. Straus WL, Ostroff SM, Jernigan DB, et al. Clinical and epidemiologic characteristics of *Mycobacterium haemophilum*, an emerging pathogen in immunocompromised patients. Ann Intern Med. 1994;120:118–25.

116. Shah MK, Sebti A, Kiehn TE, Massarella SA, Sepkowitz KA. *Mycobacterium haemophilum* in immunocompromised patients. Clin Infect Dis. 2001;33:330–7.

117. Saubolle MA, Kiehn TE, White MH, Rudinsky MF, Armstrong D. *Mycobacterium haemophilum*: microbiology and expanding clinical and geographic spectra of disease in humans. Clin Microbiol Rev. 1996;9:435–47.

118. Tan HH, Tan A, Theng C, Ng SK. Cutaneous *Mycobacterium haemophilum* infections in immunocompromised patients in a dermatology clinic in Singapore. Ann Acad Med Singapore. 2004;33:532–6.

119. Geisler WM, Harrington RD, Wallis CK, et al. Broad spectrum of dermatologic manifestations caused by *Mycobacterium haemophilum* infection. Arch Dermaol. 2002;138:229–30.

120. von Stebut E, Wiest K, Braeuninger W. Chronic infiltrates and persisting ulcerations on the arms and legs. Arch Dermatol. 2005;141: 897–902.

121. Lott JP, Werth VP, Kovarik CL. Cutaneous *Mycobacterium haemophilum* infection in iatrogenically immunocompromised patients without transplantation. J Am Acad Dermatol. 2008;59:139–42.

122. Friedli A, Krischer J, Hirschel B, et al. An annular plaque due to *Mycobacterium haemophilum* infection in a patient with AIDS. J Am Acad Dermatol. 2000;43:913–5.

123. Castro-Silva AN, Freire AO, Grinbaum RS, et al. Cutaneous *Mycobacterium haemophilum* infection in a kidney transplant recipient after acupuncture treatment. Transpl Infect Dis. 2011;13:33–7.

6

Viruses

HERPES SIMPLEX

Infections caused by herpes simplex virus (HSV) are exceedingly common. They are divided into primary and secondary (recurrent) forms, which are self-limited processes in normal hosts. The course of herpes simplex infection in immunocompromised patients may be atypical, indolent, difficult to diagnose, and respond poorly to therapy. Atypical infections in the immunocompromised patients include lesions of larger size, deeper, more invasive and painful, disabling ulcerations, satellite lesions, longer healing time, unusual locations, and atypical morphology. Untreated lesions may become deeply erosive and chronic with the development of extensive areas of necrosis and bacterial superinfection that may distort the initial appearance, resulting in misdiagnosis. Patients with human immunodeficiency virus (HIV) infection have more frequent, persistent, and severe recurrences of HSV, and are more likely to be resistant to standard antiviral medications. Lesions may remain culture positive for HSV for extended periods of time with extensive tissue destruction.

Any periorificial ulceration in the immunocompromised host should be considered herpes simplex until proven otherwise. Prompt diagnosis using Tzanck smear, rapid immunofluorescence using fluorescein-labeled monoclonal antibodies specific for HSV antigens, viral culture, and skin biopsy should be made. Recognition of chronic HSV is important in order to avoid inappropriate antibacterial and antifungal therapy, to initiate proper precautions to prevent nonvenereal transmission of HSV, and to begin effective antiviral therapy.

Chronic periorificial HSV characteristically has annular or polycyclic (scalloped border) erosions or ulcers. Upon close examination there may be a well defined, raised, friable, or minute vesicular border surrounding the polycyclic ulcerations.

Recurrent herpes labialis is the most common manifestation of HSV infection in immunosuppressed patients, similar to the clinical pattern seen in normal hosts. However, intraoral involvement, a distinctly unusual finding in immunocompetent patients, is frequently seen in the immunocompromised population. When intraoral lesions occur without herpes labialis, the correct diagnosis may be overlooked.[1] Intraoral HSV appears as single or multiple ulcers or erosions on the gingiva, palate, tongue, or buccal mucosa and display the characteristic polycyclic border. When lesions develop, they usually occur in the first four weeks after transplantation, and they often follow a serious infection or rejection episode. The patient may or may not be acutely ill. Although these ulcerations may appear in the same anatomic location as primary HSV infection in the normal host, in the majority of immunocompromised hosts, the HSV infection is not primary but rather reactivation of latent HSV.

When the tongue is involved with HSV, lesions are usually present on the lateral surface of the tongue. Linear fissures on the dorsum of the tongue due to HSV1, known as herpetic geometric glossitis, is another atypical manifestation of HSV in the compromised host.[2] The extremely tender fissures may be longitudinal, cross hatched, or branched in a striking geometric pattern.[3] The central well papillated portion of the tongue is usually involved without accompanying HSV lesions on the lips or palate. The differential diagnosis includes ulcers from trauma (dental or other), radiation- or chemotherapy-induced mucositis, neutropenia, fungal or bacterial infections, and other oral lesions, such as erythema multiforme or recurrent aphthous stomatitis, as seen in otherwise normal patients. The tongue lesions of HSV are painful and may impair nutrition. The break of mucosal integrity provides a portal of invasion by both pathogenic and normal microbial flora inhabiting the mouth.

M.E. Grossman et al., *Cutaneous Manifestations of Infection in the Immunocompromised Host,*
DOI 10.1007/978-1-4419-1578-8_6, © Springer Science+Business Media, LLC 2012

Oral HSV infections may present a myriad of morphologies: diffuse erythema mimicking bacterial mucositis; coalesced yellow papules resembling *Candida* infection; an isolated tongue ulcer appearing traumatic in origin; crateriform ulcers with white raised borders containing small vesicles; a dark red or violaceous exophytic nodule with or without ulceration on the dorsum of the tongue; or a yellow white rapidly growing nodule on the lateral tongue[4] mimicking a squamous cell carcinoma.[5]

Patients with oral and periorificial HSV may develop extension of the infection to the esophageal or respiratory tract. These usually occur in patients with HSV infection and nasogastric or endotracheal tubes, which traumatize the mucous membrane.

Chronic perianal and buttock HSV occurs as single or multiple coalescent ulcers.[6] Because of the location in the perianal area, confusion may occur with superficial ulcers secondary to pressure, maceration, heat, and irritation from urine and or feces. Frank secondary infection with bacteria and/or *Candida* may be present, which may further add to the confusion. Chronic herpetic lesions can develop into deep ulcerations requiring narcotic analgesics. The location of the ulcers may suggest a diagnosis of decubitus ulcers as well, especially in chronically ill, cachectic, debilitated, or bedridden patients. In contrast to pressure ulcers, HSV lesions are more superficial, often painful, usually multiple with scalloped borders, not confined to pressure areas, and are more often extensive with involvement in the anterior perineal region as well. Anal and perianal HSV may present as chronic ulcers, hyperkeratotic and verrucous lesions, or exophytic plaques and nodules mimicking warts (human papillomavirus) or squamous cell carcinoma. The anal HSV may be accompanied by anal or perianal pain, tenesmus, altered bowel habit, and/or mucoid or bloody anal discharge. A rare manifestation seen mainly with HIV disease or myeloproliferative disorders is a chronic polypoid vegetative plaque with erosions and ulcers on the perianal skin. Termed herpes simplex vegetans,[7] it demonstrates pseudoepitheliomatous hyperplasia, plasma cell infiltration, and is positive for herpes simplex virus 1 (HSV1) and/or herpes simplex virus 2 (HSV2).[8] Chronic herpetic ulcers in the inguinal or gluteal crease can result in "kissing," or opposing, lesions.

One variant of atypical herpes simplex virus infection is the presentation of deep linear fissures in the skin folds (inframammary, infra-abdominal, inguinal, or vulvar) termed the "knife-cut sign." Originally used to describe linear fissures seen on colonoscopy in patients with Crohn's disease, the knife-cut sign became a morphologic term used to describe metastatic Crohn's disease of the skin. Rare presentations of HSV infection as the knife-cut sign are very likely to be overlooked as a nonspecific intertrigo and therefore the infection may be undiagnosed and untreated.[9]

Atypical HSV in the immunocompromised patient presenting as nodules, tumors, verrucous growths, or hypertrophic lesions simulating neoplasms usually occur in HIV-infected patients and rarely in organ transplant recipients.[10] Hypertrophic HSV, also called herpes vegetans, occurs in the genital,[11] anal, or perianal area, clinically resembling condyloma acuminata,[12] verrucous carcinoma, or squamous cell carcinoma.[13,14] The lesions are painful, disfiguring, superficially ulcerated, and are mostly slow growing with a protracted course of months. Some of these patients received long-term or intermittent therapy with subtherapeutic doses of acyclovir leading to drug resistance. Most cases had HIV infection greater than 5 years, were male, and had a history of highly active antiretroviral therapy (HAART). The mechanism of this unusual presentation of an exaggerated tumor-like response to a very common condition (HSV in HIV patients) remains unexplained. The over-stimulated and inappropriate inflammatory response has been attributed to the immune reconstitution inflammatory syndrome (IRIS) after HAART initiation.[15] Others have correlated profound immunosuppression with the severity of cutaneous disease.

In immunocompromised patients, digital HSV may present with chronic fingertip ulcerations, painful paronychial inflammation, or bullae of the hyponychium. Herpetic whitlow may mimic a bacterial infection or paronychia and may undergo unwarranted and unnecessary treatments. The lesion may be unsuccessfully incised and drained or debrided until the atypical manifestations of infection with typical HSV is recognized. The herpetic vesicles may occur in the subungual space of the distal phalanx and cause intense pain. Most commonly only one digit of the hand is involved. Multiple herpetic whitlow, HSV infection of the fingers, was reported in a patient post chemotherapy of chronic lymphocytic leukemia (CLL) with multiple fingers affected on the same hand.[16] Herpetic whitlow is a recognized occupational hazard of medical, paramedical, and dental workers, but may also occur by autoinfection in the compromised host. In the immunocompromised patient, herpetic whitlow may progress to a chronic digital ulceration frequently lasting more than a month,[17] causing erosive crusted lesions with progressive destruction of nail structures[18] and rarely leading to gangrene necessitating amputation.[19,20]

Systemic or local immunosuppression because of the inappropriate use of a fluorinated corticosteroid cream (often in combination with an antifungal cream) produces a typical buttock eruption of HSV in the bedridden patient. The lesions appear in various stages of evolution at the same time. Groups of vesicles, erosions, scars, postinflammatory hyperpigmented macules, and rarely ulcerations are present in a nondermatomal distribution over the right and/or left cheek of the buttocks or along the midline.

Disseminated HSV types 1 or 2 infections are rare after solid organ transplantation compared to bone marrow transplant recipients.[21] It is more common in HIV disease. The HSV may result from primary infection (including transmission from the donor organ) or reactivation of the donor or recipient's viruses. HSV in the immunocompromised patient may disseminate hematogenously to visceral organs causing pneumonitis, hepatitis, pancreatitis, esophagitis, retinal necrosis, or adrenal necrosis.[22] HSV hepatitis should be suspected in any immunocompromised patient presenting with skin lesions, high fever, leukopenia, and anicteric transaminitis.[23]

Severe abdominal pain is frequently reported with HSV hepatitis.[24]

Disseminated cutaneous HSV Types 1 or 2 (Kaposi's varicelliform eruption or eczema herpeticum) may occur in immunosuppressed patients, in pregnancy, and in patients with several skin diseases including atopic dermatitis, pemphigus foliaceus, Darier's disease, Hailey and Hailey disease (benign familial pemphigus),[25] and cutaneous T-cell lymphoma.[26]

The eruption starts with small, closely grouped, monomorphic vesicles, usually but not always in areas of preexisting skin disease, and is often initially misdiagnosed as a worsening of the original disorder. The vesicles enlarge, umbilicate, and become pustular and crusted, or ulcerate, accompanied by high fever, malaise, and regional lymphademopathy. In intertriginous areas, the lesions become confluent. New lesions continue to appear for up to two weeks. The eruption is most frequently located on the head, neck, and the upper part of the body with caudal spread.

There is an increasing number of antiviral (mostly acyclovir) resistant HSV strains, especially in immunocompromised patients. Drug resistance occurs most often in HIV-infected patients but also in organ transplant recipients.[27] In patients with profound immune defects, lack of clinical response to an antiviral agent does not necessarily correlate with in vitro drug resistance.[28] The degree of immunosuppression and the prolonged use of acyclovir are considered two important factors for the development of drug resistance. Other causes of acyclovir resistance include erratic or suboptimal dosing or noncompliance with treatment regimens. Acyclovir resistant HSV should be considered whenever lesions persist for greater than one week without appreciable decrease in size, when they develop an atypical appearance, or when new satellite lesions develop after three to four days of therapy.[29] The history of prior antiviral therapy or previous resistance and incomplete or partial failure of past treatments are suspicious for antiviral resistance.[27] Resistant HSV can occur after many prior episodes with sensitive HSV.

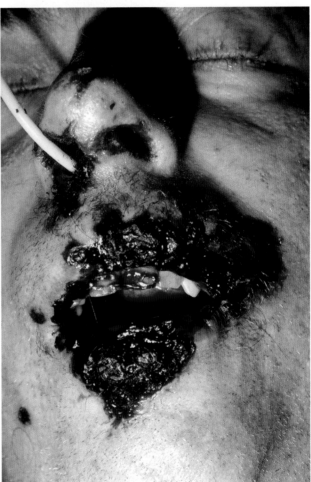

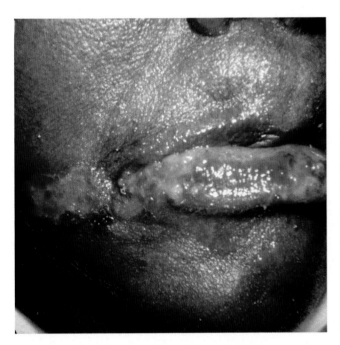

Figure 6.1. Eroded lower lip with scalloped margins due to chronic herpes simplex virus (HSV) in a renal transplant patient

Figure 6.2. Hemorrhagic crusts of the lips and nose in a heart transplant patient with chronic HSV. The black crusts have a scalloped margin on the upper lip and a vesicular margin on the chin

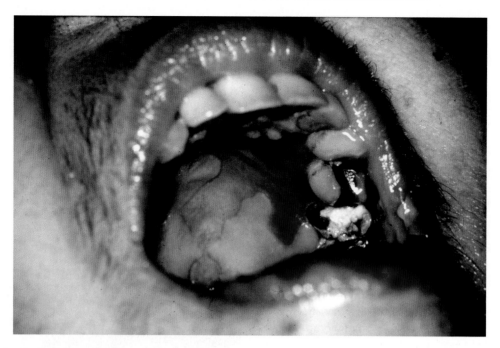

Figure 6.3.   Polycyclic HSV ulcer on the hard palate of a renal transplant patient

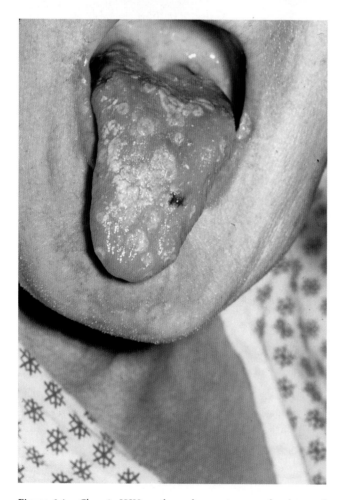

Figure 6.4.   Chronic HSV on the oral commissure, soft palate, and tongue of a patient before he died of metastatic prostate cancer

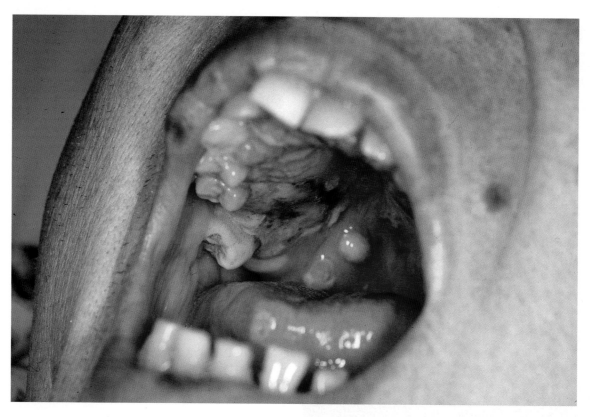

Figure 6.5. Intraoral ulcers and pustules of HSV1 in a heart transplant recipient with acute myelogenous leukemia (AML)

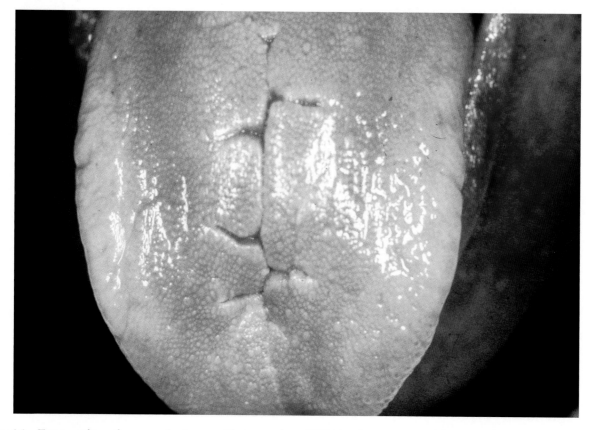

Figure 6.6. Transverse linear fissures on the dorsum of the tongue due to HSV-1 in a human immunodeficiency (HIV)-positive man

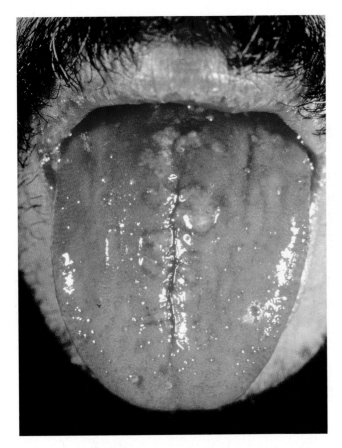

Figure 6.7.   HSV geometric glossitis with a longitudinal linear fissure

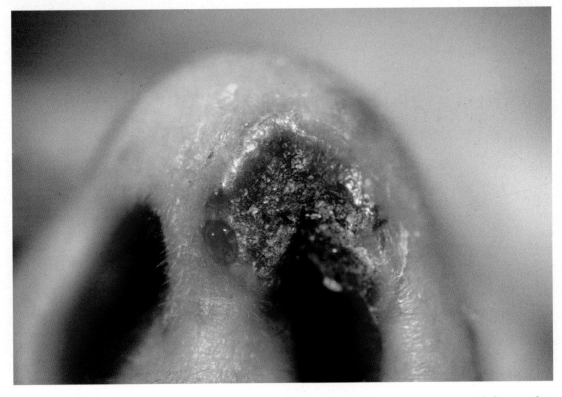

Figure 6.8.   Crusted ulceration with a vesicular margin due to chronic HSV in a patient on long-term systemic steroids for sarcoidosis

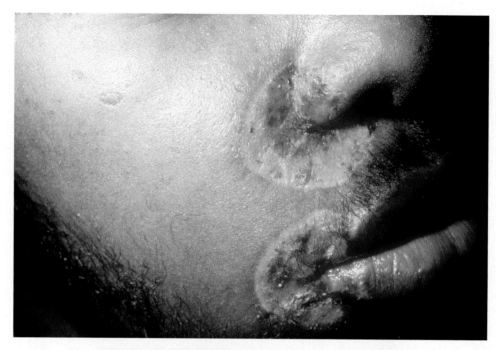

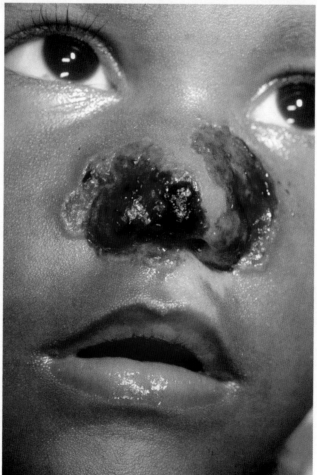

Figure 6.9. and 6.10. Scalloped ulcerations of HSV in a child and adult with human immunodeficiency virus/acquired immune deficiency syndrome (HIV/AIDS)

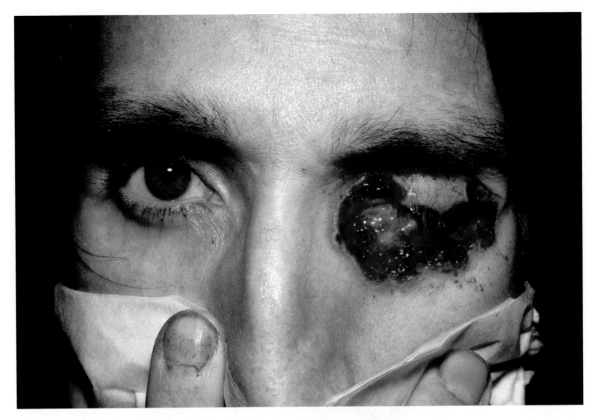

Figure 6.11. Chronic HSV of the orbit in a patient with AIDS. The annular margin is vesicular

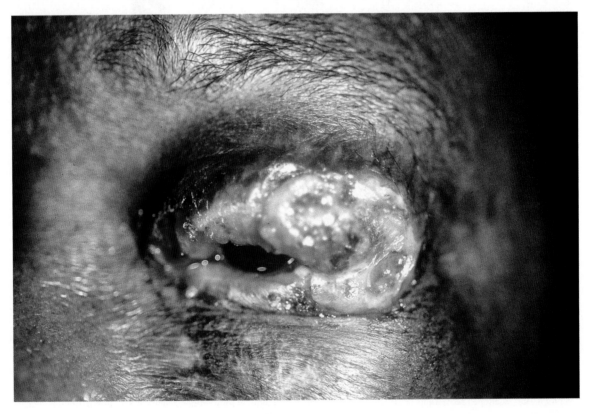

Figure 6.12. Chronic eyelid and mouth acyclovir-resistant HSV in HIV/AIDS

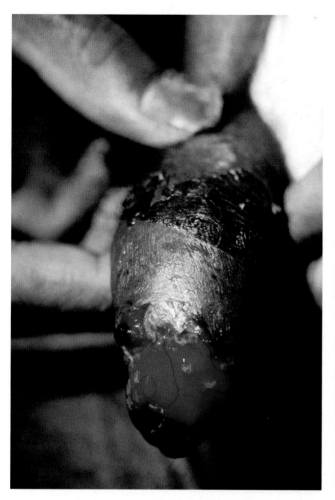

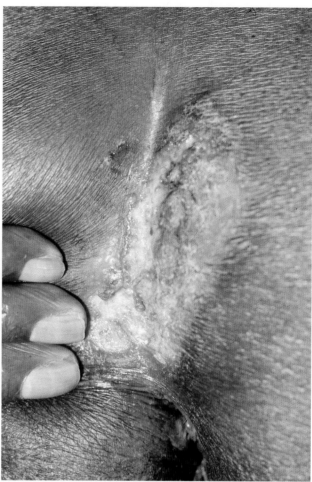

Figure 6.13. Chronic penile ulceration of a patient admitted for treatment of penile squamous cell carcinoma. Tzanck smear from the annular margin confirmed a diagnosis of HSV, and the lesion healed completely with acyclovir

Figure 6.14. Multiple coalescent ulcers with a polycyclic border in the gluteal fold of a patient with chronic lymphocytic leukemia during chemotherapy

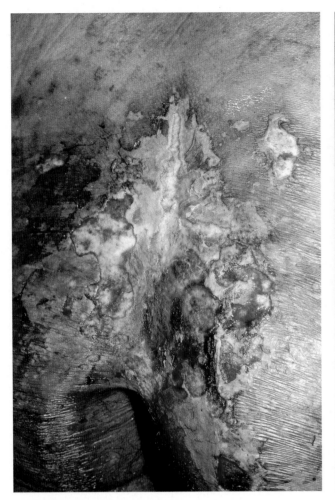

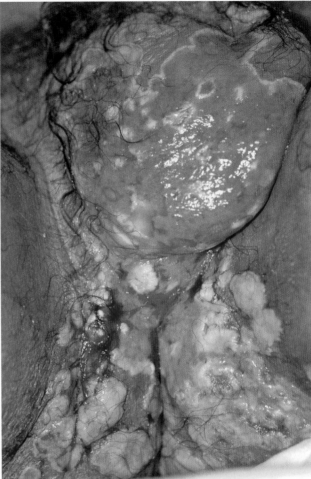

Figure 6.15. Multiple superficial ulcers on the buttock and perianal area of woman with systemic lupus erythematosus on immunosuppressants

Figure 6.16. A 30-year-old-man with a history of HIV/AIDS presented with a 3-year history of treatment-resistant ulcerative perineal herpes simplex virus II. Sensitivity testing of the virus revealed high-level acyclovir resistance. The patient was started on intravenous foscarnet but stopped because of severe myelosuppression from this treatment. He was then treated with topical cidofovir but developed acute tubular necrosis of his kidneys secondary to significant systemic absorption of the medication through his skin ulcerations. The patient also failed a trial of thalidomide

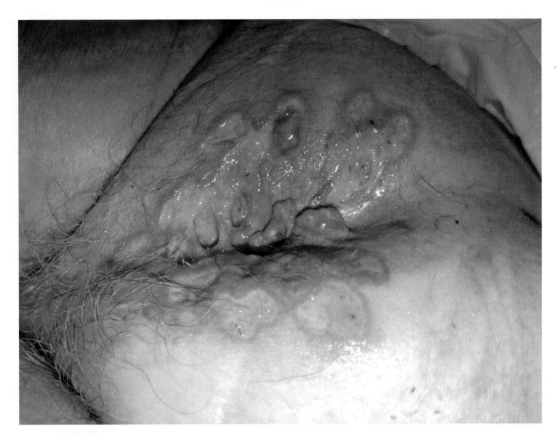

Figure 6.17. An 87-year-old-man being treated with pulse dose systemic corticosteroids for sight-threatening temporal arteritis presented with a 1-month history of painful perianal ulcerations. Skin examination revealed numerous deep, cribriform ulcerations with scalloped borders and yellow fibrinous exudates mimicking pyoderma gangrenosum. Viral culture was positive for herpes simplex virus II

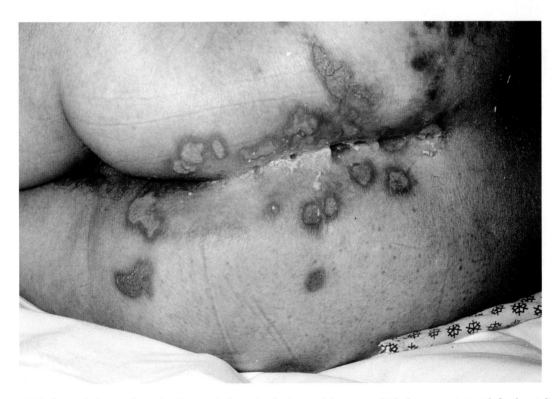

Figure 6.18. Multiple punched-out and annular ulcers on the buttocks of a 62-year-old woman on high-dose systemic steroids for chronic lung disease

Figure 6.19. Multiple groups of vesicles, pustules, and crusts due to the spread of HSV on the buttocks in a bedridden patient on high-dose systemic steroids after resection of a meningioma

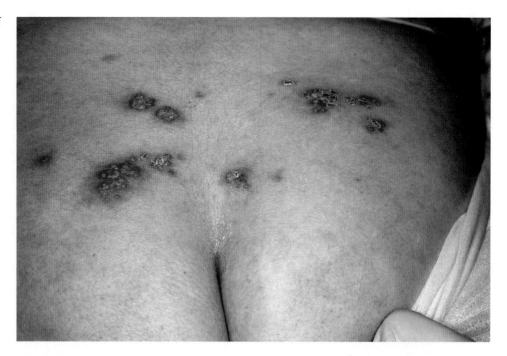

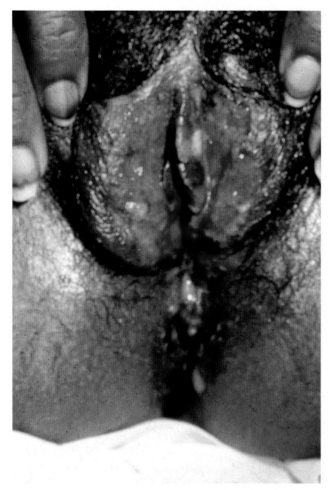

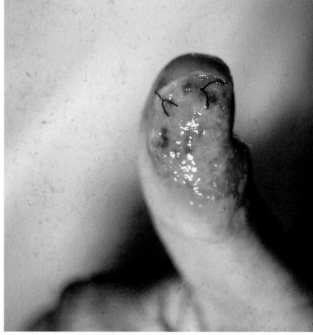

Figure 6.21. Chronic digital ulceration due to HSV in AIDS

Figure 6.20. Painful vulvar ulcerations of chronic HSV in an HIV-positive woman. Perianal HSV ulcers were also present

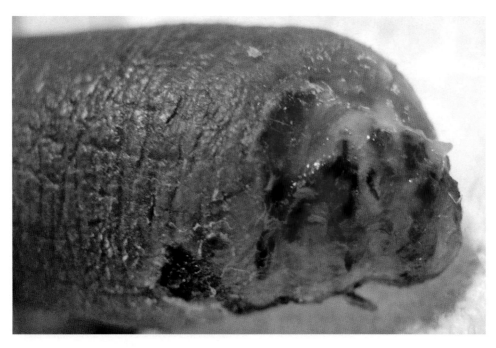

Figure 6.22. A 38-year-old man with HIV/AIDS (CD4 4 cells/μL) presented with a 7-month history of a painful lesion on his second right digit following a manicure. He was treated with doxycycline, cephalexin, and fluconazole without improvement. Viral culture was positive for herpes simplex virus II (Courtesy of Kanade Shinkai, M.D., Ph.D.)

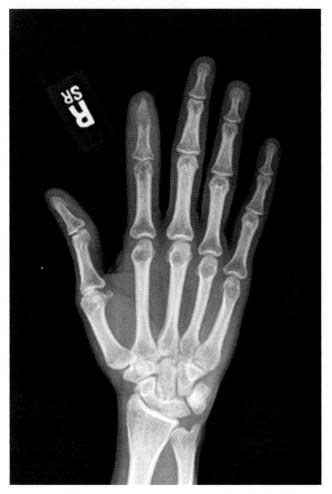

Figure 6.23. An X-ray of the patient's finger revealed extensive soft tissue swelling and erosion of the distal phalynx most consistent with soft tissue and osseus infection (Courtesy of Kanade Shinkai, M.D., Ph.D.)

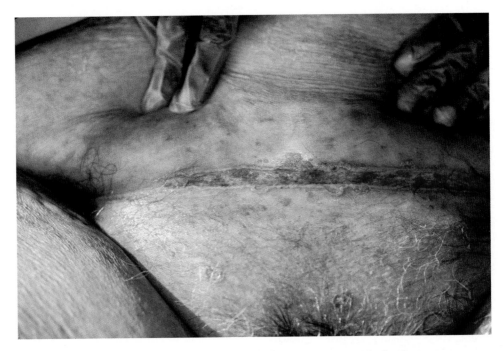

Figure 6.24. The knife-cut sign due to HSV1 in the intra-abdominal fold of an immunocompromised patient

Figure 6.25. A 40-year-old woman with HIV/AIDS and "knife-cut sign" characteristic of herpes simplex virus. Cultures of the labial linear fissures were positive for herpes simplex virus II

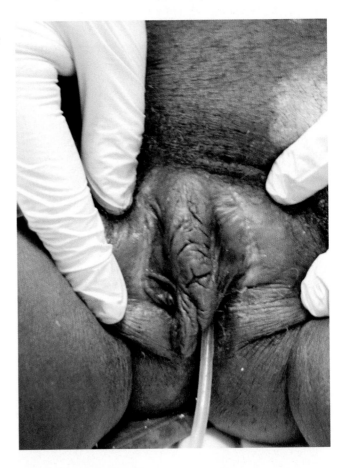

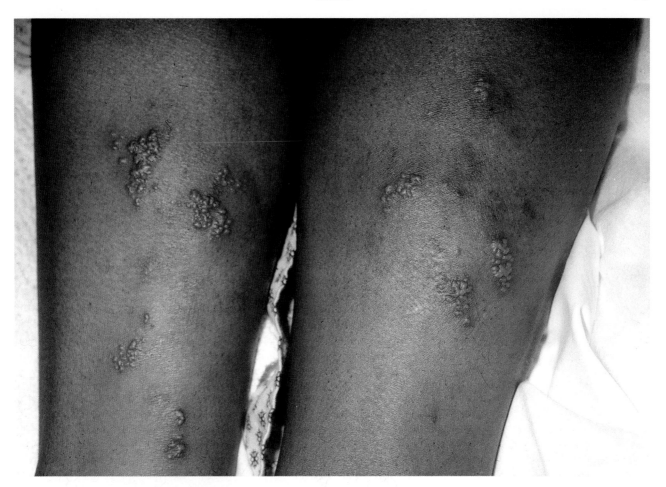

Figure 6.26. Herpes simplex infection simultaneously involving both legs in a patient with AIDS. Bilateral eyelid HSV has been observed by the authors as well

Figure 6.27. A 15×9-cm bullae of HSV on the occipital scalp with a scalloped erythematous border and central crusting in a 34-year-old HIV-positive man

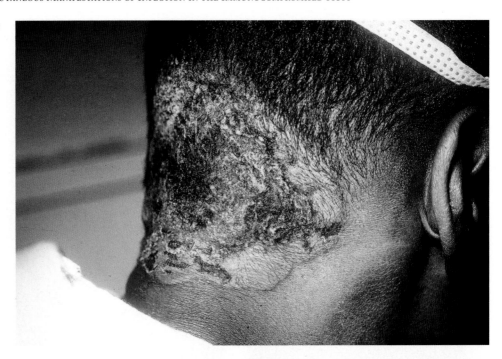

Figure 6.28. A large exophytic plaque of chronic HSV in HIV mimicking a wart or squamous cell carcinoma

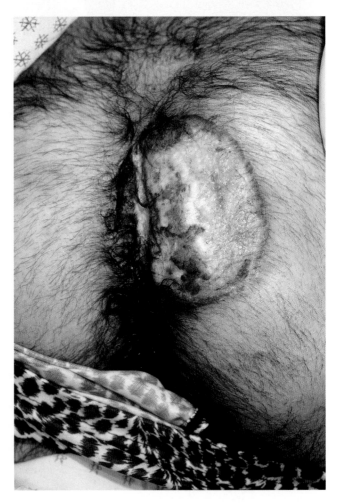

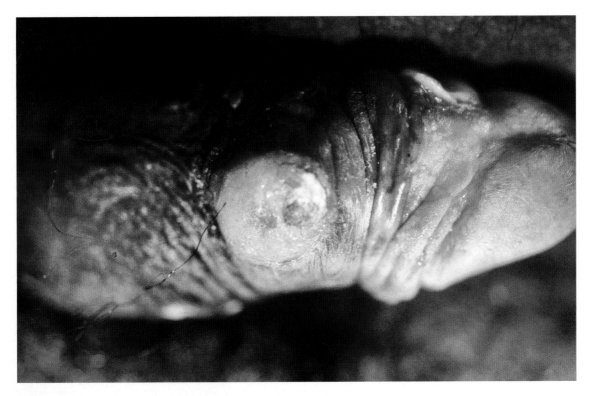

Figure 6.29.   Hypertrophic HSV or HSV vegetans in a 42-year-old with HIV/AIDS (CD4 6 cells/μL)

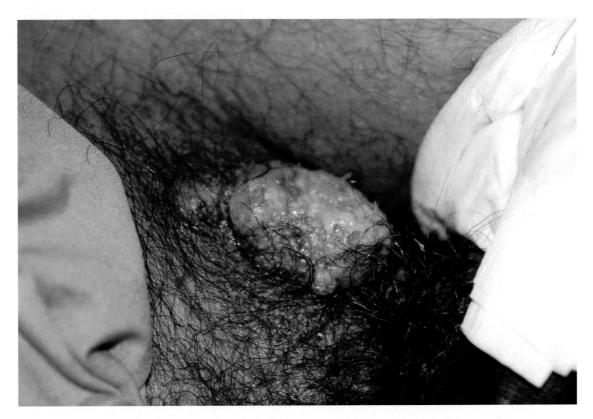

Figure 6.30.   A 46-year-old man with a history of HIV presented with a 1.5-year history of a large purulent, verrucous nodule in the left groin. The nodule was culture and direct fluorescence antibody (DFA)-positive for HSV II. Biopsy of the lesion revealed marked epithelial hyperplasia and papillomatosis with numerous multinucleated giant cells. The patient was treated with acyclovir and foscarnet with little improvement. The patient was noncompliant with home therapy

Figure 6.31. Chronic crusted hyperkeratotic herpes simplex was present in the face of this patient with AIDS for 5 months until he died. The HSV was not resistant to acyclovir

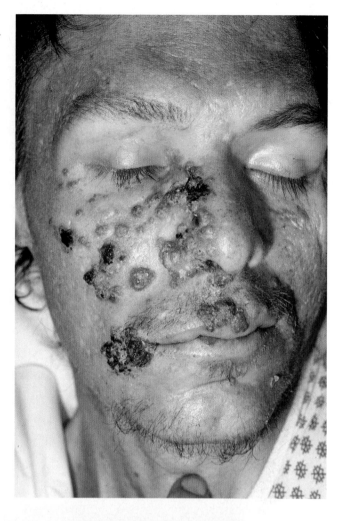

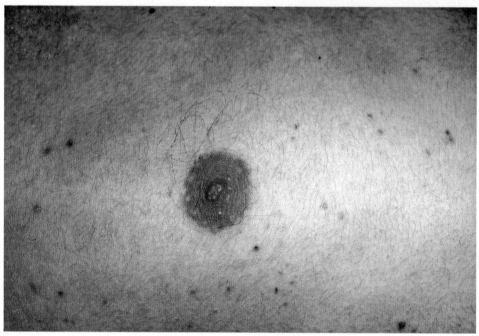

Figure 6.32. Disseminated cutaneous HSV in a patient with AIDS initially thought to be folliculitis

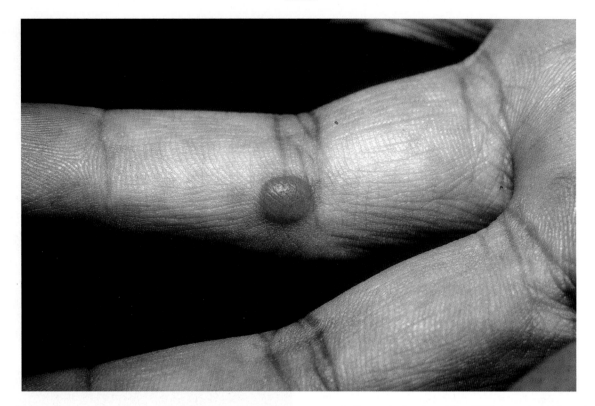

Figure 6.33. Disseminated HSV in a renal transplant patient with tense serous bullae on the hands and feet. HSV was cultured from the skin bullae and urine

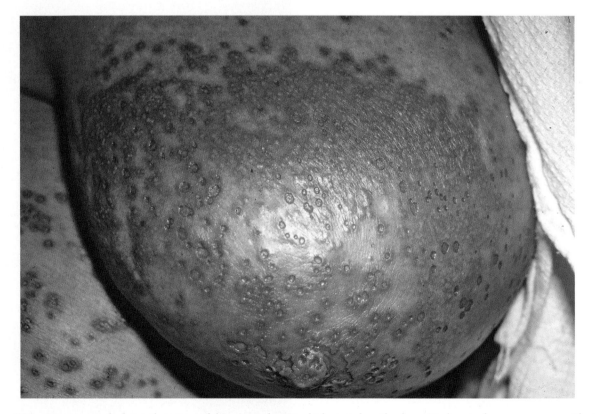

Figure 6.34. Discrete punched-out ulcerations of disseminated HSV, which started on the dermatitic breast of a young woman with atopic dermatitis

Figure 6.35. Inframammary erosions with satellite erosions and vesicles in a 64-year-old woman with chronic benign familial pemphigus

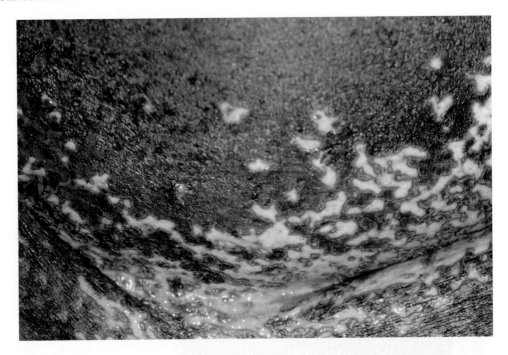

Figure 6.36. Honey-colored and hemorrhagic crusts of disseminated herpes simplex in atopic dermatitis on the third day of treatment with acyclovir. The HSV started on the right eyelid

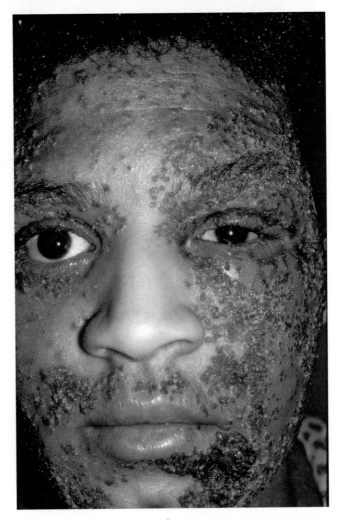

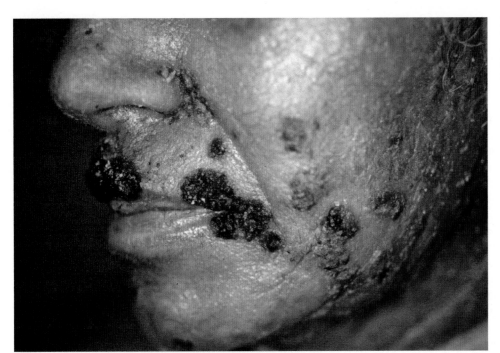

Figure 6.37. A 57-year-old woman with pemphigus foliaceus on cyclosporine and mycophenolate mofetil developed disseminated HSV1

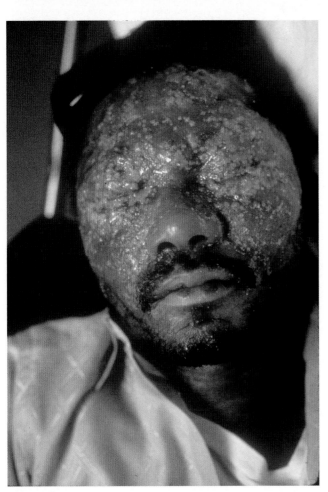

Figure 6.38. A 36-year-old man with cutaneous T-cell lymphoma (CTCL) presented to the emergency room with fever, severe pain, and an outbreak of facial vesicles and pustules. Two weeks before this, multiple new nodules of CTCL developed on his forehead and cheeks. Numerous pustules with thick yellow exudates were concentrated over erythematous plaques on the forehead and cheeks. Facial edema and erythema were present, and the eyes were swollen shut. HSV 2 was cultured from the pustules. After resolution of the disseminated HSV with acyclovir, leonine facies of CTCL became evident. Since the HSV occurred only in the newly developed tumor nodules, one may speculate that localized areas of depressed T-cell function accounted for this pattern of cutaneous infection

HUMAN HERPES 6

Human herpes virus 6 (HHV-6), known as the causal agent of exanthem subitum in infancy (sixth disease, roseola infantum), has recently been recognized as an opportunistic pathogen most often in transplant patients but also in cancer patients undergoing chemotherapy and HIV-infected patients.[30] HHV-6 is a member of the beta-herpes subfamily, which is in the Roseola virus genus along with human herpes virus 7 (HHV-7). Like other herpes viruses, after the primary infection HHV-6 establishes latency in different cells and organs, including monocytes, macrophages, salivary glands, brain, and kidneys. Reactivation of HHV-6 can occur both in normal individuals and in immunocompromised patients. Most HHV-6 infections represent reactivation infection 2–4 weeks after transplantation.[31] Use of OKT3 monoclonal antibodies (muromonab-CD3), alemtuzumab, and antithymocyte globulin for prevention of transplant rejection is associated with increased incidence of HHV-6 reactivation in solid organ transplant recipients.[32] The clinical symptoms of HHV-6 reactivation include fever, rash, pneumonitis, bone marrow suppression, and encephalitis. The rash of HHV-6 reactivation can be confused with acute skin graft versus host disease (GVHD), and HHV-6 reactivation has been associated with the development of acute severe GVHD.[33] Even with histologic examination, it is difficult to distinguish between acute GVHD exacerbated by HHV-6 infection and a viral exanthem of HHV-6 2–4 weeks post bone marrow transplantation. The exanthem of HHV-6 in acute lymphocytic leukemia was described as a relapsing centripetal macular or maculopapular eruption.[34] The temporal behavior of the eruption resembled the rash of acute lymphocyte recovery.

VARICELLA-ZOSTER

Herpes zoster (HZ) represents the second manifestation of infection with the varicella-zoster (VZ) virus. Following the primary varicella infection (chicken pox), the virus remains dormant in a dorsal root ganglion or a cranial nerve ganglion. Reactivation occurs as herpes zoster with cutaneous vesicles and dermatomal pain. The skin lesions of VZ in the immunocompromised host occur in three forms: (1) dermatomal HZ (which may be one or multiple dermatomes), (2) disseminated HZ, and (3) chronic HZ or recurrent HZ.

The factors precipitating HZ are unclear, but immunosuppression appears to be an important cause. The incidence of HZ increases with increasing age in the general population. In patients with malignant disease, the incidence of HZ is further increased: highest in lymphoreticular disorders, Hodgkin's disease, then non-Hodgkin's lymphomas, followed by solid tumors, particularly small cell carcinoma of the lung.[35] Transplant recipients (renal, cardiac, but particularly bone marrow transplants) have an increased incidence of HZ. HZ is a frequent harbinger of HIV in homosexual men.[36,37] The development of HZ in patients at risk for HIV may be a sign of the presence of HIV infection.[37] Recently the use of anti-tumor necrosis factor alpha (anti-TNF alpha) monoclonal antibodies has been associated with an increased incidence of HZ.[38]

Herpes zoster in the immunocompromised host is not just a problem of increased frequency, but the HZ is more severe.[39] Morbidity is more problematic than mortality.

DERMATOMAL HERPES ZOSTER

Dermatomal HZ is the most common presentation of HZ. A single dermatome with a few scattered erythematous patches with vesicles may be present or multiple contiguous dermatomes (usually less than three) may be involved. Large vesicles or bullae (1–2 cm) and pustules, some of which are certainly umbilicated, may coalesce. Hemorrhagic bulla and marked epidermal necrosis with extensive ulcerations and black eschars may occur. These can slough, producing extensive scarring of the entire dermatome necessitating skin grafting. The necrosis may not be restricted to skin. Hall et al. described HZ of cranial nerve five with necrosis of the underlying maxilla and alveolar bone in a patient with reticulum cell sarcoma on systemic steroids.[40]

The incidence of HZ may be increased in locally immunosuppressed sites such as the areas of primary tumors or in radiation portals. HZ may develop at skin sites overlying nodal involvement of lymphoma or other tumors.[41] HZ may develop at incision sites, suggesting that surgery may serve as a local precipitating factor.[42] Recurrent dermatomal HZ, usually at a different site, is a problem most often seen in HIV-positive patients.

Non-contiguous multidermatomal HZ is very rare in both immunocompetent and immunocompromised persons. Most cases have been limited to two non-contiguous dermatomes. This unusual presentation has been referred to as zoster duplex unilateralis or bilateralis depending on whether one or both halves of the body are involved. When more than two non-contiguous dermatomes are involved it has been termed zoster multiplex. Reported cases have described 2–7 non-contiguous widely separated dermatomes.[43] The clinical appearance of these patients is usually that of typical HZ but the lesions may be more ulcerative and necrotic, and they may scar more severely.

Monodermatomal HZ has masqueraded as disseminated HZ in a woman with breast cancer secondary to her transverse rectus abdominus myocutaneous (TRAM) flap reconstruction. The TRAM procedure realigned the nerves and created a pseudodisseminated VZV.[44]

DISSEMINATED HERPES ZOSTER

Dissemination of HZ is defined as cutaneous disease in more than three contiguous dermatomes, more than 20 lesions scattered outside of the initial dermatomal lesions, or systemic involvement. Systemic involvement usually follows the rash with pneumonitis, meningoencephalitis, and rarely hepatitis with acute liver failure which may be fatal. Visceral dissemination of VZV, as often reported in immunocompromised patients, is very uncommon in persons with acquired immune deficiency syndrome (AIDS).[45] Disseminated VZV can present with an acute abdomen, small bowel pseudo-obstruction, or pneumatosis intestinalis that precedes or occurs in the absence of skin involvement (zoster sine herpete). The clinical triad of severe abdominal pain, hyponatremia from SIADH (syndrome of inappropriate anti-diuretic hormone), and disseminated HZ has been reported after stem cell transplantation or conventional chemotherapy.[46,47]

Visceral zoster can present months after bone marrow transplantation with poorly localized abdominal pain that precedes the skin eruption by as much as 3 weeks (average is 6 days), with evolving pancreatitis, hepatitis, and paralytic ileus.[48] The pain was epigastric, occasionally involving the right upper quadrant or radiating to the back.[49] Intestinal VZV can cause mucosal necrosis and hemorrhage while invasion of the neural plexi can lead to paralytic ileus. Hemorrhagic infarction of the abdominal sympathetic ganglia with colonic dilatation, acute pseudo-obstruction of the colon (Ogilvie's syndrome), is one cause of abdominal pain with VZV reactivation.[50,51] In ten bone marrow transplant (BMT) recipients with visceral zoster who presented with abdominal pain and elevated serum transaminases with subsequent skin lesions, the case fatality rate was 50% despite antiviral therapy.[48] Early detection of blood VZV DNA by polymerase chain reaction (PCR)[50,51] in the appropriate clinical setting (unexplained abdominal pain, hepatitis, SIADH, and/or biochemical evidence of pancreatitis without biliary obstruction in the immunosuppressed patient without vesicular skin lesions) should facilitate earlier, empiric treatment with acyclovir.[46,48]

Disseminated VZV infection clinically mimicking vasculitis in a patient with rheumatoid arthritis on the TNF alpha blocking agent etanercept was reported presenting with hemorrhagic and necrotic lesions of the lower extremities.[52] Atypical varicella initially presented mimicking hand foot and mouth disease in a 35-year-old woman during chemotherapy for a diffuse large B cell lymphoma. One week later she developed a disseminated febrile vesicular eruption of VZV.[53]

The vaccine strain of varicella (attenuated Oka strain of VZV) has produced disseminated life threatening infection when inadvertently administered to immunocompromised patients.[54]

Another form of disseminated HZ seen almost exclusively in HIV-positive patients, but also in patients with leukemia, lymphoma,[55] and multiple myeloma,[56] is described oxymoronically as "recurrent primary varicella" or atypical recurrent varicella. These patients develop one or more episodes (relapsing chicken pox) of disseminated VZ in the absence of an initial dermatomal distribution which is usually painful and characteristic of HZ (shingles). This presentation is clinically indistinguishable from varicella (except for (a) the occasional paucity of lesions, (b) the larger diameter of lesions (1–4 cm), (c) the same stage of development of all lesions, and (d) the prolonged healing time) and can be separated by the presence of antibody evidence of previous VZV infection (IgG positive, IgM negative). Clinical histories of varicella may not be reliable, and the absence of varicella antibody does not necessarily confirm the infection as primary, especially in HIV-infected[57] patients or elderly immunosuppressed patients who may lose antibody over time.[58] The alternative explanation to recurrent endogenous outbreaks is exogenous reinfection with VZ virus in an immunocompromised adult. Even with a history of previous chicken pox and detectable antibodies to VZ virus, the immunosuppressed patient has a risk of chicken pox after exposure to it.[59]

CHRONIC HERPES ZOSTER

HZ persisting for more than 1 month is seen almost exclusively in HIV infected patients with low CD4 counts and occasionally in organ transplant recipients receiving immunosuppressive medications or in patients undergoing cancer chemotherapy regimens.[60] Chronic or persistent HZ occurs in three forms:

1. Hyperkeratotic HZ with persistently thickly crusted verrucous lesions which may be seen alone or in association with vesicular or ulcerated lesions.[61-63] They are usually very chronic (months or years) and are often resistant to acyclovir. The unusual appearance of the hyperkeratotic lesions may be due to coinfection with other organisms such as *Candida albicans*, *Mycobacterium-avium* complex (MAC) or *Pityrosporum* species.

2. Ecthymatous crusted punched out ulcerations with thick overlying eschar or central black eschar characteristically not surrounded by erythema. They may be surrounded by a rim of vesicles.[45] Chronic ulcerative HZ up to 10 cm has been reported.[64]

3. Disseminated cutaneous lesions described as vesicular, nodular, hyperkeratotic, necrotic, pox-like[65] or pinpoint-sized papules.[66]

In all of these forms of chronic HZ, there is continued prolonged active infection by VZ virus. These atypical chronic skin lesions can occur in HIV-positive patients who have received reduced or so-called maintenance doses (which are subtherapeutic) of acyclovir for prolonged courses. Many of the reported cases of chronic VZ are acyclovir resistant; however, the drug resistance of VZ virus isolated from one given lesion may vary over time.[67]

Chronic HZ can produce an annular translucent plaque with rolled border and pinpoint hemorrhage mimicking a basal cell carcinoma, but the histopathology demonstrates viral folliculitis.[68] In these immunosuppressed patients, chronic VZV can: (1) follow varicella (in this situation the lesions show no tendency toward healing and progressively become verrucous or hyperkeratotic in appearance), (2) develop directly from HZ, with slow progression from a zosteriform eruption to hyperkeratotic papulonodules, or (3) occur with no evidence of classic dermatomal HZ.[67]

Although chronic VZ infection in the HIV-seronegative immunosuppressed patients has been described, it is an uncommon manifestation.[69]

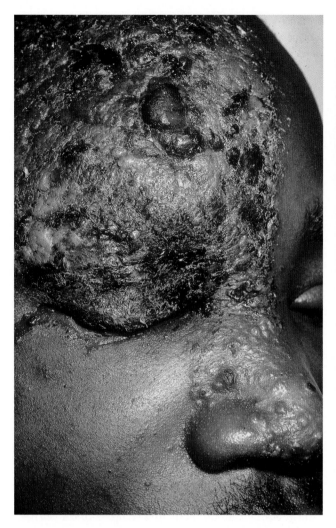

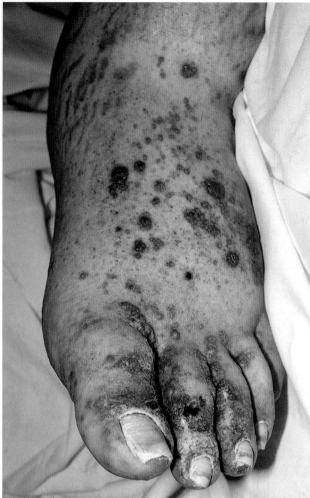

Figure 6.39. Coalescent bullae progressing to epidermal necrosis of herpes zoster involving the first division of the trigeminal nerve in a patient on systemic steroids for sarcoidosis

Figure 6.40. Hemorrhagic bullae of dermatomal herpes zoster in a 30-year-old patient receiving chemotherapy for a non-Hodgkin's lymphoma

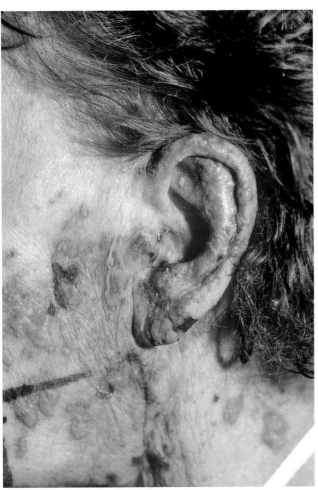

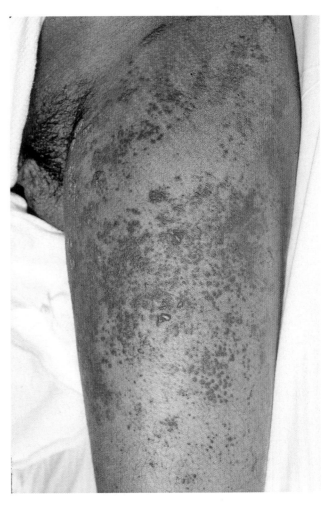

Figure 6.41. Herpes zoster developed in the radiation portal for a squamous cell carcinoma of the oropharynx

Figure 6.42. Small purpuric vesicles of dermatomal herpes zoster in a renal transplant patient

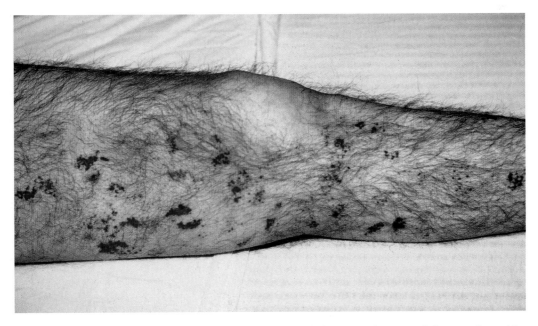

Figure 6.43. Skin biopsy-proven herpes zoster in a patient on systemic steroids for temporal arteritis. Only grouped petechiae and purpuric papules in a dermatomal distribution were visible

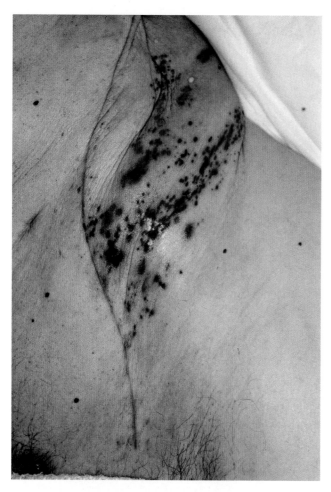

Figure 6.44. Herpes zoster stopped at the nephrectomy scar (for renal cell carcinoma)

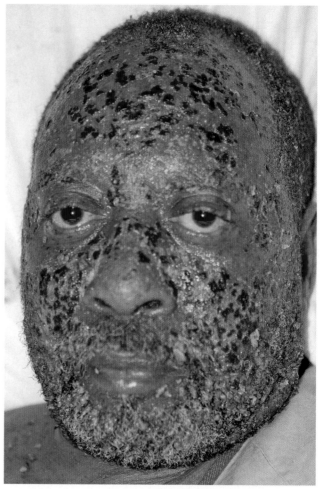

Figure 6.45. A 57-year-old man with a bilateral lung transplant and disseminated herpes zoster with fatal fulminant hepatic failure

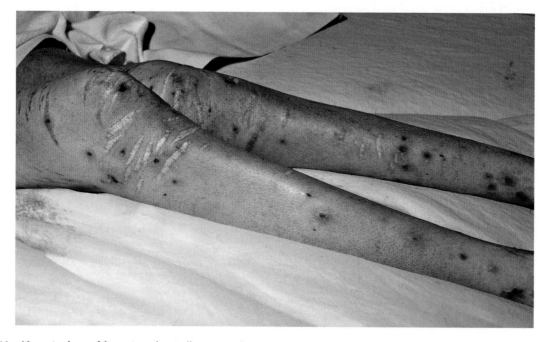

Figure 6.46. Necrotic ulcers of disseminated varicella-zoster infection in a teenager on long-term systemic steroids for glomerulonephritis

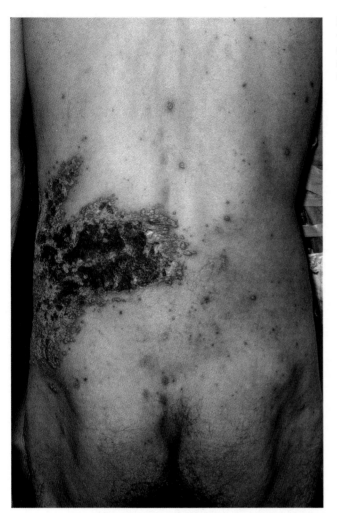

Figure 6.47. Dermatomal and disseminated cutaneous lesions of varicella-zoster (VZ) infection in an HIV-positive intravenous drug abuser. Vesicular, pustular, and ulcerative lesions involve the L1–L3 dermatomes. More than 100 discrete VZ lesions are scattered over the body

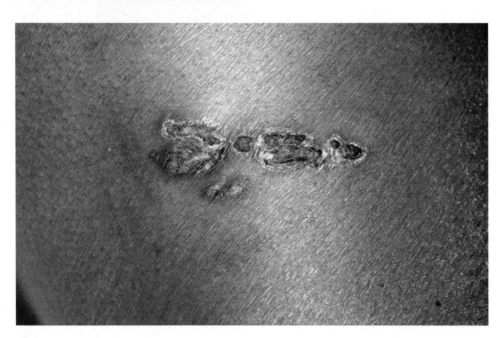

Figure 6.48. Hyperkeratotic papules of chronic varicella-zoster infection in the T11–T12 dermatome of an HIV-positive intravenous drug abuser. The lesion healed with debridement and oral acyclovir

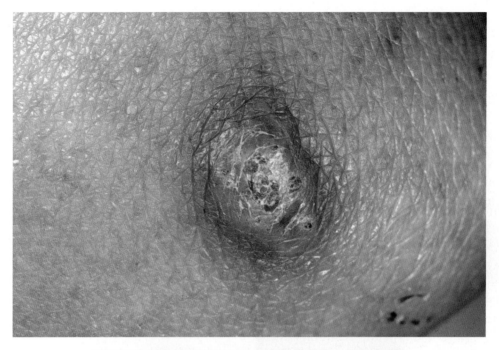

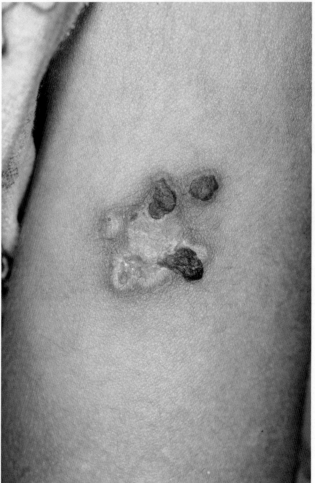

Figure 6.49.–6.51.　Chronic varicella-zoster in three HIV-positive patients. All direct fluorescent antibody and/or culture positive

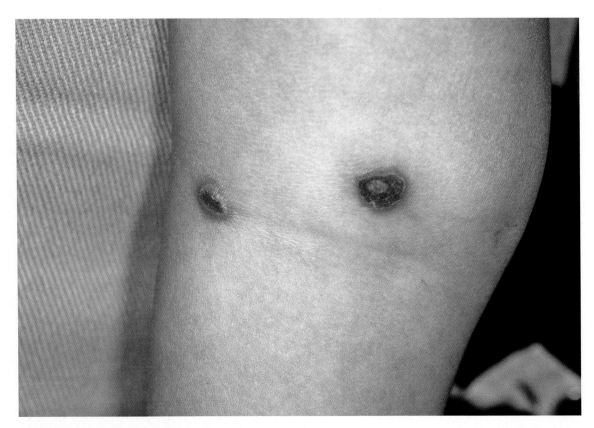

Figure 6.51.

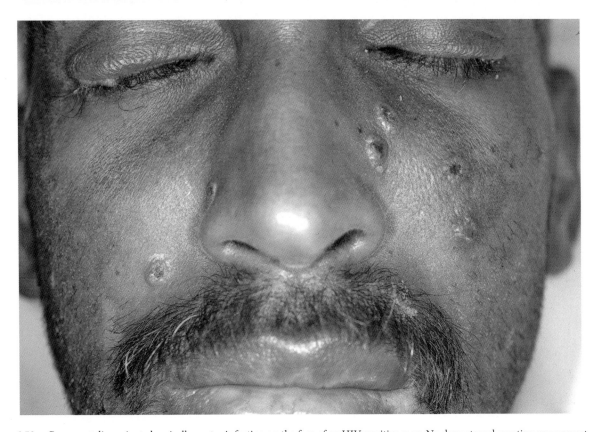

Figure 6.52. Recurrent disseminated varicella-zoster infection on the face of an HIV-positive man. No dermatomal eruption was present

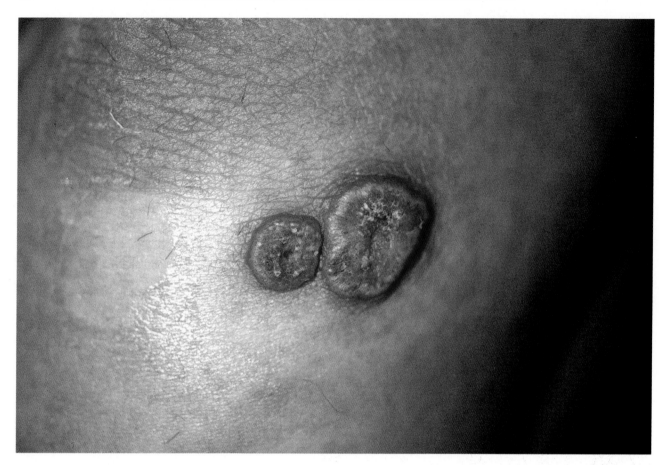

Figure 6.53. A 24-year-old woman with chronic and recurrent varicella zoster over 4 months was her initial manifestation of HIV disease. These pustular vegetative plaques of VZ were on her arm

Molluscum Contagiosum

Molluscum contagiosum (MC), a large DNA virus of the pox virus family, mainly affects children with normal immunity, sexually active adults, and immunocompromised individuals. In children, the infection occurs on the face, chest, abdomen, and extremities. The disease is often sexually transmitted in adults, and lesions occur on the genitalia, lower portion of the abdomen, and upper thighs. Typical lesions of MC are centrally umbilicated shiny papules 3–5 mm in diameter. In otherwise healthy hosts, MC is usually a self-limited cutaneous infection often with fewer than 20 lesions which may resolve spontaneously within 3–12 months.

MC should be recognized as a cutaneous marker of severe immunodeficiency. In adults whose HIV status is unknown, molluscum contagiosum may be the first sign of HIV infection. The prevalence of MC in HIV infections ranges from 5% to 18%. The severity of MC infection has been shown to be inversely related to the patient's CD4 count. Extensive MC may serve as a marker of poor prognosis or advanced stage of HIV disease.[70] Settings other than HIV disease have been reported with widespread recurrent MC in adults, including sarcoidosis; atopic dermatitis; leukemia; lymphoma; thymoma; organ transplantation; following treatment of mycosis fungoides and erythroderma with prednisone and methotrexate, idiopathic CD4 positive lymphopenia[71]; and psoriasis treated with methotrexate, TNF alpha antagonists (infliximab), or CD11A antibody (efalizumab). Giant or extensive lesions have been reported after splenectomy and in Wiskott-Aldrich syndrome. MC is a rare cutaneous complication of immunosuppressed patients but common in HIV-infected patients.

In patients immunocompromised by either their primary disease or their therapy, MC has been clinically characterized by a large number of lesions, unusual distribution, atypical appearance, large size, resistance to treatment, and rapid recurrence. The infection is not self-limited and may spread widely. Severe cases of MC may rapidly develop with hundreds of lesions. The lesions are frequently localized to the face and scalp rather than the genital area. Numerous MC may be so confluent as to give the face a cobblestone appearance or coalesce to form a large plaque. Extensive MC in the beard area is common and suggests that the infection can be spread by shaving. Viral folliculitis of the face caused by MC produced multiple flesh to red-colored papules symmetrically distributed on the chin and cheeks in a lung transplant recipient mimicking tinea barbae.[72] Facial MC may be disfiguring and recalcitrant to treatment.[73] In addition to the well-known extensive periorbital and eyelid involvement in HIV-infected patients, MC can rarely involve the conjunctival cornea.

Giant nodular lesions of MC, with a diameter greater than 10–15 mm, are frequently seen. The MC may become erythematous, lobulated, or verrucous nodules with central necrosis measuring 15–20 mm on the face or scalp. The individual lesions may become atypical in appearance and may be mistaken for a cutaneous horn, a basal cell carcinoma, or a keratoacanthoma. Disseminated cryptococcosis, histoplasmosis, and other infections (see Chap. 16, Differential Diagnosis) have also been reported mimicking MC. Biopsies should be performed for a definitive diagnosis in patients with atypical MC or what one "thinks" is atypical MC in the HIV patient, especially with signs of a systemic illness (particularly headache or pulmonary infiltrates). In contrast to the rare occurrence of two infective organisms in the same cutaneous lesion, coexistent histopathological features of both cutaneous cryptococcosis and histoplasmosis with molluscum contagiosum can be found in AIDS patients with severe immunosuppression.[74]

Other unusual manifestations of MC include: a cold facial abscess in an HIV-positive patient with a history of disseminated MC[75] and intraoral MC occurring as a gingival mass.[76]

MC in the HIV population is usually resistant to conventional therapy. MC in the immunosuppressed individual is often recalcitrant to treatment, persists, or recurs following each effort to treat, running a chronic, relapsing course.

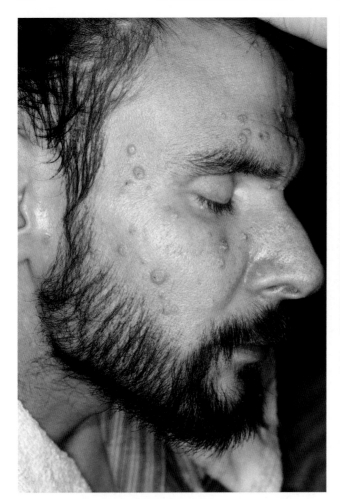

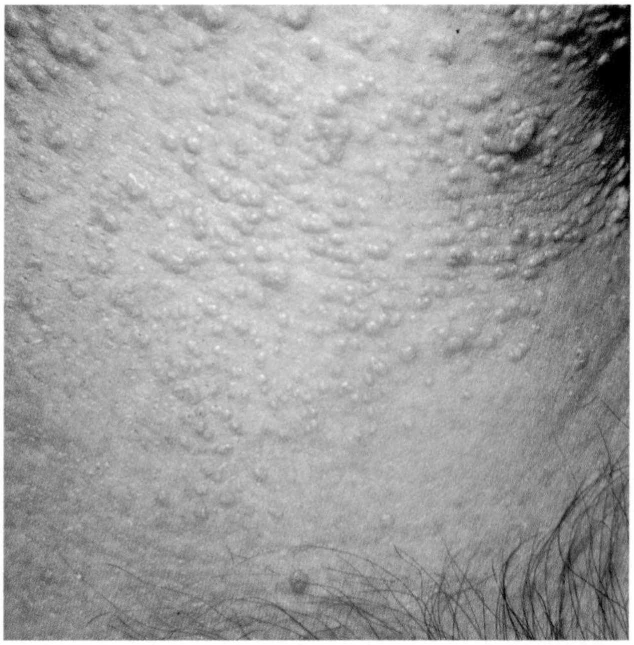

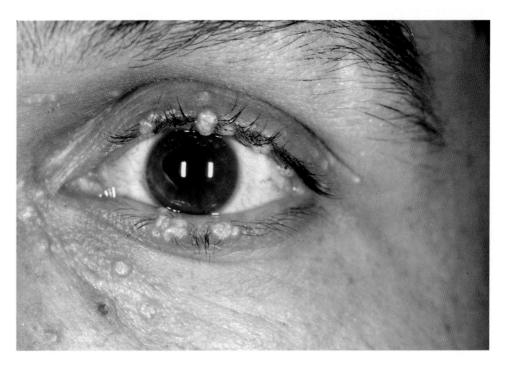

Figure 6.56. Innumerable molluscum on the neck of an HIV-positive man producing a cobblestone appearance

Figure 6.54. Multiple giant molluscum contagiosum in an HIV-positive man

Figure 6.55. Molluscum on the eyelids and periorbital region of an HIV-positive man

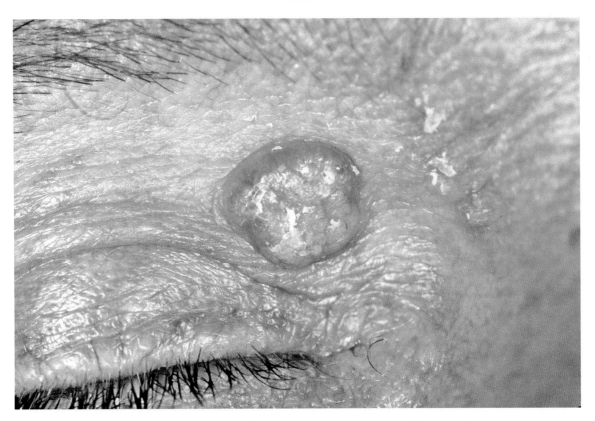

Figure 6.57. Giant molluscum mimicking a cutaneous malignancy on the upper eyelid of an HIV-positive man

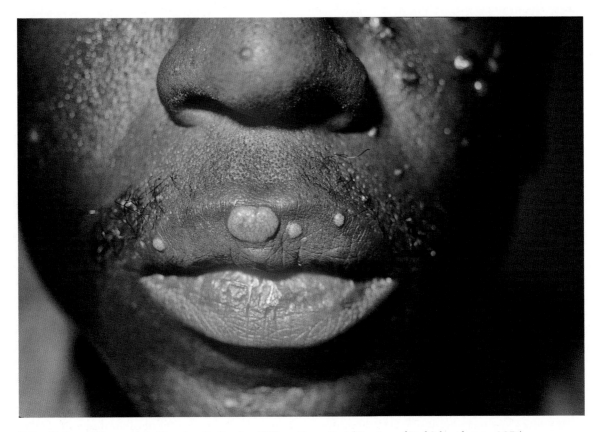

Figure 6.58. Molluscum in an atypical location, the lip of an HIV-positive patient (Courtesy of Paul Schneiderman, M.D.)

CYTOMEGALOVIRUS

Cytomegalovirus (CMV), along with herpes simplex virus (HSV), varicella-zoster virus (VZV), Epstein-Barr virus (EBV), and human herpes virus (HHV-6,7,8), belongs to the Herpesviridae family. CMV (HHV-5) is a common human viral infection affecting 40–100% of adults worldwide. Acute infections are often asymptomatic, but once the infection is acquired, there is a lifelong latency along with the risk of intermittent reactivation. CMV disease in the immunocompromised host can be the result of either a primary CMV infection in a previously uninfected (seronegative) host, reactivation of latent virus, or reinfection with a new virus subtype. Most CMV disease is due to reactivation of latent virus. CMV infections may appear rapidly following iatrogenic immunosuppression in organ transplantation, cancer chemotherapy, and steroid therapy, or insidiously in states of gradual progressive immunosuppression in HIV/AIDS. The patterns of organ involvement and clinical disease vary among different immunocompromised patient groups with some manifestations characteristic, such as retinitis in HIV-infected individuals, gastrointestinal ulceration (esophagitis and proctocolitis) and hepatitis in solid organ transplant recipients, and interstitial pneumonitis and myelosuppression in bone marrow transplant recipients.[77] Skin manifestations of CMV are rare in any setting, and diagnosis is often delayed owing to the difficulty demonstrating CMV in tissue.

CMV infection in the skin is probably more common than the paucity of reports would suggest because of a variable and confusing clinical picture, histologically occult infection, and simultaneous presence of other infectious pathogens. Cutaneous manifestations of CMV infection are not sufficiently distinctive to allow the diagnosis to be made on clinical findings alone. If one excludes patients with the rashes non-specifically associated with CMV infection (either because of failure to do a skin biopsy or because of nonspecific findings on biopsy) and those patients without skin lesions in whom CMV was inadvertently found in the skin at autopsy, the remaining patients with histologically CMV-positive skin lesions are predominantly those with ulcers and those with maculopapular exanthems. The most common manifestation of CMV infection in the skin is a chronic ulcer of the anal, perianal, or anogenital area. The ulcers may be single or multiple, some with satellite lesions, painful (occasionally non-painful), and vary in size (as large as 15 cm). The borders are sharply marginated, round, oval, or irregular, and raised or verrucous. The correct diagnosis relies on culture and histopathologic examination because of the identical appearance of chronic ulcerations caused by herpes simplex virus in the immunocompromised host. In addition, HSV may present superficially in ulcers coinfected with CMV; superficial HSV infection in perianal ulcers which appears refractory to antiviral treatment in an AIDS patient may be due to underlying CMV.[78] Deep cutaneous biopsies of ulcerated lesions with profuse exudate are needed to diagnose CMV co-infection. Perianal CMV ulcers may occur because of: (1) fecal shedding of the reactivated virus present anywhere latent along the gastrointestinal tract, particularly the colon which has a special tropism for the virus and is frequently colonized, (2) spread from contiguous CMV procto-colitis, (3) the affinity of CMV for granulation tissue in ulcers, and (4) reinfection through anal intercourse reaching the anogenital area hematogenously.[79]

The cardinal manifestation of CMV infection in the skin is a chronic ulcer.[79] Lee reported a large cutaneous ulcer of the chest (10 × 7 cm) at the site of extravasated intravenous (IV) fluid in a liver transplant recipient and multiple small ulcers in the area of a healed surgical wound in a heart transplant recipient.[80] Weiss et al. reported multiple small ulcers due to CMV that were initially confused with an exacerbation of the patient's Wegner's granulomatosis.[81] Colsky et al. reported multiple painful skin ulcerations on the arms and back misdiagnosed initially as pyodermic gangrenosum.[82] The largest ulcer (8 × 15 cm) was undermined with thick black central eschars and a purulent exudate. Husain et al. described ulcers on the thigh and hand of an HIV-infected woman with pulmonary infiltrates, hepatitis, and retinitis which resolved with ganciclovir.[83]

Although uncommon, oral manifestations of CMV infection have included painful erosions or ulcers of the tongue, buccal mucosa, and pharynx.

Similar to the chronic perianal ulcers, CMV and HSV have been documented simultaneously in the same skin ulcer of the lower lip in a patient with AIDS.[84]

Widespread exanthematous, maculopapular, or morbilliform eruptions often with petechiae or purpura[84,85] may be a specific cutaneous lesion of CMV infection. Unlike the nonspecific maculopapular eruption in patients treated with ampicillin (analogous to the eruption that occurs with ampicillin and EBV infection/infectious mononucleosis or sulfonamides and HIV infection), characteristic large intranuclear inclusions with a surrounding halo, or "owl's eye" of CMV, can be demonstrated in endothelial cells of dermal or subcutaneous vessels in the morbilliform eruptions directly due to CMV[86] and confirmed with immunoperoxidase stain. The swollen endothelial cells may evolve into an obstructive endothelitis, capillaritis, and small vessel vasculitis with accompanying evolution of skin lesions from morbilliform eruption to petechiae, palpable purpura,[87,88] or infarction and ulceration.[89]

Other morphologies of CMV in the immunocompromised host which may be the first clue to systemic CMV infection have included: hyperpigmented and indurated areas of the thighs[90]; a 4-cm verrucous plaque with central ulceration of the heel in a patient with AIDS[91]; crusted papules of the face and arms due to simultaneous CMV, *Staphylococcus aureus,* and an acid-fast bacillus in a patient with AIDS[92]; scattered verrucous cone-shaped plaques with central ulceration or necrosis associated with CMV viremia in a patient with AIDS[91]; perifollicular papulopustules on the back of a heart/lung transplant recipient with CMV pneumonitis; and a generalized vesiculobullous eruption with multinucleate giant cells on Tzanck smear and skin biopsy considered to be diagnostic of HSV or VZV in a patient with necrotizing vasculitis on cyclophosphamide and steroids. Viral cultures confirmed the diagnosis of CMV infection (skin, esophagus, lung) rather than the more likely disseminated HSV or VZV.[93]

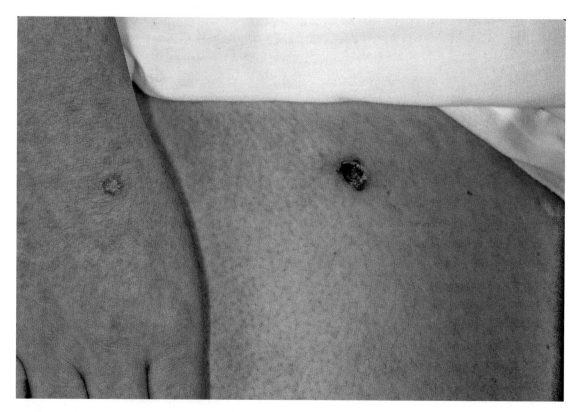

Figure 6.59. Hemorrhagic crusted ulcerations on the proximal thigh and hand due to biopsy-proven cytomegalovirus (CMV) confirmed by immunoperoxidase stain in a 27-year-old woman with AIDS

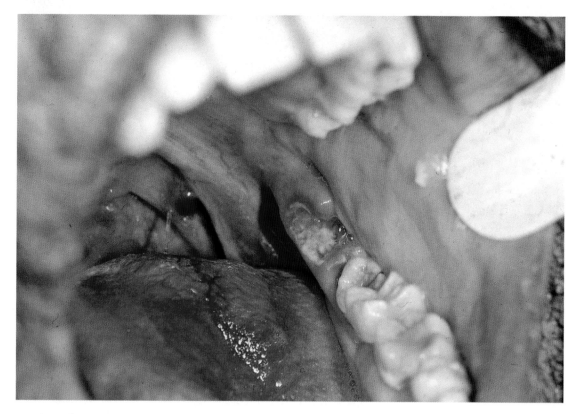

Figure 6.60. CMV ulcer on the alveolar ridge of a patient with AIDS

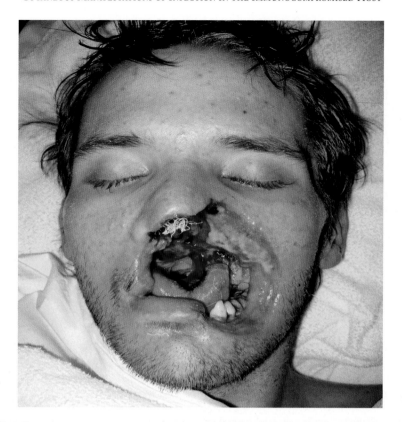

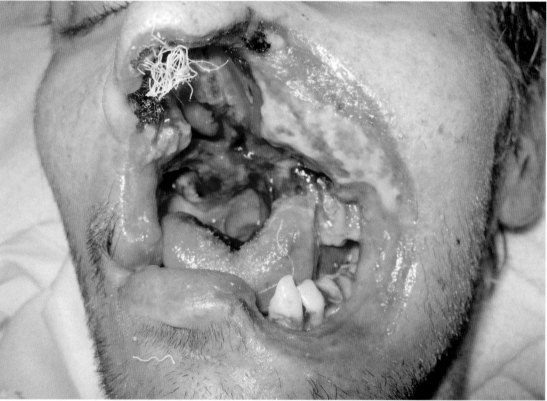

Figure 6.61.–6.64.   A 28-year-old man with HIV/AIDS (CD4 20 cells/μL) who was found at home with a 4–6 week history of painful central facial necrosis (Figs. 6.61 and 6.62). Facial cultures from debrided tissue were negative for bacterial, fungal, mycobacterial, or viral organism. Blood culture was positive for *Eggerthella lenta*. Biopsy of his hard palate revealed multinucleated giant cells with viral inclusions (Fig. 6.63). CMV staining of the hard palate biopsy was positive for cytomegalovirus (Fig. 6.64) (Figures 6.62–6.64 courtesy of Deborah Goddard, M.D.)

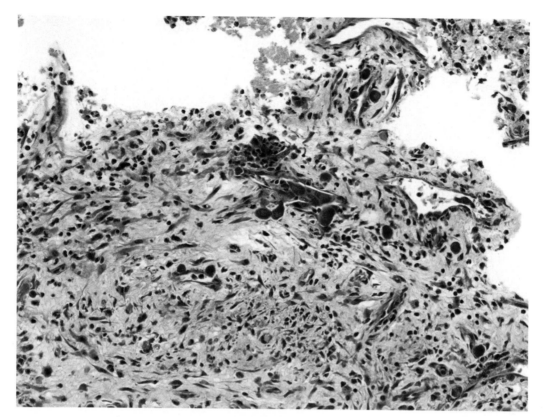

Figure 6.63.

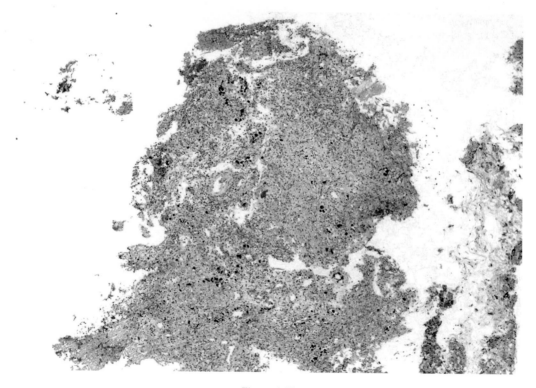

Figure 6.64.

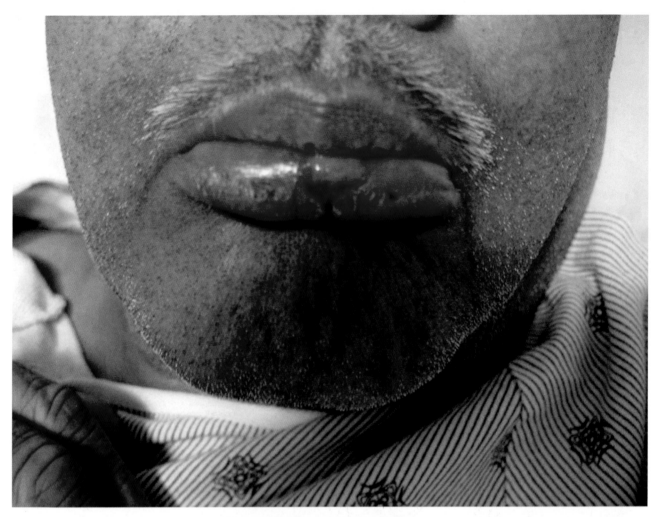

Figure 6.65.   A 58-year-old heart transplant recipient presented with a lip ulceration. Biopsy of the ulcer revealed multinucleated giant cells in the dermis with inclusion bodies and immunoperoxidase staining of cytomegalovirus (Courtesy of Deborah Goddard, M.D.)

Human Papillomavirus

Infection with human papillomavirus (HPV) is among the most common viral infections of skin and is responsible for simple warts on glabrous skin, genital warts (condyloma accuminata), and bowenoid papulosis (which is histologically indistinguishable from Bowen's disease or squamous cell carcinoma in situ). There are over 120 recognized subtypes of HPV, many with predilection for certain anatomic sites (HPV-6 and 11 cause 90% of genital warts) and some with oncogenic potential (particularly HPV 16, 18, 34, and 39 in genital lesions, HPV16 in digital and periungual skin, and HPV 5 and 8 in *epidermodysplasia verruciformis*).

Although both immunocompetent and immunosuppressed patients may be infected with HPV, lesions may be recalcitrant and difficult to control, morphologically more numerous, extensive and exuberant, painful, deeply affecting the patients' quality of life, and more numerous in the absence of a normal functioning immune system. Viral warts increase in prevalence with the duration of immunosuppression. Warts in immuno-compromised patients may be associated with novel HPV sub-types. Eighty percent of organ transplant recipients may develop some warts.[94] Immunosuppression with TOR inhibitors (target-of-rapamycin, i.e., sirolimus, everolimus) may have reduced incidence of HPV infection, and possibly CMV, compared to calcineurin inhibitors (i.e., cyclosporine, tacrolimus).[94]

HPV has the appearance of gray, brown, or flesh-colored, sessile or pedunculated, exophytic papules, plaques, or tumors on the penis, vulva, cervix, anus, perineal or perianal areas, glabrous skin, or anal cavity. They may present as one lesion or multifocal lesions ranging in size from millimeters to centimeters. Increased proliferation of lesions is associated with pulse immunosupression during transplant rejection, progressive immunosuppression, or during immune reconstitution after initiation of HAART in HIV disease.

Genital warts (condyloma accuminata, CA) are common. It is estimated that 1–2% of all sexually active individuals in the USA have CA, and the incidence has been increasing steadily since the 1950s. In the immunocompromised host,[95] CA may be recurrent, recalcitrant to therapy, become widespread, and form large confluent disfiguring cauliflower-like masses becoming several centimeters in size. While common CA are benign, HPV associated giant CA also known as Buschke-Lowenstein tumor (BLT) on the penis or perianal area may manifest clinically as malignant disease (verrucous carcinoma). BLTs do not metastasize and have a benign histology. However, BLTs have the potential for expansive and destructive growth with malignant transformation occurring in up to 50% of cases.[96] The destruction of local tissues by BLT can cause pain, bleeding, pruritus, fistulae, mechanical obstruction interfering with defecation, and bacterial colonization of the fistulae with abscess formation and sepsis. Paradoxical worsening of BLT as a consequence of immune reconstitution syndrome after the start of HAART has been reported.

Reports of unusual morphologies and HPV subtypes associated with immunosuppression have included:

- Generalized gingival enlargement which appeared typical of drug-induced gingival hypertrophy with extensive papillomatosis of the palate exhibiting dysplasia and HPV in a renal transplant patient.[97]
- HPV type 7, the cause of "butcher's wart" and normally not associated with persons who are not meat handlers, being commonly found in the oral mucosa and facial skin of HIV-seropositive patients.[98]
- Tinea versicolor–like lesions of acquired epidermodysplasia verruciformis, which are positive mainly for HPV types 5 and 8 in HIV-positive patients.[99]
- Urethral and bladder condylomata caused by HPV 6 presenting as hematuria in an HIV-seropositive man.[100]
- Disseminated HPV type 11 (a mucosal type of virus that infects the genital tract or larynx) involving the arms, hands, axillae, chest, abdomen, thighs, and genitalia in a patient with pemphigus vulgaris receiving systemic steroids, cyclophosphamide, and IVIg.[101]

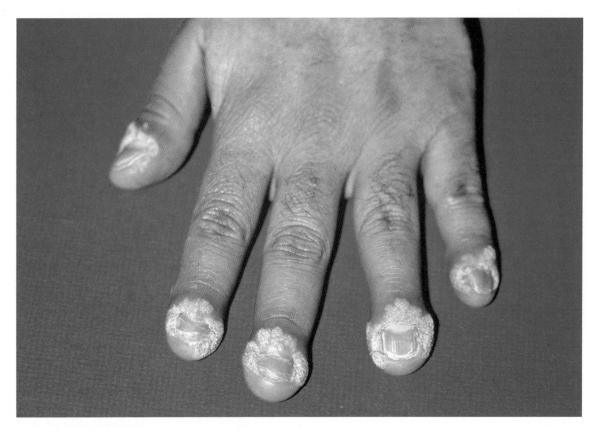

Figure 6.66. Extensive periungual warts in an HIV-positive patient

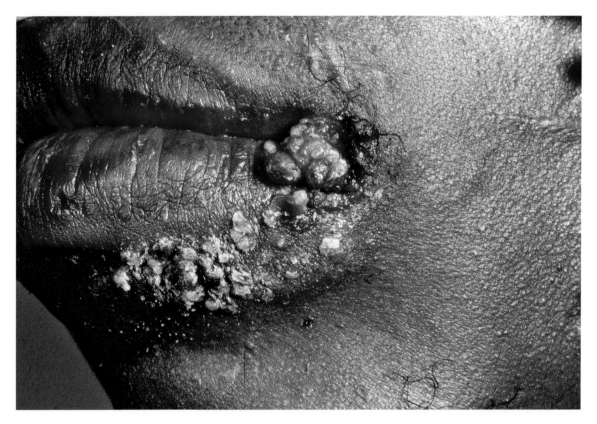

Figure 6.67. A plaque of warts involving the oral commissure of a patient with AIDS

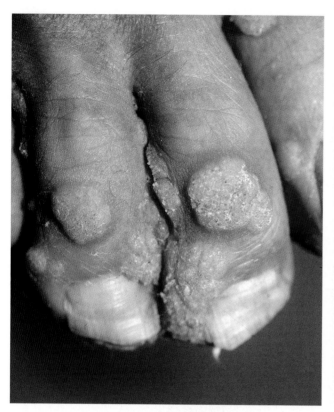

Figure 6.68. Multiple digital and kissing interdigital warts in a renal transplant patient (Courtesy of Robert Kalb, M.D.)

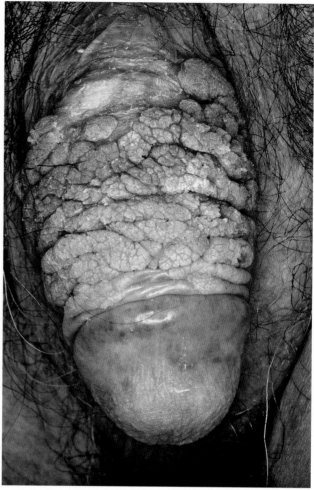

Figure 6.69. Warts coalescing to cover the shaft of the penis of an HIV-positive man (Courtesy of Robert Kalb, M.D.)

Figure 6.70. Profuse anal warts in an HIV-positive man (Courtesy of Robert Kalb, M.D.)

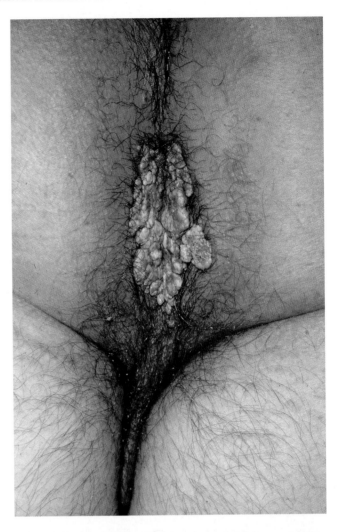

Figure 6.71. Multiple intraoral warts involving the gingival and labial mucosa of a man with a 20-year history of chronic lymphocytic leukemia (Courtesy of David J. Zegarelli, D.D.S.)

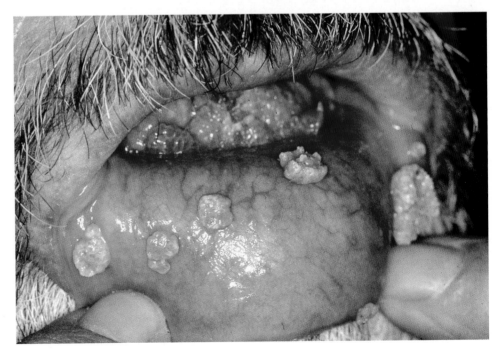

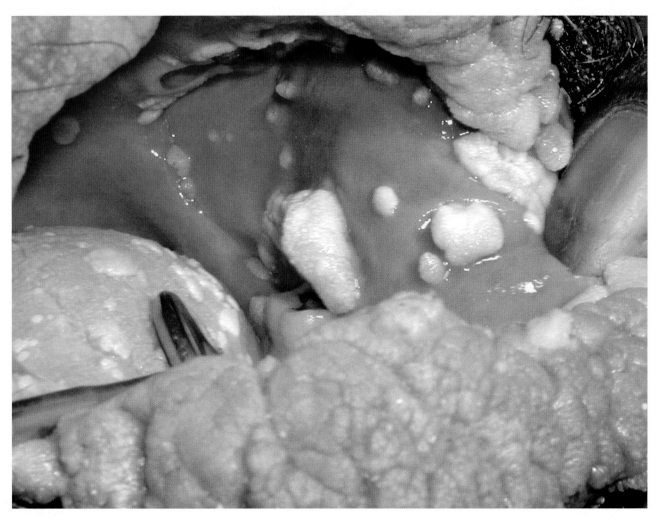

Figure 6.72. Florid oral warts of the lips, tongue, and mucosal epithelium in a 49-year old African American male with HIV (Courtesy of Eric Stoopler, D.M.D.)

WEST NILE VIRUS INFECTION

West Nile Virus infection (WNV) is caused by a neurotropic RNA virus that belongs to the genus flavivirus. WNV is maintained and amplified in nature in wild birds (Passerine birds, sparrows) and American crows (*Corvus brachyrynchos*). These birds are the principal host, and the infection is transmitted to humans by the *Culex* mosquito bird-feeding species, its main vectors. WNV can be transmitted through organ transplantation, blood transfusion, breast feeding, and intrauterine transmission from mother to fetus. WNV was first isolated from the blood of a febrile woman in the West Nile district of Uganda in 1937. In 1999, WNV caused an outbreak for the first time in the western hemisphere in New York City. Since then WNV has rapidly expanded geographically to nearly all areas of the USA and Canada. WNV infection typically occurs from July through December, peaking from late August to early September.

WNV infection in the normal host is characterized by asymptomatic infection or the acute onset of fever, headache, fatigue, malaise, muscle pain, weakness, gastrointestinal symptoms, and rash lasting up to 1 week.[102] Neuroinvasive disease develops in less than 1% of WNV-infected persons.

Differences between the course of WNV infection in immunocompromised patients versus normal individuals include: (1) the average incubation period tends to be longer in immunocompromised patients, with an average of 13.5 days versus 8 days for a normal host, but can be up to 21 days in immunocompromised patients; (2) immunosuppressed patients may have prolonged viremia, delayed development of antibodies, and increased likelihood of severe disease, particularly neuroinvasive disease[103] (the serious neurologic manifestations in immunocompromised patients include aseptic meningitis, acute flaccid paralysis (similar to that seen with acute poliomyelitis), and encephalitis which can be fatal); (3) a higher mortality rate; and (4) a decreased incidence of skin rash.[104] The rash has most often been described as a generalized maculopapular, macular, or morbilliform eruption, sparing the palms, soles, face, and mucosa. The incidence of rash in the normal population with WNV infection was up to 60–80%. Rash was infrequently reported or not reported at all in the small published series of immunocompromised patients and not described with dysesthesias (generalized tingling or burning), hyperesthesia, or severe pain as reported in the normal population.[105] Pruritus was infrequently mentioned.

REFERENCES

Herpes Simplex

1. Toback AL, Grossman ME. Chronic intraoral herpes simplex infection in renal transplant recipients. Transplant Proc. 1986;18:966–9.
2. Grossman ME, Stevens AW, Cohen PR. Herpetic geometric glossitis. N Engl J Med. 1993;329:1859–60.
3. Cohen PR, Kazi S, Grossman ME. Herpetic geometric glossitis: a distinctive pattern of lingual herpes simplex virus infection. South Med J. 1995;88:1231–5.
4. Burgoyne M, Burke W. Atypical herpes simplex infection in patients with acute myelogenous leukemia recovering from chemotherapy. J Am Acad Dermatol. 1989;20:1125.
5. Husak R, Tebbe B, Goerdt S, et al. Pseudotumour of the tongue caused by herpes simplex virus type 2 in an HIV-1 infected immunosuppressed patient. Br J Dermatol. 1998;139:118–21.
6. Kalb RE, Grossman ME. Chronic perianal herpes simplex in immunocompromised hosts. Am J Med. 1986;80:486–90.
7. Patel AB, Rosen T. Herpes vegetans as a sign of HIV infection. Dermatol Online J. 2008;14(4):6.
8. Römer A, Greiner A, Enk A, Hartschuh W. Herpes simplex vegetans: atypical genital herpes infection with prominent plasma cell infiltration in B-cell chronic lymphocytic leukemia. J Dtsch Dermatol Ges. 2008;6:865–7.
9. Lieb JA, Brisman S, Herman S, Macgregor J, Grossman ME. Linear erosive herpes simplex virus infection in immunocompromised patients: the "knife-cut sign". Clin Infect Dis. 2008;47:1440–1.
10. Hanjani NM, Foster DC, Scott GA, Mercurio MG. A genital mass due to herpes simplex virus in a renal transplant recipient. J Low Genit Tract Dis. 2007;11:173–6.
11. Holmes A, McMenamin M, Mulcahy F, Bergin C. Thalidomide therapy for the treatment of hypertrophic herpes simplex virus-related genitalis in HIV-infected individuals. Clin Infect Dis. 2007;44: e96–9.
12. Tong P, Mutasim DF. Herpes simplex virus infection masquerading as condyloma acuminate in a patient with HIV disease. Br J Dermatol. 1996;134:797–800.
13. Nadal SR, Calore EE, Manzione CR, et al. Hypertrophic herpes simplex simulating anal neoplasia in AIDS patients: report of five cases. Dis Colon Rectum. 2005;48(12):2289–93.
14. Gubinelli E, Cocuroccia B, Lazzarotto T, Girolomoni G. Nodular perianal herpes simplex with prominent plasma cell infiltration. Sex Transm Dis. 2003;30:157–9.
15. Mosunjac M, Park J, Wang W, et al. Genital and perianal herpes simplex simulating neoplasia in patients with AIDS. AIDS Patient Care STDS. 2009;23(3):153–8.
16. Smith E, Hallman JR, Pardasani A, McMichael A. Multiple herpetic whitlow lesions in a patient with chronic lymphocytic leukemia. Am J Hematol. 2002;69:285–8.
17. Mahmood K, Afzal S. Ulcerating lesions on forearm, fingertips and tongue in a liver-transplant recipient. Clin Exp Dermatol. 2007;33:91–3.
18. Robayna MG, Herranz P, Rubio FA, et al. Destructive herpetic whitlow in AIDS: report of three cases. Br J Dermatol. 1997;137:812–5.
19. Zuretti AR, Schwartz IS. Gangrenous herpetic whitlow in a human immunodeficiency virus-positive patient. Am J Clin Pathol. 1990;93: 828–30.
20. Khera P, Haught JM, McSorley J, English III JC. Atypical presentations of herpesvirus infections in patients with chronic lymphocytic leukemia. J Am Acad Dermatol. 2009;60(3):484–6.
21. Basse G, Mengelle C, Kamar N, et al. Disseminated herpes simplex type-2 (HSV-2) infection after solid-organ transplantation. Infection. 2008;36:62–4.
22. Dinotta F, De Pasquale R, Nasca MR, Tedeschi A, Micali G. Disseminated herpes simplex infection in a HIV+ patient. G Ital Dermatol Venereol. 2009;144:205–9.
23. Arkin LM, Castelo-Soccio L, Kovarik C. Disseminated herpes simplex virus (HSV) hepatitis diagnosed by dermatology evaluation. Int J Dermatol. 2009;48:1017–29.
24. Sevilla J, Fernández-Plaza S, González-Vicent M, et al. Fatal hepatic failure secondary to acute herpes simplex virus infection. J Pediatr Hematol Oncol. 2004;26:686–8.
25. Almeida L, Grossman ME. Benign familial pemphigus complicated by herpes simplex virus. Cutis. 1989;44:261.
26. Masessa JM, Grossman ME, Knobler EH, Bank DE. Kaposi's varicelliform eruption in cutaneous t-cell lymphoma. J Am Acad Dermatol. 1989;21(1):133–5.

27. Castelo-Soccio L, Bernardin R, Stern J, Goldstein SA, Kovarik C. Successful treatment of acyclovir-resistant herpes simplex virus with intralesional cidofovir. Arch Dermatol. 2010;146(2):124–6.

28. Sims CR, Thompson K, Chemaly RF, et al. Oral topical cidofovir: novel route of drug delivery in a severely immunosuppressed patient with refractory multidrug-resistant herpes simplex virus infection. Transpl Infect Dis. 2007;9(3):256–9.

29. Bacon TH, Levin MJ, Leary JJ, Sarisky RT, Sutton D. Herpes simplex virus resistance to acyclovir and penciclovir after two decade of antiviral therapy. Clin Microbiol Rev. 2003;16:114–28.

Human Herpes 6

30. Abdel-Haq NM, Asmar BI. Human herpesvirus 6 (HHV6) infection. Indian J Pediatr. 2004;71:89–96.

31. Ljungman P, Singh N. Human herpesvirus-6 infection in solid organ and stem cell transplant recipients. J Clin Virol. 2006;37 Suppl 1:S87–91.

32. Razonable RR, Zerr DM. AST Infectious Diseases Community of Practice. HHV-6, HHV-7 and HHV-8 in solid organ transplant recipients. Am J Transplant. 2009;9 Suppl 4:S97–100.

33. Yoshikawa T, Goshima F, Akimoto S, et al. Human herpesvirus 6 infection of human epidermal cell line: pathogenesis of skin manifestation. J Med Virol. 2003;71:62–8.

34. Fujita H, Maruta A, Tomita N, et al. Human herpesvirus-6-associated exanthema in a patient with acute lymphocytic leukaemia. Brit J Haematol. 1996;92:947–9.

Varicella Zoster

35. Feld R, Evans WK, DeBoer G. Herpes zoster in patients with small-cell carcimona of the lung receiving combined modality treatment. Ann Intern Med. 1980;93:282–3.

36. Friedman-Kien AE, Lafleur FL, Gendler E, et al. Herpes zoster: a possible early clinical sign for development of acquired immunodeficiency syndrome in high-risk individuals. J Am Acad Dermatol. 1986;14(6): 1023–8.

37. Cohen PR, Grossman ME. Clinical features of human immunodeficiency virus-associated disseminated herpes zoster virus infection – a review of the literature. Clin Exp Dermatol. 1989;12:273–6.

38. Strangfeld A, Listing J, Herzer P, et al. Risk of herpes zoster in patients with rheumatoid arthritis treated with anti-TNF-α agents. JAMA. 2009;301(7):737–44.

39. Dolin R, Reichman RC, Mazur MH, Whitley RJ. Herpes zoster-varicella infections in immunosuppressed patients. Ann Intern Med. 1978;89:375–88.

40. Hall HD, Jacobs JS, O'Malley JP. Necrosis of maxilla in patients with herpes zoster. Oral Surg. 1974;37(5):657–62.

41. Rusthoven JJ, Ahlgren P, Elhakim T, et al. Varicella-zoster infection in adult cancer patients. Arch Intern Med. 1988;148(7):1561–6.

42. Mazur MH, Dolin R. Herpes zoster at the NIH: a 20 year experience. Am J Med. 1978;65(5):738–44.

43. Vu AQ, Radonich MA, Heald PW. Herpes zoster in seven disparate dermatomes (zoster multiplex): Report of a case and review of the literature. J Am Acad Dermatol. 1999;40:868–9.

44. Tuchman M, Weinberg JM. Monodermatomal herpes zoster in a pseudodisseminated distribution following breast reconstruction surgery. Cutis. 2008;81:71–2.

45. Gnann JW. Varicella-Zoster Virus: Atypical presentations and unusual complications. J Infect Dis. 2002;186 Suppl 1:S91–8.

46. Rau R, Fitzhugh CD, Baird K, et al. Triad of severe abdominal pain, inappropriate antidiuretic hormone secretion, and disseminated varicella-zoster virus infection preceding cutaneous manifestations after hematopoietic stem cell transplantation: utility of PCR for early recognition and therapy. Pediatr Infect Dis J. 2008;27(3):265–8.

47. Au WY, Ma SY, Cheng VC, Ooi CG, Lie AK. Disseminated zoster, hyponatraemia, severe abdominal pain and leukaemia relapse: recognition

of a new clinical quartet after bone marrow transplantation. Br J Dermatol. 2003;149:862–5.

48. David DS, Tegtmeier BR, O'Donnell MR, Paz IB, McCarty TM. Visceral varicella-zoster after bone marrow transplantation: report of a case series and review of the literature. Am J Gastroenterol. 1998;93: 810–3.

49. Leena M, Ville V, Veli-Jukka A. Visceral varicella zoster virus infection after stem cell transplantation: a possible cause of severe abdominal pain. Scand J Gastroentero. 2006;41:242–4.

50. Nomdedéu JF, Nomdedéu J, Martino R, et al. Ogilvie's syndrome from disseminate varicella-zoster infection and infracted celiac ganglia. J Clin Gastroenterol. 1995;20(2):157–9.

51. Ishizawa J, Fujita H, Iguchi M, et al. Quantification of circulating varicella-zoster virus DNA for follow-up in a case of visceral varicella-zoster infection ameliorated with intravenous acyclovir. Int J Hematol. 2007;85(3):242–5.

52. Tresch S, Trüeb RM, Kamarachev J, French LE, Hofbauer GFL. Disseminated herpes zoster mimicking rheumatoid vasculitis in a rheumatoid arthritis patient on Etanercept. Dermatology. 2009;219(4): 347–9.

53. Osawa M, Umemoto N, Tajima N, et al. Atypical varicella mimicking hand-foot-mouth disease in an adult patient with malignant lymphoma during chemotherapy. Br J Dermatol. 2004;151:254–5.

54. Levy O, Orange JS, Hibberd P, et al. Disseminated varicella infection due to the vaccine strain of varicella-zoster virus, in a patient with a novel deficiency in natural killer T cells. J Infect Dis. 2003;188(7): 948–53.

55. Nikkels AF, Simonart T, Kentos A, et al. Atypical recurrent varicella in 4 patients with hemopathies. J Am Acad Dermatol. 2003;48(3): 442–7.

56. Baxter JD, DiNubile MJ. Relapsing chickenpox in a young man with non-Hodgkin's lymphoma. Clin Infect Dis. 1994;18:785–8.

57. Gulick R, Heath-Chiozzi M, Crumpacker CS. Varicella-zoster virus disease in patients with human immunodeficiency virus infection. Arch Dermatol. 1990;127:1086–8.

58. Shelley WB, Shelley ED, Talanin NY, et al. "Chickenpox redux" in elderly patients presenting with a "pox tongue". J Geriatr Dermatol. 1995;3(2):34–7.

59. McNamara MP, LACrosse S, Piering WF, Rytel MW. Exogenous reinfection with varicella-zoster virus. N Engl J Med. 1987;317(8):511.

60. Jeyaratnam D, Robson AM, Hextall JM, Wong W, MacMahon E. Concurrent verrucous and varicelliform rashes following renal transplantation. Am J Transplant. 2005;5:1777–80.

61. Berger AA, Bonnez W, Evans T. Diagnosis: chronic cutaneous verrucous varicella-zoster infection. Clin Infect Dermatol. 1998;27: 380–1.

62. Hoppenjans WB, Bibler MR, Orme RL, Solinger AM. Prolonged cutaneous herpes zoster in acquired immunodeficiency syndrome. Arch Dermatol. 1990;126(8):1048–50.

63. Grossman MC, Grossman ME. Chronic hyperkeratotic herpes zoster and HIV infection. J Am Acad Dermatol. 1993;28:306–8.

64. Leibovitz E, Kaul A, Rigaud M, et al. Chronic varicella zoster in a child infected with human immunodeficiency virus: case report and review of the literature. Cutis. 1992;49:27–31.

65. Janier M, Hillion B, Baccard M, et al. Chronic varicella zoster infection in acquired immunodeficiency syndrome. J Am Acad Dermatol. 1988;18:584–5.

66. Castanet J, Rodot S, Lacour J, et al. Chronic varicella presenting as disseminated pinpoint-sized papules in a man infected with the human immunodeficiency virus. Dermatology. 1996;192:84–6.

67. Nikkels AF, Snoeck R, Rentier B, Pierard GE. Chronic verrucous varicella zoster virus skin lesions: clinical, histological, molecular and therapeutic aspects. Clin Exp Dermatol. 1999;24:346–53.

68. Tsao H, Tahan SR, Johnson RA. Chronic varicella zoster infection mimicking a basal cell carcinoma in an AIDS patient. J Am Acad Dermatol. 1997;36:831–3.

69. Gallagher JG, Merigan TC. Prolonged herpes-zoster infection associated with immunosuppressive therapy. Ann Intern Med. 1979;91(6): 842–6.

Molluscum Contagiosum

70. Mansur AT, Göktay F, Gündüz S, Serdar ZA. Multiple giant molluscum contagiosum in a renal transplant recipient. Transpl Infect Dis. 2004;6:120–3.

71. Bohm M, Luger TA, Bonsmann G. Disseminated giant molluscum contagiosum in a patient with idiopathic CD4+ lymphocytopenia. Dermatology. 2008;217:196–8.

72. Feldmeyer L, Kamarashev J, Boehler A, et al. Molluscum contagiosum folliculitis mimicking tinea barbae in a lung transplant recipient. J Am Acad Dermatol. 2010;63(1):169–71.

73. Yoshinaga I, Conrado LA, Schainberg SC, Grinblat M. Recalcitrant molluscum contagiosum in a patient with AIDS: combined treatment with CO$_2$ laser, trichloroacetic acid, and pulsed dye laser. Lasers Surg Med. 2000;27(4):291–4.

74. Annam V, Inamadar AC, Palit A, Yelikar BR. Co-infection of molluscum contagiosum virus and cryptococcosis in the same skin lesion in a HIV-infected patient. J Cutan Pathol. 2008;35 Suppl 1:29–31.

75. Bates CM, Carey PB, Dhar J, Hart CA. Molluscum contagiosum – a novel presentation. Int J STD AIDS. 2001;12(9):614–5.

76. Fornatora ML, Reich RF, Gray RG, Freedman PD. Intraoral molluscum contagiosum: a report of a case and a review of the literature. Oral Surg Oral Med Oral Pathol Oral Radiol Endod. 2001;92: 318–20.

Cytomegalovirus

77. Kaisar MO, Kirwan RM, Strutton GM, et al. Cutaneous manifestations of cytomegalovirus disease in renal transplant recipients: a case series. Transpl Infect Dis. 2008;10:209–13.

78. Ramdial PK, Dlova NC, Sydney C. Cytomegalovirus neuritis in perineal ulcers. J Cutan Pathol. 2002;29(7):439–44.

79. Daudén E, Fernández-Buezo G, Fraga J, Cardeñoso L, García-Díez A. Mucocutaneous presence of cytomegalovirus associated with human immunodeficiency virus infection. Arch Dermatol. 2001;137(4):443–8.

80. Lee JY. Cytomegalovirus infection involving the skin in immunocompromised hosts. Am J Clin Pathol. 1989;92:96–100.

81. Weiss DJ, Greenfield Jr JW, O'Rourke KS, McCune WJ. Systemic cytomegalovirus infection mimicking exacerbation of Wegener's granulomatosis. J Rheumatol. 1993;20(1):155–7.

82. Colsky AS, Jegasothy SM, Leonardi C, Kirsner RS, Kerdel FA. Diagnosis and treatment of a case of cutaneous cytomegalovirus infection with a dramatic clinical presentation. J Am Acad Dermatol. 1998;38:349–51.

83. Husain S, Evans L, Rabinowitz AD, Grossman M. CMV inclusion disease presenting as a cutaneous ulcer in AIDS. Arch Dermatol. 1994;130:1312–3, 1315.

84. Lee JY, Peel R. Concurrent cytomegalovirus and herpes simplex virus in skin biopsy specimens from two AIDS patients with fatal CMV infection. Am J Dermatopathol. 1989;11:136–43.

85. Trimarchi H, Casas G, Jordan R, et al. Cytomegalovirus maculopapular eruption in a kidney transplant patient. Transpl Infect Dis. 2001;3(1):47–50.

86. Rees AP, Meadors M, Ventura HO, Pankey GA. Diagnosis of disseminated cytomegalovirus infection and pneumonitis in a heart transplant recipient by skin biopsy: case report. J Heart Lung Transplant. 1991;10:329–32.

87. Konstadt JW, Gatusso P, Eng A, et al. Disseminated cytomegalovirus infection with cutaneous involvement in a heart transplant patient. Clin Cases Dermatol. 1990;2:3.

88. Curtis JL, Egbert BM. Cutaneous cytomegalovirus vasculitis: an unusual presentation of a common opportunistic pathogen. Hum Pathol. 1982;13:1138–41.

89. Golden MP, Hammer SM, Wanke CA, Albrecht MA. Cytomegalovirus vasculitis. Medicine (Baltimore). 1994;73:246–55.

90. Feldman PS, Walker AN, Baker R. Cutaneous lesions heralding disseminated cytomegalovirus infection. J Am Acad Dermatol. 1982;7: 545–8.

91. Bournérias I, Boisnic S, Patey O, et al. Unusual cutaneous cytomegalovirus involvement in patients with acquired immunodeficiency syndrome. Arch Dermatol. 1989;125(9):1243–6.

92. Horn TD, Hood AF. Clinically occult cytomegalovirus present in skin biopsy specimens in immunosuppressed hosts. J Am Acad Dermatol. 1989;21:781–4.

93. Bhawan J, Gellis S, Ucci A, Chang TW. Vesiculobullous lesions caused by cytomegalovirus infection in an immunocompromised adult. J Am Acad Dermatol. 1984;11:743–7.

Human Papillomavirus

94. Dharancy S, Catteau B, Mortier L, et al. Conversion to sirolimus: a useful strategy for recalcitrant cutaneous viral warts in liver transplant recipient. Liver Transpl. 2006;12(12):1883–7.

95. Gormley RH, Kovarik CL. Dermatologic manifestations of HPV in HIV-infected individuals. Curr HIV/AIDS Rep. 2009;6(3):130–8.

96. Mudrikova T, Jaspers C, Ellerbroek P, Hoepelman A. HPV-related anogenital disease and HIV infection: not always 'ordinary' condylomata acuminate. Neth J Med. 2008;66:98–102.

97. Al-Osman A, Perry JB, Birek C. Extensive papillomatosis of the palate exhibiting epithelial dysplasia and HPV 16 gene expression in a renal transplant recipient. J Can Dent Assoc. 2006;72:331–4.

98. De-Villiers EM. Prevalence of HPV 7 papillomas in the oral mucosa and facial skin of patients with human immunodeficiency virus. Arch Dermatol. 1989;125:1590.

99. Rogers HD, Macgregor JL, Nord KM, et al. Acquired epidermodysplasia verruciformis. J Am Acad Dermatol. 2009;60(2):315–20.

100. Asvesti C, Delmas V, Dauge-Geffroy MC, et al. Condylomes multiples de l'urethre et de la vessie relevant une infection par HIV. Ann Urol (Paris). 1991;25:146–9.

101. Ko MJ, Chu CY. Disseminated human papillomavirus type 11 infection in a patient with pemphigus vulgaris: confirmed by DNA analysis. J Am Acad Dermatol. 2004;51:S190–3.

West Nile Virus Infection

102. Ferguson DD, Gershman K, LeBailly A, Petersen LR. Characteristics of the rash associated with West Nile virus fever. Clin Infect Dis. 2005;41(8):1204–7.

103. Ravindra KV, Freifeld AG, Kalil AC, et al. West Nile virus-associated encephalitis in recipients of renal and pancreas transplants: case series and literature review. Clin Infect Dis. 2004;38(9):1257–60.

104. Hayes EB, Sejvar JJ, Zaki SR, et al. Virology, pathology and clinical manifestations of West Nile virus disease. Emerg Infect Dis. 2005;11:1174–9.

105. Kleinschmidt-DeMasters BK, Marder BA, Levi ME, et al. Naturally acquired West Nile virus encephalomyelitis in transplant recipients. Arch Neurol. 2004;61(8):1210–20.

7

Rickettsiae

The Rickettsiae are small gram negative intracellular bacteria which target vascular endothelial cells, monocytes, and polymorphonuclear leukocytes. They are divided into *Rickettsia*, *Ehrlichia*, and *Anaplasma*. The Rickettsiae are traditionally divided into three groups: the spotted fever group, the typhus group, and the scrub typhus group (*Orienta tsutsugamushi* only).

Immunosuppression may result in an altered appearance of the rash and behavior of the infectious disease. Reports of infections due to Rickettsiae in immunocompromised patients are rare so that generalizations cannot be drawn from the few case reports in this patient population.

RICKETTSIA

Rickettsial pox presented in the usual fashion in a 47-year-old human immunodeficiency virus (HIV)-positive woman with fever, headache, an eschar, and a generalized papulovesicular eruption. The atypical finding was the relative abundance of *R. akari* in the papulovesicles by immunohistochemical staining and few lesions in the eschar. This tissue distribution of *Rickettsia* differs from the normal host.[1]

The unusual feature of scrub typhus caused by *Orienta tsutsugamushi*, a gram negative intracellular bacillus characterized by fever, eschar, lymphadenopathy, and a maculopapular rash in HIV-infected patients, is the dramatic drop in their retroviral load.[2] Unlike many other intracellular pathogens, scrub typhus disease severity is not increased in individuals co-infected with HIV.[2]

EHRLICHIA

Human ehrlichiosis is caused by *E. chaffeensis* which infect macrophages and monocytes and by *E. ewingii*. In contrast to *E. chaffeensis*, *E. ewingii* infects granulocytes and most cases have been described in immunocompromised patients. *E. ewingii* may be more common among transplant recipients than immunocompetent patients. In a series of human ehrlichiosis in transplant patients, none had a rash compared to the 17–36% incidence in immunocompetent patients.[3] However the clinical manifestations are more severe in the immunocompromised host. The diagnosis of ehrlichiosis should be considered in any patient with fever, rash, transaminase elevations, and new onset thrombocytopenia or leukopenia who has had potential tick exposures in an endemic area.[4] Most cases occur between April and September.

Thirteen cases of *E. chaffeensis* in HIV infected patients diagnosed serologically or by the presence of characteristic intracellular bacterial aggregates (morulae) in patient leukocytes presented with a febrile illness. Six of thirteen (46%) had a rash described as diffusely erythematous or morbilliform or scattered petechiae or macules. The distribution varied from localized to the extremities or to extensive involvement of the trunk.[5]

HUMAN GRANULOCYTIC ANAPLASMOSIS

Human granulocytic anaplasmosis (HGA) is a tick-borne zoonotic infection caused by *Anaplasma phagocytophilum*. HGA presents as a febrile illness, with headache, myalgias, pancytopenia, transaminitis, and rash uncommonly.[6]

REFERENCES

Rickettsia

1. Sanders S, Di Costanzo D, Leach J, et al. Rickettsialpox in a patient with HIV infection. J Am Acad Dermatol. 2003;48:286–9.
2. Watt G, Kantipong P, de Souza M, et al. HIV-1 suppression during acute scrub-typhus infection. Lancet. 2000;356:475–9.

M.E. Grossman et al., *Cutaneous Manifestations of Infection in the Immunocompromised Host*,
DOI 10.1007/978-1-4419-1578-8_7, © Springer Science+Business Media, LLC 2012

Ehrlichia

3. Thomas LD, Hongo I, Bloch KC, Tang TW, Dummer S. Human ehrlichiosis in transplant recipients. Am J Transplant. 2007;7(6): 1641–7.

4. Safdar N, Love RB, Maki DG. Sever *Ehrlichia chaffeenisis* infection in a lung transplant recipient: a review of ehrlichiosis in the immunocompromised patient. Emerg Infect Dis. 2002;8:320–3.

5. Paddock CD, Folk SM, Shore GM, et al. Infections with *Ehrlichia chaffeenisis* and *Ehrlichia ewingii* in person coinfected with human immunodeficiency virus. Clin Infect Dis. 2001;33:1586–94.

Human Granulocytic Anaplasmosis

6. Bakken JS, Dumler S. Clinical diagnosis and treatment of human granulocytotropoic anaplasmosis. Ann NY Acad Sci. 2006;1078: 236–47.

8

Crusted Scabies

Hyperkeratotic or crusted scabies, formerly called Norwegian scabies, is caused by the same mite, *Sarcoptes scabiei*, as common scabies.[1] When it was first described by Danielssen and Boeck in 1848 in Norwegian lepers, it was not appreciated as a manifestation of immunodeficiency. Norwegian scabies was seen in those with Down's syndrome (trisomy 21) or severe mental retardation. It is increasingly being seen in immunocompromised patients of varying types including those with human immunodeficiency virus (HIV) disease, acquired immune deficiency syndrome (AIDS), human T-lymphotropic virus-1 (HTLV-1) associated adult T-cell leukemia/lymphoma,[2] chronic lymphocytic leukemia, organ transplantation, patients on treatment with immunosuppressants or systemic steroids, physical debilitation (critical illness, kwashiorkor), and neurological disorders with decreased cutaneous sensation and reduced ability to mechanically remove the mites and destroy the burrows by scratching (tabes dorsalis, syringomyelia, and Parkinson's disease).

Hyperkeratotic scabies localized to areas treated with potent flourinated topical steroids (local immunosuppression) in otherwise immunocompetent hosts have been reported.[3] Preexisting atopic or contact dermatitis and the use of topical steroids may mask the infestation and promote transmission of scabies.

Hyperkeratotic scabies is characterized by thickly crusted plaques on the palms, soles, scalp, ears, buttocks, and extensor surfaces of the extremities. The creamy, grey, yellow-brown, yellow-green, or grey-white scaly crusted or hyperkeratotic plaques may be deeply fissured and/or cover the entire body. The plaques vary in thickness from 3 to 15 mm.[4] Plaques may resemble the hide of a pachyderm (elephant, rhinoceros, or hippopotamus).[5] Removal of the crusted plaque leaves a smooth, red, moist, velvety undersurface. The nails are often thickened and dystrophic with subungual debris and periungual crusting. The nails are the frequent source of relapsed infection. Acral distribution is typical with a variable erythematous scaly eruption which may be generalized. Rarely crusted scabies may involve the entire body including the face, head, and scalp looking like an exfoliative erythroderma. Widespread scaly yellowish-brown papules may mimic Darier's disease.[6] In addition, crusted scabies is often difficult to recognize clinically and can mimic or may be mistaken for psoriasis,[7] keratoderma blenorrhagicum or reactive arthritis, adverse drug reaction,[8] systemic lupus erythematosus, severe contact dermatitis, and dermatitis herpetiformis. Bullous scabies mimics the eruption of bullous pemphigoid in patients over 65 years of age. Although not widely recognized, scabies may involve the scalp and can be confused with seborrheic dermatitis or may be overlooked during routine clinical examination, neglected during treatment, and lead to treatment failure and puzzling relapses.[9] HIV-infected individuals may present with atypical forms of crusted scabies with disease localized to the penis, vulva, face,[10] or plaques on the toes, toenails, and toewebs.[11] Generalized lymphadenopathy, elevated IgE levels, and eosinophilia may be present in crusted scabies.

A particularly misleading feature associated with crusted scabies is the absence of burrows and pruritus of classic scabies. Together with the atypical appearance of the rash, the diagnosis is frequently delayed and only recognized when typical scabies develops in secondary cases. Hyperkeratotic scabies, like common scabies, is transmitted by close personal contact. Classic scabies is often sexually transmitted and considered a "disease of passion" requiring prolonged skin to skin contact. Hyperkeratotic scabies may be spread by casual contact including nursing care and fomites. The scale of crusted scabies flakes off and contaminates clothing, bed linen, curtains, floors, walls, furniture, and toys, and remains infective for prolonged periods.

Most nosocomial outbreaks of scabies result from unrecognized crusted scabies at admission.[12] In the hospital setting,

M.E. Grossman et al., *Cutaneous Manifestations of Infection in the Immunocompromised Host*,
DOI 10.1007/978-1-4419-1578-8_8, © Springer Science+Business Media, LLC 2012

early diagnosis is essential to prevent dissemination of this highly contagious form of scabies and large outbreaks or explosive epidemics of ordinary scabies among healthcare workers, hospital employees, patients, family members, and other caretakers. Healthcare workers often develop the initial scabetic lesions on the forearms, the areas in immediate contact with the patient being cared for. The mean incubation period is 15 days (range 12–27 days).[13] The high contagiousness of Norwegian scabies is related to the extremely large number of mites in the skin. The typical case of scabies in the immunocompetent patient is generally associated with a low mite load, an average of 10–15 mites on the body surface. In contrast, hundreds of thousands to millions of viable mites are present in the hyperkeratotic skin of Norwegian scabies. Crusted scabies results from the failure of the host immune response to control the proliferation of the scabies mite in the skin with resulting hyperinfestation. Norwegian scabies is the clinical manifestation of immunodeficiency. Immunosuppressed patients may present with what appears to be common scabies but still harbor a higher burden of mites and be more infective than an immunocompetent host. These patients may have a dramatic number of burrows on their hands or even their face. Normal immunocompetent hosts exposed to crusted scabies develop classic scabies which suggests that both ectoparasitic infections are caused by the same organism and that the host response accounts for the difference in clinical presentation.

The unusually widespread skin involvement in crusted scabies can provide a portal of entry for fatal bacteremia due to *Staphylococcus aureus*, *Streptococcus pyogenes*, and *Enterobacter cloacae*.[14-16] The severe skin damage from this infestation removes one of the last defense mechanisms against infection in the immunocompromised host and allows repetitive bacterial seeding of the bloodstream. Most patients with crusted scabies and bacteremia have prominent fissures of the hands and feet.

The diagnosis of crusted scabies can be readily confirmed with a skin biopsy or microscopic examination of skin scrapings for the presence of mites, eggs, or scybala (fecal pellets).

The treatment of crusted scabies is with ivermectin, a systemic antiparasitic drug. It is administered as an oral dose of 0.2mg/kg weekly until clear. The optimum number of doses of ivermectin is not standardized. The concomitant use of topical scabicides and keratolytics is justified because of concern that the drug alone may not penetrate the hyperkeratosis.[17]

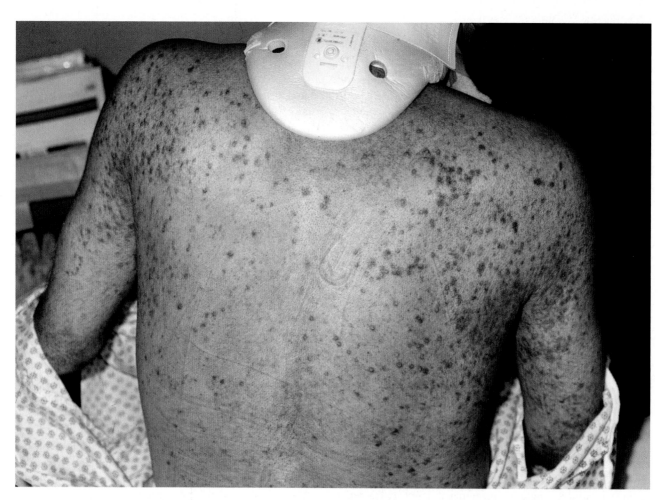

Figure 8.1. A 33-year-old Dominican man with human T-cell lymphotropic virus type I (HTLV-I) associated T-cell leukemia developed gray-brown papules over the flanks and periaxillary areas

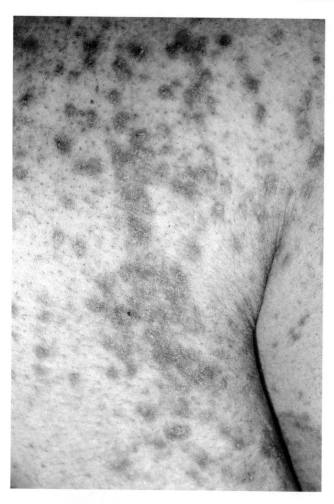

Figure 8.2. Close-up shows multiple gray-brown papules with scale and/or crust. Mineral oil preparation had a multitude of adult mites

Figure 8.3. Yellow crusted plaque of the second toe due to localized crusted scabies in acquired immune deficiency syndrome (AIDS) (From Arico et al.[18])

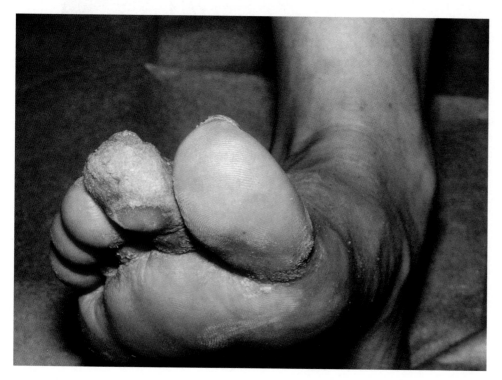

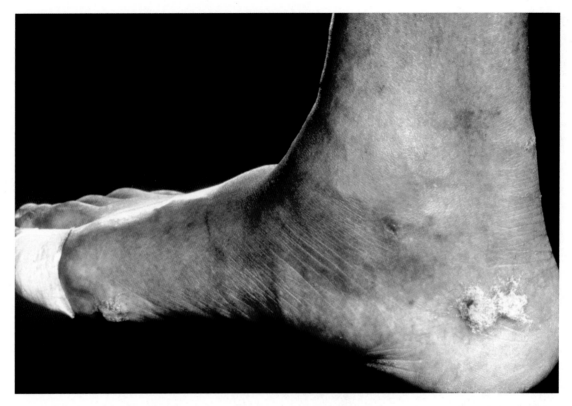

Figure 8.4.   Hyperkeratotic plaques of crusted scabies on the foot of a patient with AIDS (Courtesy of Mary Ruth Buchness, M.D.)

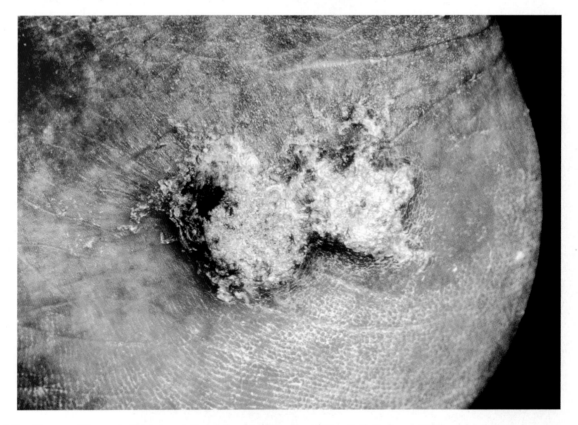

Figure 8.5.   Close-up of the crusted heel plaque of crusted scabies (Courtesy of Mary Ruth Buchness, M.D.)

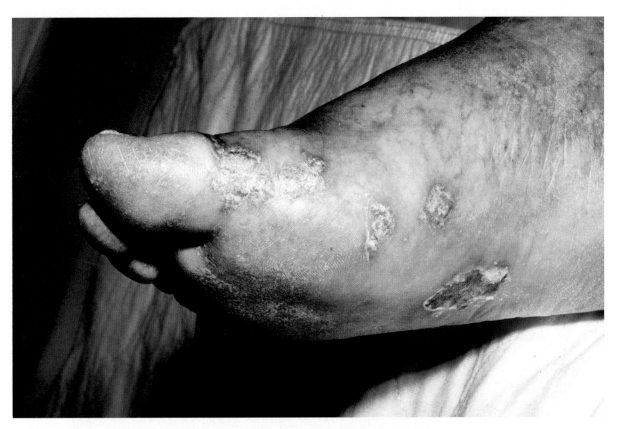

Figure 8.6. Plaques of crusted scabies on the foot of a 38-year-old with refractory acute myelogenous leukemia (Courtesy of Mary Ruth Buchness, M.D.)

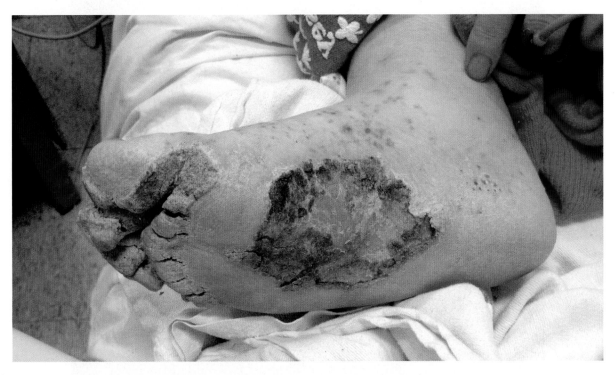

Figure 8.7. Plantar plaques of crusted scabies in HTLV-I positive acute T-cell leukemia

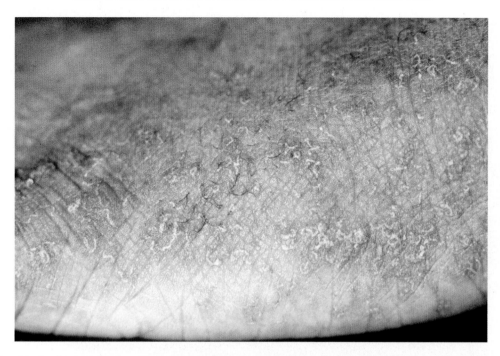

Figure 8.8. A multitude of scabetic burrows on the hand of a human immunodeficiency virus (HIV)-positive patient (Courtesy of Mary Ruth Buchness, M.D.)

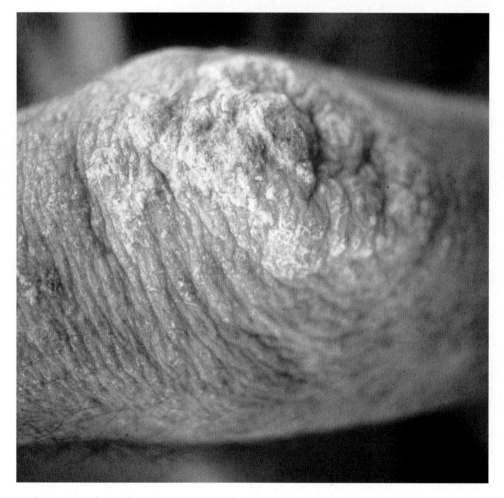

Figure 8.9. Psoriasisform plaque of crusted scabies on the elbow of an HIV-positive homosexual (From Donabedian and Khazan[8])

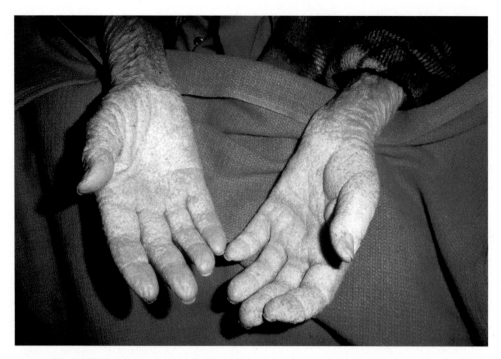

Figure 8.10. Gray-white hyperkeratotic plaques due to crusted scabies on both hands of an HIV-positive patient

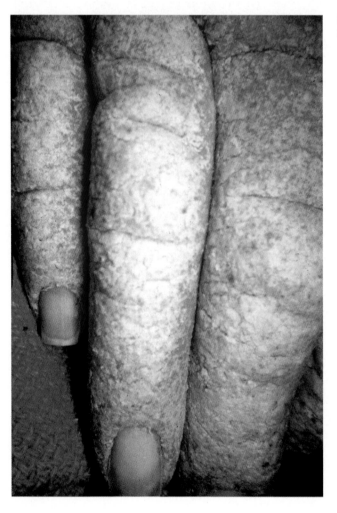

Figure 8.11. Thick yellow-white hyperkeratotic plaques of crusted scabies on the hands of an HIV-positive patient

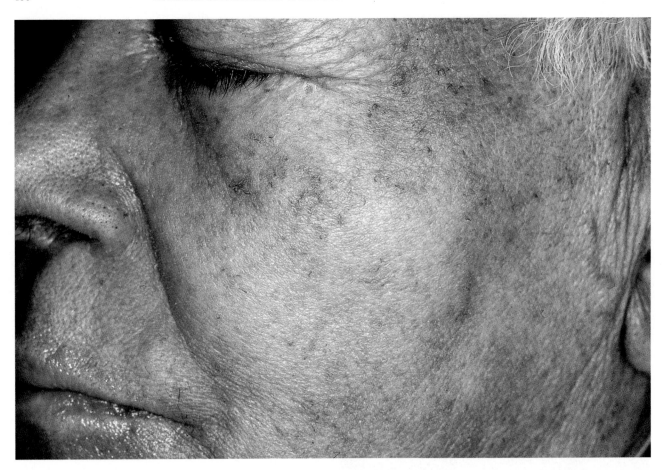

Figure 8.12. Multitude of facial burrows of scabies in a 72-year-old Dominican woman with HTLV-I associated T-cell leukemia and WBC count of 261,000 cells/mm³

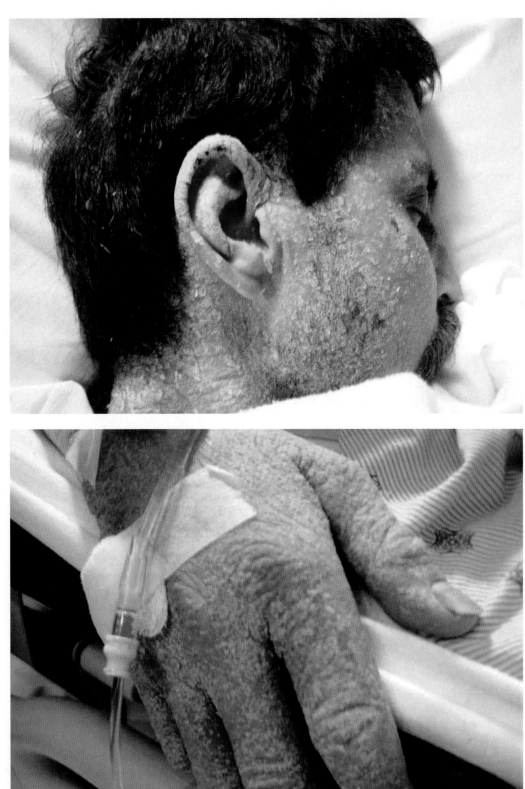

Figure 8.13. and 8.14. A 29-year-old man with a history of renal transplantation presented with a 5-month history of scaly, pruritic eruptions seen on the face, ears, neck, and hands. Skin scrapings confirmed hyperkeratotic or crusted scabies

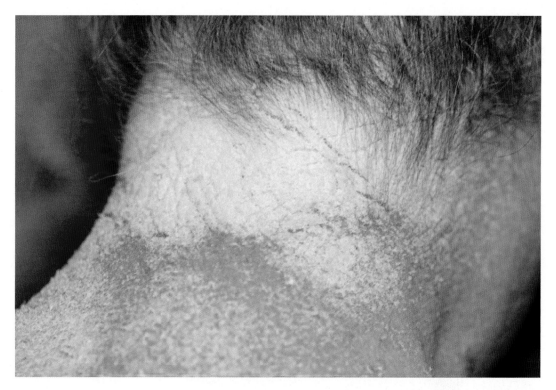

Figure 8.15. Thick white fissured plaque of crusted scabies on the neck of a 60-year-old woman with a history of lung transplantation

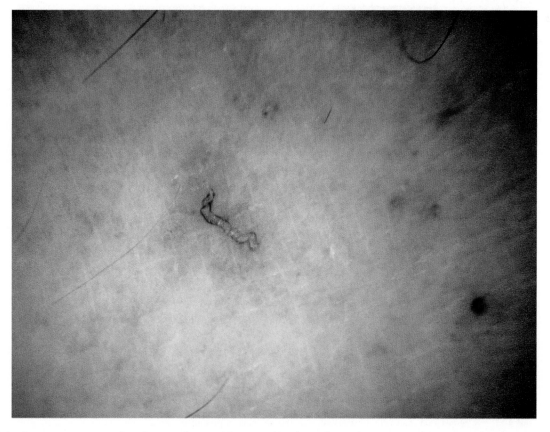

Figure 8.16. Dermatoscopic view of a scabies mite burrow (Courtesy of Jocelyn Lieb, M.D.)

REFERENCES

1. Hengge U, Currie BJ, Jäger G, Lupi O, Schwartz RA. Scabies: a ubiquitous neglected skin disease. Lancet Infect Dis. 2006;6:769–79.

2. del Giudice P, Sainte Marie D, Gérard Y, Couppié P, Pradinaud R. Is crusted (Norwegian) scabies a marker of adult T cell leukemia/lymphoma in human T lymphotropic virus type I-seropositive patients? J Infect Dis. 1997;176(4):1090–2.

3. Binić I, Janković A, Janković D, Ljubenovic M. Crusted (Norwegian) scabies following systemic and topical corticosteroid therapy. J Korean Med Sci. 2010;25(1):188–91.

4. Karthikeyan K. Crusted scabies. Indian J Dermatol Venereol Leprol. 2009;75:340–7.

5. Khera P, English JC. Pachyderma. N Engl J Med. 2009;361(15):e29.

6. Anolik MA, Rudolf RI. Scabies simulating Darier disease in an immunocompromised host. Arch Dermatol. 1976;112(1):73–4.

7. Inserra DW, Bickley LK. Crusted scabies in acquired immunodeficiency syndrome. Int J Dermatol. 1990;29:287–9.

8. Donabedian H, Khazan U. Norwegian scabies in a patient with AIDS. Clin Infect Dis. 1992;14:162–4.

9. Anbar TS, El-Domyati MB, Mansour HA, Ahmad HM. Scaly scalp associated with crusted scabies: case series. Dermatol Online J. 2007;13(3):18.

10. Tibbs CJ, Wilcox DJ. Norwegian scabies and herpes simplex in a patient with chronic lymphatic leukemia and hypogammaglobulinemia. Br J Dermatol. 1992;126:523–4.

11. Bakos L, Reusch MC, D'Elia P, Aquino V, Bakos RM. Crusted scabies of the vulva. J Eur Acad Dermatol Venereol. 2007;21:682–4.

12. Varou R, Remoudaki HD, Maltezou HC. Nosocomial scabies. J Hosp Infect. 2007;65:9–14.

13. Fajardo-Velázquez R, Urdez-Hernández E, Ysita-Morales A. Nosocomial outbreak of scabies from a Norwegian scabies case. Salud Publica Mex. 2004;46(3):251–4.

14. Glover R, Young L, Goltz RW. Norwegian scabies in acquired immunodeficiency syndrome: report of a case resulting in death from associated sepis. J Am Acad Dermatol. 1987;16:396–9.

15. Hulbert TV, Larsen RA. Hyperkeratotic (Norwegian) scabies with gram-negative bacterium as the initial presentation of AIDS. Clin Infect Dis. 1992;14:1164–5.

16. Bonomo RA, Jacobs M, Jacobs G, Graham R, Salata RA. Norwegian scabies and a toxic shock syndrome toxin 1-producing strain of *Staphylococcus aureus* endocarditis in a patient with trisomy 21. Clin Infect Dis. 1998;27:645–6.

17. del Giudice P. Ivermectin in scabies. Curr Opin Infect Dis. 2002;15:123–6.

18. Arico M et al. Localized crusted scabies in the acquired immunodeficiency syndrome. Clin Exp Dermatol. 1992;17:339–41.

9

Protozoa

TRYPANOSOMA CRUZI (CHAGAS' DISEASE)

Reactivation of Chagas' disease (American trypanosomiasis) in immunocompromised hosts presents as a constellation of symptoms and may include skin signs.[1] Patients with Chagas' cardiomyopathy who have undergone cardiac transplantation experience Chagas' disease reactivation 28.8–33.8% of the time within weeks to 3 months of initiating immunosuppressive therapy.[2,3] Reactivation Chagas' disease may present with fever, heart failure, myocarditis, and painful skin lesions. The skin lesions most commonly present on the lower extremities or trunk.[3] Erythematous painful, indurated plaques resemble cellulitis. Sometimes they are crusted or ulcerated, involve the lower extremities or the extensor surfaces of the elbows or hips.[4] Reactivation chagoma is a tender nodule or multiple painful subcutaneous nodules.[5] Patients may present with cutaneous lesions before any systemic sign of reactivation Chagas' disease, so skin biopsy is essential for diagnosis. Unlike the active stage of the natural course of Chagas' disease, there is usually no lymphadenopathy or hepatosplenomegaly. Diagnosis can be made by examination of a skin biopsy specimen from the areas of cutaneous involvement, which often reveal abundant *Trypanosoma cruzi* organisms without the use of special stains. Immunohistochemical stains can be used if the organisms are not readily identified or they need to be distinguished from other similar appearing protozoa, such as *Leishmania*, particularly in endemic areas.[6,7] The parasitologic and serologic methods usually used to detect *Trypanosoma cruzi* infection are not sensitive detectors of reactivation, which is best diagnosed by identification of parasites in the tissue obtained by biopsies of the endomyocardium or skin.

Chronic Chagas' disease can also reactivate in conjunction with other immunosuppressed states, such as human immunodeficiency virus (HIV) infection, hematological malignancies, and bone marrow or solid organ transplantation.[8] The most common manifestations of reactivation in HIV patients are myocarditis and meningoencephalitis. The majority of HIV infected patients that experience reactivation are severely immunosuppressed with a CD4 count of less than 200 cells/mL and have already developed another opportunistic infection.[8] Skin lesions have been described in HIV patients with Chagas' disease reactivation, and the most common cutaneous manifestation is erythema nodosum-like nodules which demonstrate amastigotes on skin biopsy.[8,9] Patients who have received solid organ transplantation, including heart and kidney, for indications other than Chagas' disease have also been reported with reactivation syndromes. Cutaneous manifestations include edematous and indurated erythematous plaques, crusted or scaly plaques, erythema nodosum-like lesions associated with panniculitis in both legs,[10] and erythematous nodules, which may be present on the trunk, lower limbs, or, less commonly, upper limbs.[4,5,11]

Acute Chagas' disease may also occur in nonendemic areas from infected blood products transfused to immunosuppressed patients or transplanted organs from chagasic donors. Chronic infection with Chagas' disease is not usually detected in the blood or organs donated by immigrants from endemic areas.

M.E. Grossman et al., *Cutaneous Manifestations of Infection in the Immunocompromised Host*, DOI 10.1007/978-1-4419-1578-8_9, © Springer Science+Business Media, LLC 2012

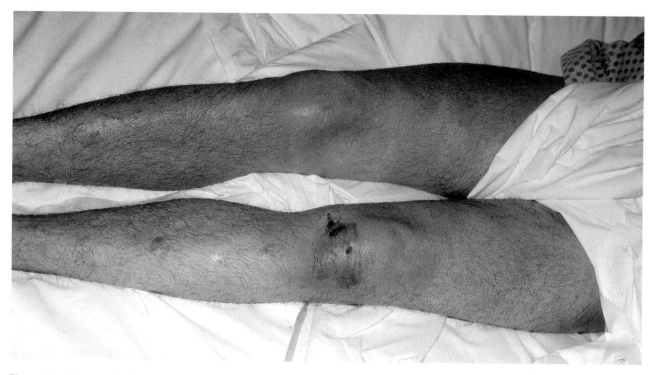

Figure 9.1. Five months after a heart transplant for Chagas' cardiomyopathy, a 22-year-old Honduran man presented to the emergency room with fever, shortness of breath, and "cellulitis" involving the knees and thighs. The left knee was red with necrotic eschars

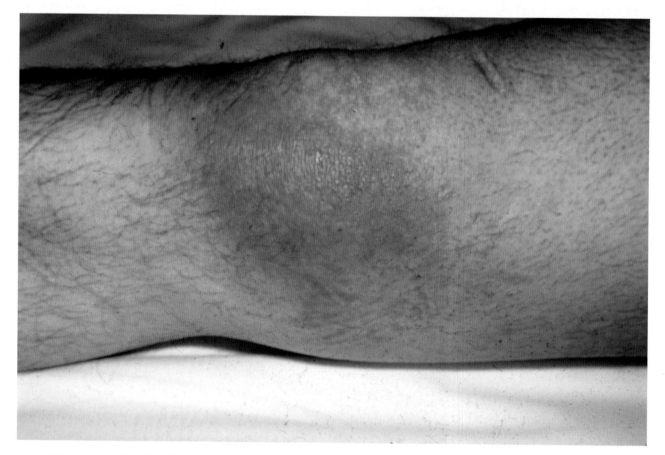

Figure 9.2. Warm tender red patches were present over both knees

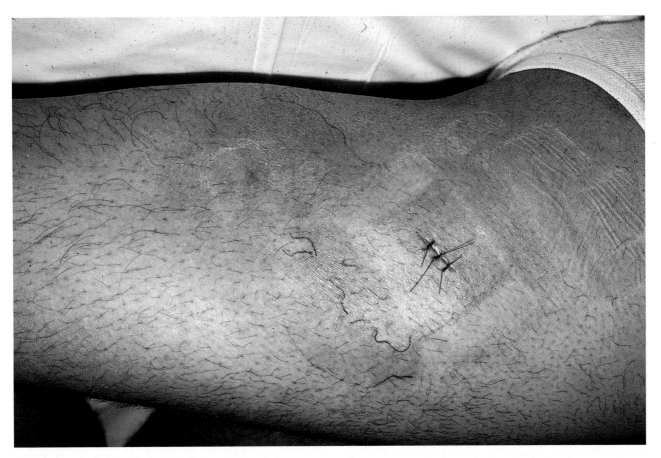

Figure 9.3. Over the lateral aspect of the right thigh was a tender irregularly shaped erythematous indurated plaque. Skin biopsy demonstrated numerous intracellular organisms consistent with the amastigote form of *T. cruzi*. Reactivated Chagas' disease responded to nifurtimox

Leishmania

Leishmaniasis is a protozoan infection whose clinical characteristics depend on the species of the infecting parasite and the immune response of the host. The species that cause cutaneous leishmaniasis have geographic variation, with *Leishmania tropica* or *Leishmania major* causing disease in the eastern hemisphere (Old World), and *Leishmania mexicana, Leishmania panamensis*, or *Leishmania (Viannia) braziliensis* as the etiologic agents in the western hemisphere (New World). Visceral leishmaniasis, most often caused by *Leishmania infantum* or *L. donovani*, may present with fever, hepatosplenomegaly, and bone marrow involvement (pancytopenia), but can rarely have skin manifestations.

Leishmaniasis can occur weeks to months after a sandfly bite in an endemic region. Cutaneous leishmaniasis typically begins as an erythematous papule on exposed skin, which may expand to indurated plaques or ulcerations over months. Associated lymphadenopathy or sporotrichoid spread of the lesions may be present. In immunocompetent patients, cutaneous lesions usually heal spontaneously in 1 month to 3 years, whereas lesions of mucocutaneous leishmaniasis and visceral leishmaniasis rarely if ever heal without treatment. Certain species in the New World can progress to mucocutaneous leishmaniasis years later or the infection can remain dormant with reactivation because of immunosuppression.

The clinical presentation of leishmaniasis varies widely in immunocompetent patients, in acquired immune deficiency syndrome (AIDS) patients and in solid organ transplant recipients. The risk of developing leishmaniasis among transplant patients is associated with the geographical region in which they and their organ donors reside.[12] Leishmaniasis occurs as a late complication of organ transplantation, with a median delay of 18 months between transplantation and disease onset. It is earlier for liver transplantation than kidney transplantation. Cutaneous infection in the immunocompromised host may represent reactivation of an unrecognized latent *Leishmania* infection induced by the immunosuppressive drugs, recent development of clinically overt disease (e.g., primary infection) in the susceptible host or iatrogenic acquisition of *Leishmania* directly from the transplanted organ or from transfusion of infected blood products. Cutaneous leishmaniasis in the immunocompromised host may have unusual clinical features,[13,14] a high parasite load,[15] and/or a slow response to treatment.[16] Concomitant opportunistic infections can mask the clinical presentation of *Leishmania*. Lesions can be present in clinically unaffected skin or within concomitant skin disease, such as a lesion of Kaposi's sarcoma.[17] In HIV positive patients with

visceral *Leishmania*, coincidental *Leishmania* can be found in other[18] skin lesions including Kaposi's sarcoma, herpes simplex, herpes zoster, bacillary angiomatosis, dermatofibroma, tattoos,[19] and in the healthy skin of HIV positive patients. Immunosuppressed patients also appear to have a higher incidence of cutaneous and mucosal involvement and disseminated cutaneous disease at presentation.[14] Extensive ulcers in unusual locations such as the lips, tongue, and genital areas may occur.[14,20] Multiple slow growing, painless skin ulcers involving all extremities were reported in a 60-year-old Saudi Arabian man with leukemia.[21] Some of the atypical presentations in HIV infected patients include: a diffusely infiltrative plaque on the face with associated coalescing papules, a large necrotic genital ulcer, diffuse erythematous verrucous, ulcerated, or psoriasiform plaques on the face, trunk, and/or extremities, diffuse purpuric erythematous plaques on the trunk, and extensive erythematous infiltration in the plantar region of the foot.[14,22]

Visceral leishmaniasis (VL) has been described as the most common form of *Leishmania* infection associated with AIDS and immunosuppression for organ transplantation. Epidemiologic data from the World Health Organization indicate that 50% of all adult cases of VL are HIV positive.[18,23] HIV infection increases the risk of developing VL by 100–2,320 times in areas of endemicity, reduces the cure rate, increases the relapse rate and the mortality rate, and makes the leishmaniasis more resistant to treatment.[24] Visceral infection in transplant patients, most commonly kidney transplant recipients, can develop as a result of reactivation of a latent infection, as a primary opportunistic infection, or from transplantation of an infected organ.[12] VL can develop in HIV-infected individuals after a long latent infection from the immune reconstitution inflammatory syndrome after initiation of highly active antiretroviral therapy (HAART).[25] VL in HIV positive patients generally does not differ clinically from classical VL caused by *L. donovani* (kala-azar) but tends to have a more severe and protracted course, more prone to relapse and is often resistant to antimonial therapy.[18] Secondary cutaneous manifestations are rare but are much more common in the HIV-infected population. When cutaneous dissemination occurs the skin lesions do not present a uniform or characteristic appearance but tend to localize symmetrically on acral zones. They include erythematous nodules on the trunk and extremities, Kaposi's sarcoma like nodules, linear brown macules on the fingers and palms,[26] dermatomyositis-like erythematous macules and papules on the dorsal hands and arms, mucosal ulcerations, and erythematous papules on the legs.[12,27-29] In leishmaniasis and HIV disease, cutaneous lesions of leishmaniasis are sometimes the first sign of visceral involvement.

AMOEBA

The genera of amoebae identified as human pathogens include *Naegleria*, *Acanthamoeba*, *Balamuthia*, and *Sappinia*.[30,31] *Acanthamoeba* species, *Balamuthia mandrillaris,* and *Naegleria fowleri* are the primary pathogenic and opportunistic free-living amoeba which can all cause fatal central nervous system infections. *Acanthamoeba* and *Balamuthia* can affect immunocompromised patients, and disseminated disease may present with skin lesions.[30]

Acanthamoeba is a free-living amoeba that is ubiquitous and occurs worldwide. They have been isolated from soil, water (fresh water, seawater, tap water, bottled mineral water, sewage), buildings and instrumentation (air-conditioning, heating, ventilating and humidifier units, Jacuzzi tubs, hydrotherapy pools in hospitals and dialysis machines, and dental irrigation units), and humans (nasal cavities, throat, cornea, skin).[32] Infected patients often give a history of exposure to a pond or swimming pool.[33] *Acanthamoeba* is part of normal nasopharyngeal and oral flora in healthy individuals. In the immunocompromised, including HIV-infected patients and transplant recipients, *Acanthamoeba* can disseminate after primary infection of the nasal sinuses or lungs by hematogenous spread to the skin and central nervous system (CNS), causing granulomatous amoebic meningoencephalitis (GAM). The mortality rate for cases of disseminated disease with GAM approaches 100%, and early diagnosis is essential. Primary cutaneous disease, likely from external inoculation, has also been described.[34] Widespread disseminated extracerebral disease has been reported primarily in immunocompromised patients, with cutaneous lesions often as the presenting sign, and other organ involvement including bone, liver, adrenal gland, kidney, pancreas, thyroid, and lungs.[35]

Skin lesions of *Acanthamoeba* most commonly begin as firm papulonodules that drain purulent material and then develop non-healing indurated ulcerations.[36] Other cutaneous manifestations of disseminated *Acanthamoeba* include infiltrative plaques, pustules, papules, panniculitic nodules, and cellulitis/abscess-like lesions.[30,35,37,38] Skin lesions are most often multiple, and commonly involve the limbs, although there have been reports of thoracic, abdominal, and periorbital involvement.[30] Some patients, especially those with HIV/AIDS, develop chronic ulcerative skin lesions, abscesses, or erythematous nodules especially of the chest and limbs. These nodules are usually firm and nontender but sometimes they become ulcerated and purulent. Reports of several cases with multiple skin ulcers without dissemination to the CNS have been published.[39,40] A profoundly immunosuppressed 63-year-old liver transplant recipient with graft-versus-host disease (GVHD) had a dramatic presentation with over 100, 2–10 mm papulopustules localized to the head covering his face, scalp, and neck.[41] He also had approximately 10 subcutaneous ulcerated and non-ulcerated nodules on the lower extremities before his demise of disseminated *Acanthamoeba*. Typically, after all cultures and stains for bacteria and fungi are negative, a diagnosis of cutaneous *Acanthamoeba* is made by skin biopsy. Microscopic examination demonstrates amoebic trophozoites (10–60 μm in diameter, eccentrically placed nucleus, and a prominent nucleolus) and cysts (round to oval, with a distinctive, wrinkled double wall). *Acanthamoeba* species can be readily cultivated from clinical specimens on non-nutrient agar plates coated with bacteria such as *Escherichia coli* or *Enterobacter aerogenes*. Definitive identification of the amebic genus is based on the visualization with immunofluorescence-stained tissue (i.e., skin or brain).

Although the majority of cases of *Balamuthia* amebic encephalitis (BAE) occur in immunocompetent patients, immunocompromised patients appear to be at risk. The predisposing factors include HIV infection, immunosuppressive medications, substance abuse, and malnutrition.[42] Risk factors for developing disease include contact (nasal inhalation or exposure to open skin) with contaminated soil (from gardening or playing with dirt) or water, with hematogenous spread of infection and dissemination to the brain. Skin lesions are present in approximately half of the cases of disseminated disease, which may present as violaceous to purple infiltrative papules and nodules.[42] The characteristic skin lesions are asymptomatic infiltrative and violaceous plaques on the central face, usually involving the nose.[43] A solitary lesion is more common than multiple lesions or smaller satellite lesions. Many patients with BAE exhibit single or multiple skin ulcerations on the face, trunk, hands, or feet. The skin ulcerations usually precede the CNS involvement and provide an opportunity for early diagnosis.

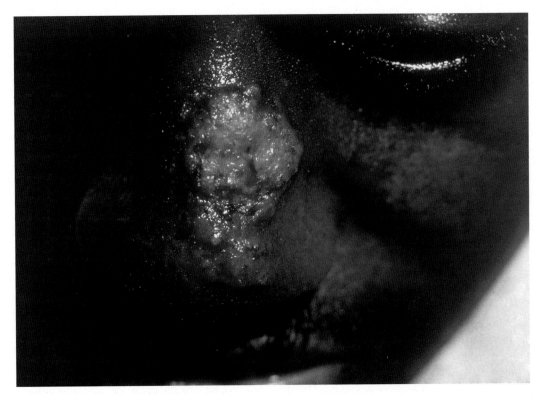

Figure 9.4. A 38-year-old human immunodeficiency virus (HIV)-positive man presented with skin lesions on the face and body, fatigue, and headache. An indurated 3-cm ulceration on the dorsum of the nose was biopsied. Histopathologic examination demonstrated a mixed inflammatory cell infiltrate with *Acanthamoeba* trophozoites and cysts scattered throughout the dermis (Courtesy of Mary Ruth Buchness, M.D. From May et al.[36], p. 352)

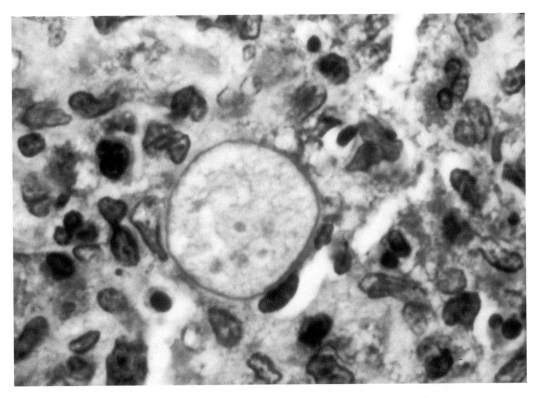

Figure 9.5. *Acanthamoeba* cyst with wrinkled double cyst wall on skin biopsy (Courtesy of Mary Ruth Buchness, M.D.)

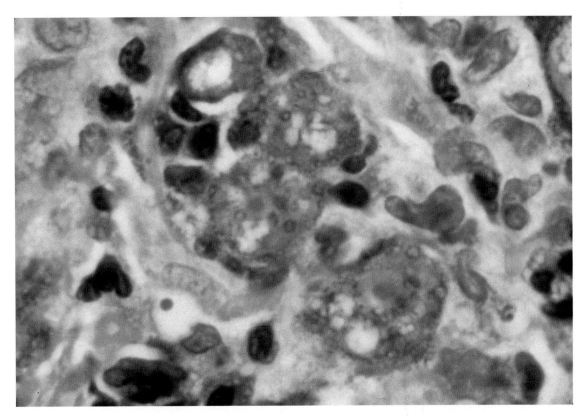

Figure 9.6. *Acanthamoeba* trophozoites on skin biopsy. Large round trophozoites with a large eccentrically placed nucleus, a prominent central nucleolus, a perinuclear vacuole, and cytoplasmic granular material positive to periodic acid-Schiff stain (Courtesy of Mary Ruth Buchness, M.D.)

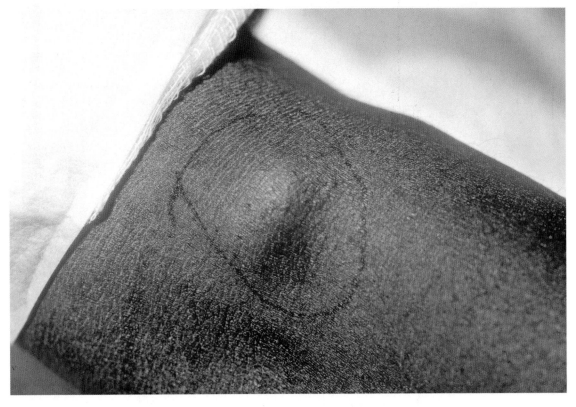

Figure 9.7. A subcutaneous nodule of *Acanthamoeba culbertsoni* (Courtesy of Mary Ruth Buchness, M.D.)

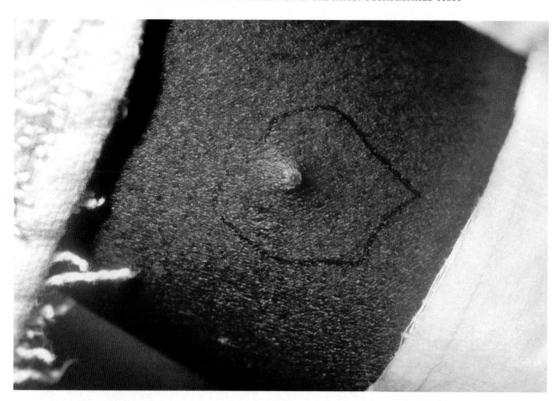

Figure 9.8.   A papulonodule of *Acanthamoeba* developed a purulent surface (Courtesy of Mary Ruth Buchness, M.D.)

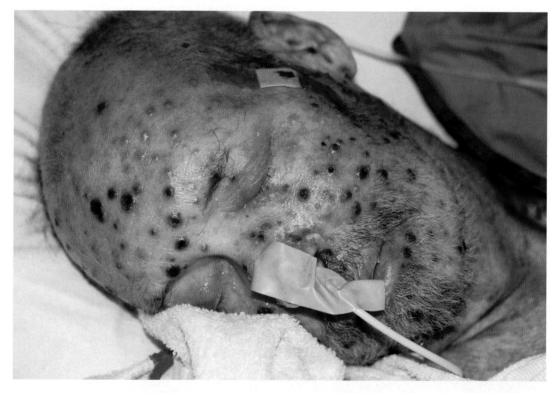

Figure 9.9.   A 64-year-old man with primary sclerosing cholangitis received a liver transplant complicated by Epstein-Barr virus (EBV) positive post-transplant lymphoproliferative disorder and acute graft versus host disease. He received multiple combination immunosuppressive regimens and day 366 post liver transplant developed innumerable erythematous papulopustules with necrotic central black eschars covering his face, head, and neck

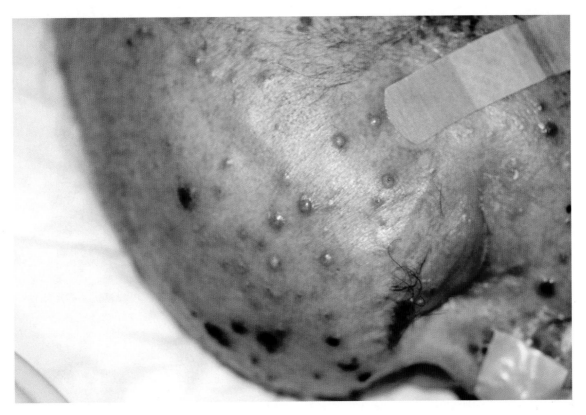

Figure 9.10. Close-up of the deep seated 4–6-mm forehead pustules

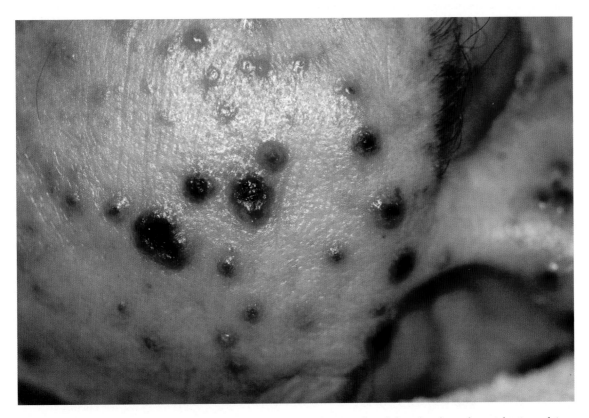

Figure 9.11. Pustules with central necrotic eschars and crusts on the forehead. Bacterial, viral, fungal, and mycobacterial stains and tissue cultures were negative

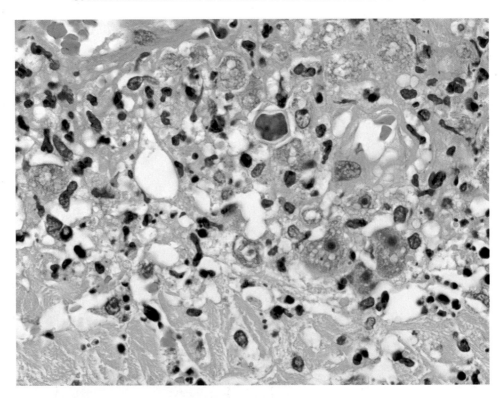

Figure 9.12. Skin biopsy demonstrated numerous *Acanthamoeba* trophozoites. The trophozoites have a single nucleus with a centrally placed, large, densely, staining nucleolus and numerous cytoplasmic vacuoles. Direct immunofluorescence and polymerase chain reaction (PCR) testing at the Centers for Disease Control (CDC) were positive for *Acanthamoeba* species and negative for *Balamuthia* and *Naegleria fowleri* (Courtesy of Sameera Husain, M.D.)

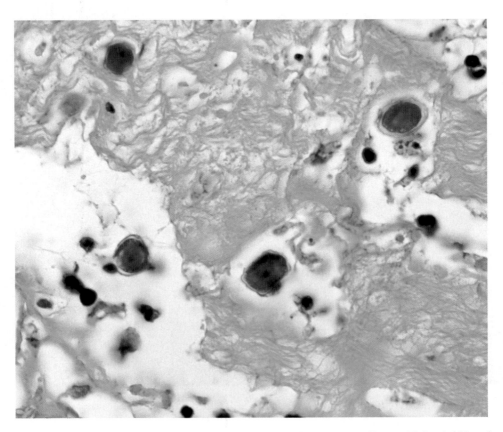

Figure 9.13. Skin biopsy with numerous double-walled cysts, 10–25 mm in size. The outer cyst wall is wrinkled with folds and ripples (Courtesy of Sameera Husain, M.D.)

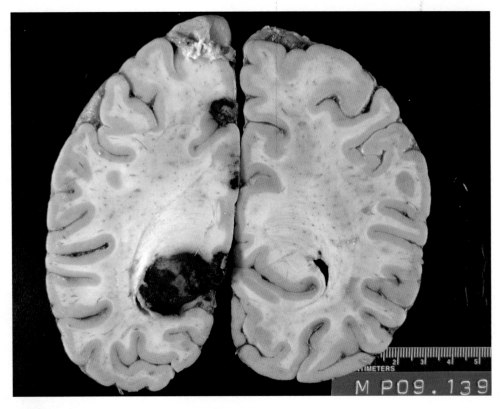

Figure 9.14. Postmortem examination revealed the presence of numerous *Acanthamoeba* trophozoite and cyst forms in the skin, lungs, liver, and brain. Numerous hemorrhagic nodules were present in the brain (Courtesy of Sameera Husain, M.D.)

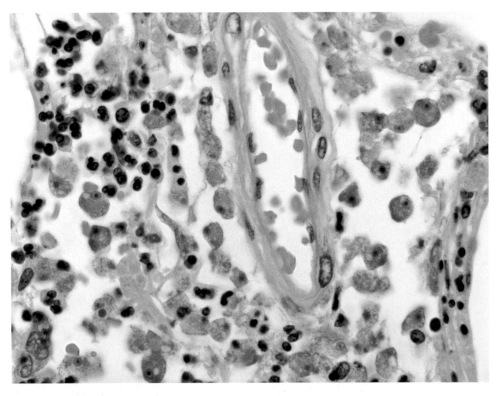

Figure 9.15. Brain postmortem section demonstrated numerous *Acanthamoeba* trophozoites lining up along a vein in the patient's brain. The organism spread hematogenously to the central nervous system across the blood–brain barrier (Courtesy of Sameera Husain, M.D.)

Pneumocystis

Pneumocystis (*carinii*) *jirovecii* pneumonia is the most common opportunistic infection in patients with HIV infection. Extrapulmonary cutaneous pneumocystis is very rare. Most cases occur with active concurrent pulmonary infection or had received pneumocystis pneumonia prophylaxis. The skin findings most frequently described consist of friable reddish papules, nodules, or polypoid lesions involving the external auditory canal.[44,45] Other manifestations include diffuse papules of the flank, back, limbs, and face clinically mimicking Kaposi's sarcoma,[46] in a 35-year-old male with AIDS. Hennessey et al. described bluish gray chest macules and molluscum contagiosum-like papules on the head and neck due to *P. jirovecii*

in two patients with AIDS.[47] Another patient developed skin ulceration, digital necrosis, and gangrene of the foot because of extensive *P. jirovecii* within the dermal arterioles and capillaries.[48] Nontender bilateral axillary firm, erythematous nonfluctuant, non-painful nodules developed in a 29-year-old HIV-positive man despite prophylaxis with high dose dapsone.[49] Concurrent infections with *P. jirovecii* and *Staphylococcus aureus* botryomycosis[50] and *P. jirovecii* and *Cryptococcus* necrotic and skin-colored umbilicated facial papules and nodules[51] have been reported in AIDS.

Cutaneous pneumocystosis may precede the onset of *P. jirovecii* pneumonia (PCP). Recognition of this extrapulmonary infection at an early stage may lead to earlier treatment and reduced morbidity from PCP.

Figure 9.16. A 31-year-old HIV-positive man with prior episodes of *Pneumocystis carinii* pneumonia (PCP) developed multiple, crusted translucent papules on the trunk and neck. The appearance was that of traumatized molluscum contagiosum. Biopsy confirmed the diagnosis of cutaneous pneumocystosis before the acute onset of PCP. The skin lesions and pneumonia resolved with intravenous pentamidine (From Hennessey et al.[47] Copyright 1991, American Medical Association)

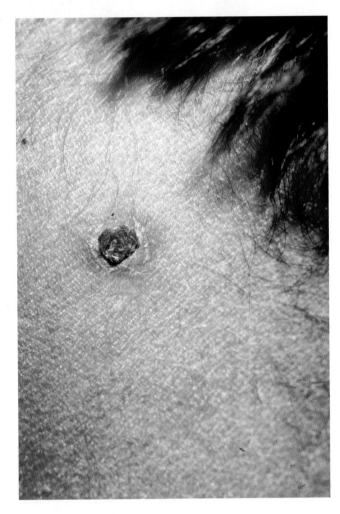

TOXOPLASMOSIS

Cutaneous toxoplasmosis is rare. Toxoplasmosis in the immunocompromised host occurs from recrudescence of a latent infection (from the cyst of the organism) acquired in the distant past (in the setting of AIDS or bone marrow transplantation) or recently acquired acute infection with the parasite, usually through the transplanted organ. When the allograft of a seropositive organ is given to a seronegative recipient, toxoplasmosis will commonly develop. In transplant patients, fever is the most common first manifestation followed by signs in the central nervous system and the lungs. Toxoplasmosis in AIDS patients commonly manifest as encephalitis, pneumonitis, and chorioretinitis. Skin involvement has been described post bone marrow transplant for acute lymphocytic leukemia (ALL) as greater than 50 disseminated discrete pleomorphic papules which demonstrated *T. gondii* bradyzoites within keratinocytes and dermal blood vessels on skin biopsy.[52] Subtle erythematous papules over the chest and back developed in a febrile 16-year-old post cord blood transplant for ALL. Skin biopsy revealed *T. gondii* bradyzoites and tachyzoites within epidermal keratinocytes with a cell–poor interface dermatitis. The resemblance to graft versus host disease clinically and histologically caused by cutaneous toxoplasmosis highlights the need for a timely skin biopsy.[53] Purple papules on the legs of a 31-year-old woman in blast crisis after a stem cell transplant for acute myelogenous leukemia (AML) demonstrated bradyzoites in the epidermis,

follicular epithelium, sweat glands and ducts, and endothelium. Polymerase chain reaction examination of the skin biopsy confirmed the presence of *Toxoplasma gondii*. Skin lesions in hematopoietic stem cell transplant recipients should undergo skin biopsy in the setting of neurologic or pulmonary disease and/or following treatment of GVHD.[54]

ENTAMOEBA

Entamoeba histolytica is a common infection worldwide and primarily causes colitis or liver abscesses. Cutaneous disease, amebiasis cutis, is very rare. It can be sexually transmitted or result from direct extension of colorectal disease to involve the anus, perianal skin, or vulva.[43] Contiguous spread of the parasite from the bowel to around a fistula, around a colostomy orifice, or around laparotomy incisions after surgery on infected bowel can also result in cutaneous infection. Cutaneous amebiasis has rarely been reported in HIV-infected patients, but there does not appear to be a clear association with the immunocompromised state. Amebiasis cutis presents as painful perianal or genital ragged ulcerations with necrotic slough and purulent exudates at the base.[55] A biopsy from the margin of the ulceration or a wet drop preparation of the skin ulcer discharge may reveal *E. histolytica* trophozoites (round or oval cells measuring 20–50 mm, basophilic with a 4–7 mm nucleus) with phagocytosed red blood cells.

REFERENCES

Trypanosoma cruzi (Chagas' Disease)

1. Kirchhoff LV. American trypanosomiasis (Chagas' disease) – a tropical disease now in the United States. N Engl J Med. 1993;329(9):639–44.

2. Stolf NA, Higushi L, Bocchi E, et al. Heart transplantation in patients with Chagas' disease cardiomyopathy. J Heart Transplant. 1987;6(5):307–12.

3. Godoy HL, Guerra CM, Viegas RF, et al. Infections in heart transplant recipients in Brazil: the challenge of Chagas' disease. J Heart Lung Transplant. 2010;29(3):286–90.

4. Hall CS, Fields K. Cutaneous presentation of Chagas' disease reactivation in a heart-transplant patient in Utah. J Am Acad Dermatol. 2008;58(3):529–30.

5. La Forgia MP, Pellerano G, de las Mercedes Portaluppi M, Kien MC, Chouela EN. Cutaneous manifestation of reactivation of Chagas disease in a renal transplant patient: long-term follow-up. Arch Dermatol. 2003;139(1):104–5.

6. Tomimori-Yamashita J, Deps PD, Almeida DR, et al. Cutaneous manifestation of Chagas' disease after heart transplantation: successful treatment with allopurinol. Br J Dermatol. 1997;137(4):626–30.

7. Libow LF, Beltrani VP, Silvers DN, Grossman ME. Post-cardiac transplant reactivation of Chagas' disease diagnosed by skin biopsy. Cutis. 1991;48(1):37–40.

8. Sartori AM, Ibrahim KY, Nunes Westphalen EV, et al. Manifestations of Chagas disease (American trypanosomiasis) in patients with HIV/AIDS. Ann Trop Med Parasitol. 2007;101(1):31–50.

9. Sartori AM, Sotto MN, Braz LM, et al. Reactivation of Chagas disease manifested by skin lesions in a patient with AIDS. Trans R Soc Trop Med Hyg. 1999;93(6):631–2.

10. Riarte A, Luna C, Sabatiello R, et al. Chagas' disease in patients with kidney transplants: 7 years of experience, 1989–1996. Clin Infect Dis. 1999;29:561–7.

11. Gallerano V, Consigli J, Pereyra S, et al. Chagas' disease reactivation with skin symptoms in a patient with kidney transplant. Int J Dermatol. 2007;46(6):607–10.

Leishmania

12. Antinori S, Cascio A, Parravicini C, Bianchi R, Corbellino M. Leishmaniasis among organ transplant recipients. Lancet Infect Dis. 2008;8(3):191–9.

13. Rosenthal PJ, Chaisson RE, Hadley WK, Leech JH. Rectal leishmaniasis in a patient with acquired immunodeficiency syndrome. Am J Med. 1988;84(2):307–9.

14. Lindoso JA, Barbosa RN, Posada-Vergara MP, et al. Unusual manifestations of tegumentary leishmaniasis in AIDS patients from the New World. Br J Dermatol. 2009;160(2):311–8.

15. Da-Cruz AM, Machado ES, Menezes JA, Rutowitsch MS, Coutinho SG. Cellular and humoral immune responses of a patient with American cutaneous leishmaniasis and AIDS. Trans R Soc Trop Med Hyg. 1992;86(5):511–2.

16. Smith D, Gazzard B, Lindley RP, et al. Visceral leishmaniasis (kala azar) in a patient with AIDS. AIDS. 1989;3(1):41–3.

17. Yebra M, Segovia J, Manzano L, et al. Disseminated-to-skin kala-azar and the acquired immunodeficiency syndrome. Ann Intern Med. 1988;108(3):490–1.

18. Puig L, Pradinaud R. Leishmania and HIV co-infection: dermatological manifestations. Ann Trop Med Parasitol. 2003;97 Suppl 1:107–14.

19. López-Medrano F, Costa JR, Rodriguez-Peralto JL, Aguado JM. An HIV-positive man with tattoo induration. Clin Infect Dis. 2007;45(2):220–1, 267–8.

20. Iborra C, Caumes E, Carrière J, et al. Mucosal leishmaniasis in a heart transplant recipient. Br J Dermatol. 1998;138(1):190–2.

21. Al-Qattan MM. Extensive cutaneous leishmaniasis of the upper limb in a patient with leukemia. Ann Plast Surg. 2002;48(6):670–1.

22. Mattos M, Caiza A, Fernandes O, et al. American cutaneous leishmaniasis associated with HIV infection: report of four cases. J Eur Acad Dermatol Venereol. 1998;10(3):218–25.

23. Choi CM, Lerner EA. Leishmaniasis: recognition and management with a focus on the immunocompromised patient. Am J Clin Dermatol. 2002;3(2):91–105.

24. Alvar J, Aparicio P, Aseffa A, et al. The relationship between leishmaniasis and AIDS: the second 10 years. Clin Microbiol Rev. 2008;21(2):334–59.

25. van der Spek BW, Hillebrand-Haverkort ME, Stam F, Kager PA. One of the many faces of immune reconstitution inflammatory syndrome. Clin Infect Dis. 2009;48(6):764–5, 836–8.

26. Colebunders R, Depraetere K, Verstraeten T, et al. Unusual cutaneous lesions in two patients with visceral leishmaniasis and HIV infection. J Am Acad Dermatol. 1999;41(5 Pt 2):847–50.

27. González-Beato MJ, Moyano B, Sánchez C, et al. Kaposi's sarcoma-like lesions and other nodules as cutaneous involvement in AIDS-related visceral leishmaniasis. Br J Dermatol. 2000;143(6):1316–8.

28. Ara M, Maillo C, Peón G, et al. Visceral leishmaniasis with cutaneous lesions in a patient infected with human immunodeficiency virus. Br J Dermatol. 1998;139(1):114–7.

29. Daudén E, Peñas PF, Rios L, et al. Leishmaniasis presenting as a dermatomyositis-like eruption in AIDS. J Am Acad Dermatol. 1996;35 (2 Pt 2):316–9.

Amoeba

30. Visvesvara GS, Moura H, Schuster FL. Pathogenic and opportunistic free-living amoebae: Acanthamoeba spp., Balamuthia mandrillaris, Naegleria fowleri, and Sappinia diploidea. FEMS Immunol Med Microbiol. 2007;50(1):1–26.

31. Ma P, Visvesvara GS, Martinez AJ, et al. Naegleria and Acanthamoeba infections: review. Rev Infect Dis. 1990;12(3):490–513.

32. Marciano-Cabral F, Cabral G. Acanthamoeba spp. as agents of disease in humans. Clin Microbiol Rev. 2003;16(2):273–307.

33. Galarza C, Ramos W, Gutierrez EL, et al. Cutaneous acanthamebiasis infection in immunocompetent and immunocompromised patients. Int J Dermatol. 2009;48(12):1324–6.

34. Torno Jr MS, Babapour R, Gurevitch A, Witt MD. Cutaneous acanthamoebiasis in AIDS. J Am Acad Dermatol. 2000;42(2 Pt 2):351–4.

35. Steinberg JP, Galindo RL, Kraus ES, Ghanem KG. Disseminated acanthamebiasis in a renal transplant recipient with osteomyelitis and cutaneous lesions: case report and literature review. Clin Infect Dis. 2002;35(5):e43–9.

36. May LP, Sidhu GS, Buchness MR. Diagnosis of Acanthamoeba infection by cutaneous manifestations in a man seropositive to HIV. J Am Acad Dermatol. 1992;26(2 Pt 2):352–5.

37. Rosenberg AS, Morgan MB. Disseminated acanthamoebiasis presenting as lobular panniculitis with necrotizing vasculitis in a patient with AIDS. J Cutan Pathol. 2001;28(6):307–13.

38. Barete S, Combes A, de Jonckheere JF, et al. Fatal disseminated Acanthamoeba lenticulata infection in a heart transplant patient. Emerg Infect Dis. 2007;13(5):736–8.

39. Slater CA, Sickel JZ, Visvesvara GS, Pabico RC, Gaspari AA. Brief report: successful treatment of disseminated acanthamoeba infection in an immunocompromised patient. N Engl J Med. 1994;331(2):85–7.

40. Visvesvara GS, Stehr-Green JK. Epidemiology of free-living ameba infections. J Protozool. 1990;37(4):25S–33S.

41. Young AL, Leboeuf NR, Tsiouris SJ, Husain S, Grossman ME. Fatal disseminated Acanthamoeba infection in a liver transplant recipient immunocompromised by combination therapies for graft-versus-host disease. Transpl Infect Dis. 2010;12(6):529–37.

42. Siddiqui R, Khan NA. *Balamuthia* amoebic encephalitis: an emerging disease with fatal consequences. Microb Pathog. 2008;44(2):89–97.

43. Lupi O, Bartlett BL, Haugen RN, et al. Tropical dermatology: tropical diseases caused by protozoa. J Am Acad Dermatol. 2009;60(6): 897–925; quiz 926–8.

Pneumocystis

44. Coulman CU, Greene I, Archibald RW. Cutaneous pneumocystosis. Ann Intern Med. 1987;106(3):396–8.

45. Schinella RA, Breda SD, Hammerschlag PE. Otic infection due to *Pneumocystis carinii* in an apparently healthy man with antibody to the human immunodeficiency virus. Ann Intern Med. 1987;106(3): 399–400.

46. Litwin MA, Williams CM. Cutaneous *Pneumocystis carinii* infection mimicking Kaposi sarcoma. Ann Intern Med. 1992;117(1):48–9.

47. Hennessey NP, Parro EL, Cockerell CJ. Cutaneous *Pneumocystis carinii* infection in patients with acquired immunodeficiency syndrome. Arch Dermatol. 1991;127(11):1699–701.

48. Davey Jr RT, Margolis D, Kleiner D, Deyton L, Travis W. Digital necrosis and disseminated *Pneumocystis carinii* infection after aerosolized pentamidine prophylaxis. Ann Intern Med. 1989;111(8):681–2.

49. Bundow DL, Aboulafia DM. Skin involvement with Pneumocystis despite dapsone prophylaxis: a rare cause of skin nodules in a patient with AIDS. Am J Med Sci. 1997;313(3):182–6.

50. Saadat P, Ram R, Sohrabian S, Vadmal MS. Botryomycosis caused by *Staphylococcus aureus* and *Pneumocystis carinii* in a patient with acquired immunodeficiency disease. Clin Exp Dermatol. 2008;33(3): 266–9.

51. Sandler B, Potter TS, Hashimoto K. Cutaneous *Pneumocystis carinii* and *Cryptococcus neoformans* in AIDS. Br J Dermatol. 1996;134(1): 159–63.

Toxoplasmosis

52. Lee SA, Diwan AH, Cohn M, Champlin R, Safdar A. Cutaneous toxoplasmosis: a case of confounding diagnosis. Bone Marrow Transplant. 2005;36(5):465–6.

53. Vidal CI, Pollack M, Uliasz A, del Toro G, Emanuel PO. Cutaneous toxoplasmosis histologically mimicking graft-versus-host disease. Am J Dermatopathol. 2008;30(5):492–3.

54. Amir G, Salant H, Resnick IB, Karplus R. Cutaneous toxoplasmosis after bone marrow transplantation with molecular confirmation. J Am Acad Dermatol. 2008;59(5):781–4.

Entamoeba

55. Bumb RA, Mehta RD. Amoebiasis cutis in HIV positive patient. Indian J Dermatol Venereol Leprol. 2006;72(3):224–6.

10

Helminth

Strongyloides stercoralis, an intestinal nematode commonly known as the human threadworm, affects millions of people worldwide.[1] It is endemic in Southeast Asia, Latin America, sub-Saharan Africa, and parts of the southeastern USA.[2] In the USA, the highest prevalence rates are found in eastern Kentucky and rural Tennessee. A unique feature of *Strongyloides stercoralis* infection is the occurrence of an autoinfection cycle which permits persistence of the parasite years after the normal host has left an endemic area. In this cycle, the rhabditiform larvae in the duodenojujenal portion of the small intestine transform directly into filariform (infective) larvae. The filariform larvae without leaving the body can reinfect the patient by penetrating the intestinal mucosa. This distinctive characteristic of *Strongyloides*, to persist and replicate within the host for decades, produces minimal or no symptoms. Immunocompromised patients may develop a fulminant illness due to a unique process in the life cycle of *Strongyloides* in which there are dramatic increases in the number of filariform larvae. In the hyperinfection syndrome, massive numbers of larvae migrate through the intestinal mucosa and into the lungs (the usual migration pattern) and disseminate to involve other organ systems not ordinarily a part of the life cycle of the parasite. Larvae may be found in the central nervous system, kidneys, liver, and almost any other organ.

Strongyloides stercoralis hyperinfection syndrome usually develops in the setting of compromised cell-mediated immunity such as severe malnutrition, chronic infection (lepromatous leprosy, human immunodeficiency virus [HIV], tuberculosis, or human T-cell lymphotropic virus type 1 [HTLV]), leukemia, lymphoma, malignancy, or organ transplantation associated with the administration of systemic steroids or other immunosuppressive drugs.[3,4] Hyperinfection syndrome can occur after augmentation of steroids or pulse steroids and other immunosuppressive drugs for treatment of transplant graft rejection. Immunosuppressive regimens including cyclosporine for organ

transplant recipients have been reported to have a decreased incidence of hyperinfection *Strongyloides*. This has been attributed to the anti-helminthic properties cyclosporine demonstrated in mouse models.[5] Organ transplant recipients can develop hyperinfection syndrome from endogeneous reactivation and by acquisition of *Strongyloides* from the transplanted organ and obligatory immunosuppression.[6]

The diagnosis of *Strongyloides* hyperinfection syndrome requires physician awareness of this infection and the clinical setting in which it occurs. There are several clues to the diagnosis:

1. Eosinophilia may be modest or absent. It may be marginal and transient so that it is not recognized. Systemic steroids and host debilitation may suppress this characteristic finding. The presence of eosinophilia should initiate a vigorous search for parasites.

2. Unexplained or persistent bacteremia with enteric organisms despite administration of appropriate antibiotics; gram negative or polymicrobial sepsis.

3. Serious infection (pneumonia, meningitis or bacteremia) from a suspected intraabdominal source. Gram negative bacteria follow the parasite through the intestinal wall or piggyback on the larvae. These bacteria produce the peculiar winding trails or serpiginous tracks on blood agar plates from culture of a body fluid with *Strongyloides* larvae.[7,8]

4. Nonspecific gastrointestinal symptoms (abdominal pain and distention, diarrhea, nausea and vomiting, constipation, gastrointestinal [GI] bleeding, or ulceration). The clinical picture may mimic ulcerative colitis.

5. Nonspecific pulmonary symptoms and signs (cough, wheezing, hemoptysis [massive in some cases], transient interstitial infiltrates); severe pulmonary disease and acute respiratory distress syndrome (ARDS).

6. Concurrent infection or prior therapy for other intestinal parasites.

M.E. Grossman et al., *Cutaneous Manifestations of Infection in the Immunocompromised Host*,
DOI 10.1007/978-1-4419-1578-8_10, © Springer Science+Business Media, LLC 2012

7. History of residence or travel to an endemic area even many years previously.

In any of these clinical settings, the thumbprint sign of periumbilical purpura is pathognomonic of hyperinfection *Strongyloides*.[9,10] Most of the multiple purpuric lesions appear as small ecchymoses, as if caused by the pressure of thumbs or other fingers during physical examination of the abdomen. The purpura radiates from the umbilicus and progresses to involve the flanks and proximal lower extremities. Innumerable fine petechiae rapidly develop over 24–48 h as a reticulated pattern of linear and serpiginous purpuric streaks.[11,12]

The vascular distribution of the lesions of hyperinfection *Strongyloides* closely parallels that of the caput medusa seen in chronic liver disease with portal hypertension. In that setting, increased portal pressure leads to retrograde flow through the periumbilical portosystemic anastomoses. The patients reported with periumbilical purpura had been placed on respirators before the development of their skin lesions. Positive pressure ventilation produces a rise in portal pressure. It is hypothesized that numerous larvae leave the host's bowel through the superior and inferior mesenteric veins entering the liver. Patients receiving respiratory assistance have transient rises in portal pressure, shunting portal blood through the periumbilical portal systemic shunt. This blood carries numerous larvae that, on reaching the dermal vascular plexus, cause extravasation of red blood cells.[9] A subtle case of two faint periumbilical purpuric patches was seen by one of the authors in a patient with mild gastrointestinal and pulmonary symptoms who was not on mechanical ventilation. Skin biopsy revealed the filariform larvae of *Strongyloides* supporting the hypothesis that while the larvae may migrate through the skin during hyperinfection, positive pressure mechanical ventilation is required to produce the classically described periumbilical thumbprint purpura. A 25-year-old Mexican man with acquired immune deficiency syndrome (AIDS) (CD4 count 70) was hospitalized with GI complaints, weight loss, and numerous 2–3 mm purpuric papules on his abdomen. Skin biopsy demonstrated filariform larvae of *Strongyloides*.[13]

Strongyloides hyperinfection syndrome can be confirmed by microscopic examination of the nasogastric aspirates, bronchopulmonary lavage specimens, or skin biopsy. The filariform larvae are immediately infective, so gloves must be worn when handling these specimens to prevent the larvae from entering mucocutaneous surfaces of the health care worker. The skin biopsy from a purpuric patch readily demonstrates *Strongyloides* filariform larvae in and around blood vessels and throughout the dermis in association with extravasated red blood cells. Multiple longitudinal and cross-sections of the larvae are usually seen. There is a significant absence of any inflammatory cell infiltrate. Serologic tests are useful in patients with negative stool exams but may not be reliable for immunocompromised hosts.[7]

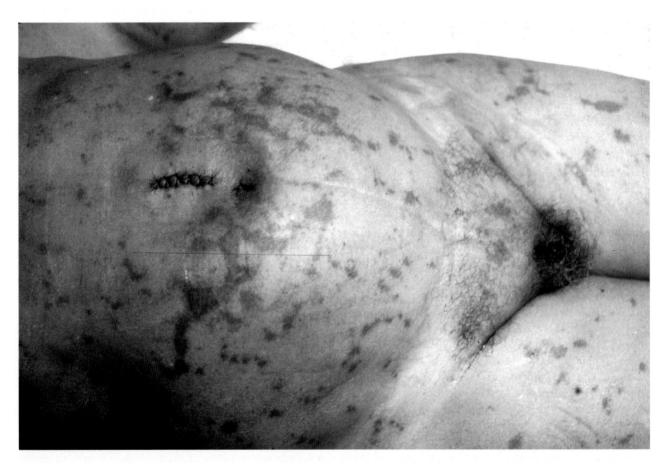

Figure 10.1. A 62-year-old woman with polymyositis on systemic steroids was from the Dominican Republic and had lived in the USA for 10 years. She presented with fever, abdominal pain, and bilateral interstitial pulmonary infiltrates. Nonpalpable periumbilical purpura appeared 24 h after a normal exploratory laparotomy

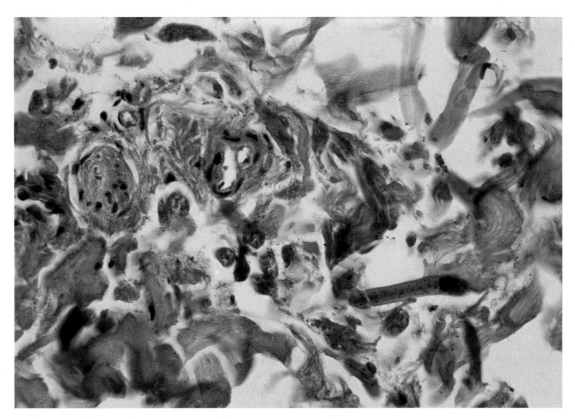

Figure 10.2. Skin biopsy of the purpura showed multiple longitudinal and cross sections of the larvae of *Strongyloides*. There was a significant absence of an inflammatory response to the larvae, which accounted for the eruption being nonpalpable

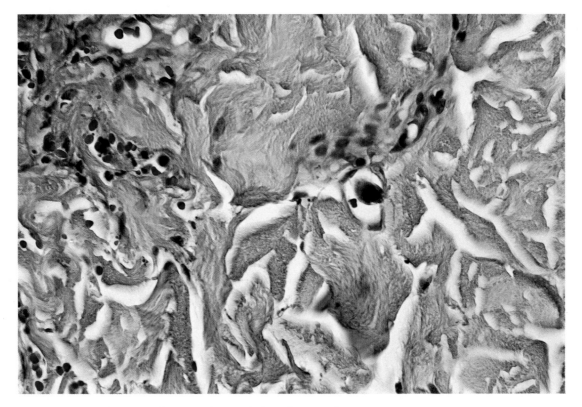

Figure 10.3. Skin biopsy with intravascular larvae of *Strongyloides* without an inflammatory response

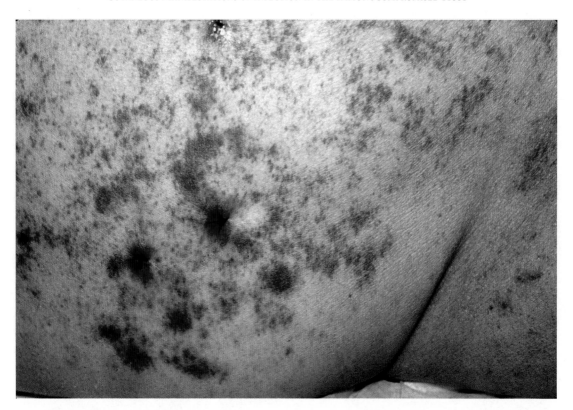

Figure 10.4. A 60-year-old man, born in Ecuador, had been treated for 7 years for asthma with many courses of systemic steroids. Blood eosinophilia was often greater than 15% and attributed to asthma after a negative stool for ova and parasites. On his last hospital admission because of respiratory distress he was intubated. Less than 12 h later he developed periumbilical purpura

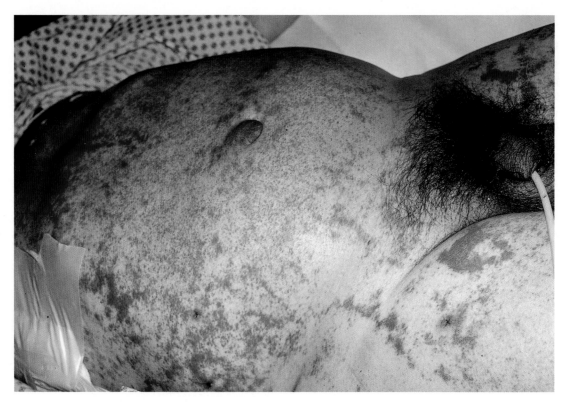

Figure 10.5. Multiple purpuric thumbprints appeared on the abdomen, flanks, and proximal thighs

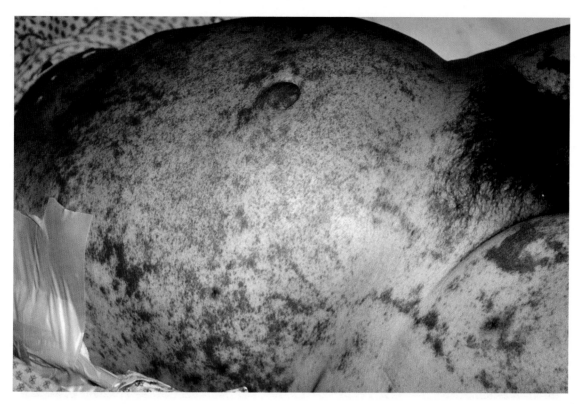

Figure 10.6. Over the next 24 h, innumerable petechiae developed in the same areas. Skin biopsy of purpura demonstrated larvae throughout the dermis both inside and outside of blood vessels

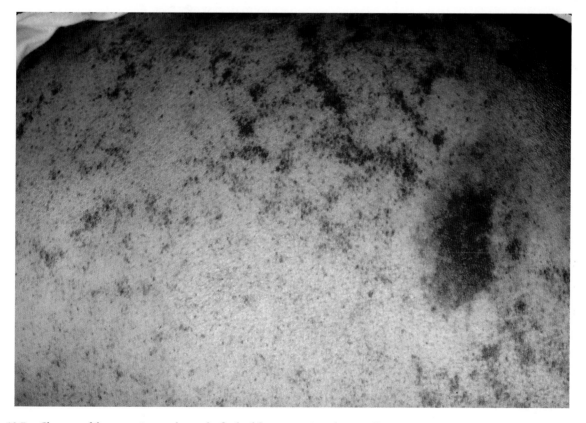

Figure 10.7. Close-up of the purpuric macules on the flank of the same patient shown in Figs. 10.3–10.6

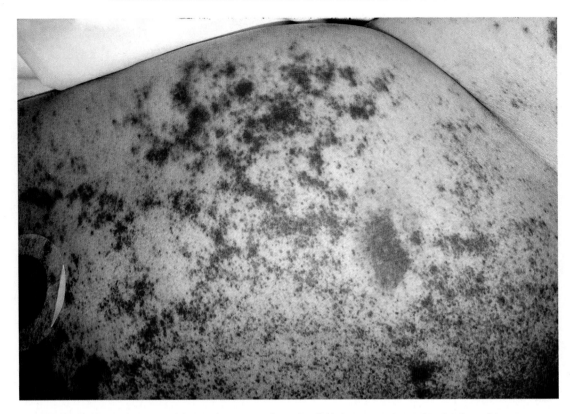

Figure 10.8. Within 48 h, the purpuric macules spread into a vascular network-like pattern with a multitude of petechiae

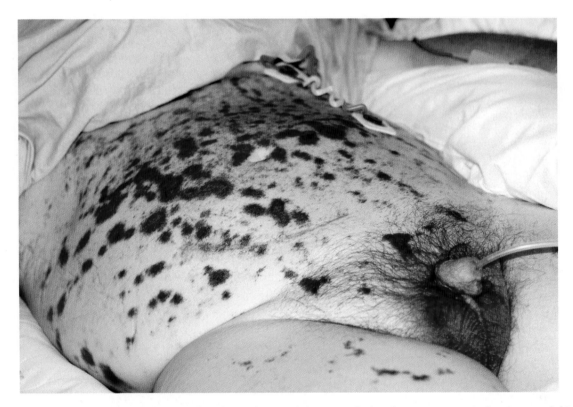

Figure 10.9. A 67-year-old man with a history of renal transplantation with a linear array thumbprint purpura from hyperinfection *Strongyloides*. The organism was acquired from the donor transplanted kidney. Bronchial washings, gastrointestinal aspirates, and skin biopsy were positive for *Strongyloides*

REFERENCES

1. Roxby AC, Gottlieb GS, Limaye AP. Strongyloidiasis in transplant patients. Clin Infect Dis. 2009;49(9):1411–23.

2. Gordon SM, Gal AA, Solomon AR, Bryan JA. Disseminated strongyloidiasis with cutaneous manifestations in an immunocompromised host. J Am Acad Dermatol. 1994;31:255–9.

3. Keiser PB, Nutman TB. *Strongyloides stercoralis* in the immunocompromised population. Clin Microbiol Rev. 2004;17(1):208–17.

4. Krishnamurthy R, Dincer HE, Whittemore D. *Strongyloides stercoralis* hyperinfection in a patient with rheumatoid arthritis after anti-TNF-alpha therapy. J Clin Rheumatol. 2007;13(3):150–2.

5. Schad GA. Cyclosporine may eliminate the threat of overwhelming strongyloidiasis in immunosuppressed patients. J Infect Dis. 1986; 153(1):178.

6. Weiser JA, Scully BE, Bulman WA, Husain S, Grossman ME. Periumbilical parasitic thumbprint purpura: *Strongyloides* hyperinfection syndrome acquired from a cadaveric renal transplant. Transpl Infect Dis. 2011;13(1):58–62.

7. Abdalla J, Saad M, Myers JW, Moorman JP. An elderly man with immunosuppression, shortness of breath, and eosinophilia. Clin Infect Dis. 2005;40(10):1464. 1535–6.

8. Raffalli J, Friedman C, Reid D, et al. Photo quiz. Clin Infect Dis. 1995;21(6):1377. 1459.

9. Bank DE, Grossman ME, Kohn SR, Rabinowitz AD. The thumbprint sign: rapid diagnosis of disseminated strongyloidiasis. J Am Acad Dermatol. 1990;23(2 Pt 1):324–6.

10. Salluh JI, Bozza FA, Pinto TS, et al. Cutaneous periumbilical purpura in disseminated strongyloidiasis in cancer patients: a pathognomonic feature of potentially lethal disease? Braz J Infect Dis. 2005;9(5): 419–24.

11. Kalb RE, Grossman ME. Periumbilical purpura in disseminated strongyloidiasis. JAMA. 1986;256(9):1170–1.

12. von Kuster LC, Genta RM. Cutaneous manifestations of strongyloidiasis. Arch Dermatol. 1988;124(12):1826–30.

13. Kao D, Murakawa GJ, Kerschmann R, Berger T. Disseminated strongyloidiasis in a patient with acquired immunodeficiency syndrome. Arch Dermatol. 1996;132(8):977–8.

11

Spirochete

TREPONEMA PALLIDUM (SYPHILIS)

Syphilis is a sexually transmitted disease of worldwide distribution that shares a particularly strong association with human immunodeficiency virus (HIV) infection. The incidence of primary and secondary syphilis decreased in the 1990s to 2.1 cases per 100,000 by the year 2000,[1] perhaps in part due to high fatality rates in acquired immune deficiency syndrome (AIDS) patients.[2] However, by 2007, the incidence of syphilis increased to 3.3 cases per 100,000, almost exclusively in men, with 64% of all cases of early syphilis occurring in men who have sex with men.[1]

Reasons for the association between syphilis and HIV include a shared mode of transmission (including unprotected oral sex), the increased risk for transmission of HIV disease in the setting of genital ulcerative disease such as syphilis, and a compromised ability of HIV-infected individuals to combat infection with *Treponema pallidum*. For this last reason, clinical presentations of syphilis in HIV disease are often exaggerated and may not correlate with serologic titer (Venereal Disease Research Laboratory (VDRL) or rapid plasma reagin (RPR) test).

In the normal host, untreated syphilis passes through relatively predictable stages: primary syphilis, manifested by a painless chancre on the genitals, hands, or mouth; secondary syphilis, following the primary chancre by approximately 6 weeks, which involves pharyngitis and a generalized maculopapular eruption that may include palms, soles, and mucous membranes (mucous patches or condyloma lata); and tertiary syphilis, which may occur years later and include cardiovascular or neurologic disease and mucocutaneous gummas. Serologic titers are predicable, being highest in secondary syphilis, and usually correlate with the flagrancy of the secondary eruption.

In the HIV-infected host, the presentation of syphilis may be wildly different and the skin lesions are often unusually exuberant. Primary syphilis is more likely to present with multiple chancres than in non-HIV-infected patients (70% vs. 34%).[1] Chancres may be giant,[3] become more locally destructive, causing perforations in the labia or prepuce, and take longer to heal than in non HIV-infected patients.[4] HIV-infected patients more frequently present with concomitant chancre and rash. Clinical manifestations of syphilis with HIV infection may be atypical with a wide range of presentations including ocular and central nervous system involvement, more frequent progression to neurosyphilis and failure of penicillin treatment to prevent the development of neurosyphilis, rapid progression from stage to stage leading to earlier symptoms of secondary to tertiary syphilis, altered histopathologic manifestations, and unreliable serology.[5]

Secondary syphilis in the HIV-infected patient may follow the initial inoculation by a very brief period, may be the initial presentation of infection, or may present concomitantly with the primary chancre.[1] Chancres may remain unrecognized because of their asymptomatic character and frequently hidden location (anal, rectal, or oral).[6] HIV-positive patients present with secondary disease that is more aggressive with greater constitutional symptoms, more organ involvement, and atypical florid rashes.[7] Glover et al. reported widespread shiny, erythematous, hairless plaques reminiscent of a lymphoreticular malignancy.[8] Varioliform, lichenoid,[9] and frambesiform lesions,[10] indurated red plaques,[11] tuberous plaques,[12] and cervical adenitis[13] have all been described. A case of secondary syphilis mimicking the signs of reactive arthritis with keratoderma and chorioretinitis was described.[14,15] Fonseca et al. reported secondary syphilis presenting as uveitis, madarosis, and diffuse 1–2 cm violet-brown plaques, some with anetoderma-like changes, on the face, trunk, and extremities, but sparing the palms, soles, and mucous membranes with histopathologic findings mimicking leprosy.[16] Secondary syphilis has also presented as a pruritic hyperkeratotic, lichenoid plaque

M.E. Grossman et al., *Cutaneous Manifestations of Infection in the Immunocompromised Host*,
DOI 10.1007/978-1-4419-1578-8_11, © Springer Science+Business Media, LLC 2012

on the scrotum and base of the penis mimicking eczema.[17] Gregory et al. reported a papulosquamous eruption of secondary syphilis with palatal perforation.[18] The telescoping of disease with an oral gummatous perforation characteristic of tertiary syphilis with secondary syphilis demonstrated the rapid progression of syphilis in the HIV-infected host. Atypical secondary syphilis in the immunocompromised patient may mimic tinea imbricata and erythema annulare centrifugum[19] or severe wart-like hyperkeratotic plaques.[20] An HIV-positive man presented with unusual oral lesions, indurated, painless, nodules in triangular array on the dorsal central tongue. The same case was reported twice as secondary syphilis.[21] A similar firm well-demarcated indurated nodule with superficial erosion, 20 mm in diameter on the dorsal central tongue was reported as primary syphilis in an HIV-positive man.[22]

Noduloulcerative cutaneous syphilis, or lues maligna, once a rare form of secondary syphilis seen in alcoholics and in those malnourished with self-neglect and poor health, is becoming increasingly common in the HIV-infected patient[23,24] and may be the initial sign of HIV infection.[25] The risk of lues maligna has been associated with declining immune status.[4] Patients with noduloulcerative syphilis present with a prodrome of fever, headache, and myalgias followed by papulopustules that centrally ulcerate.[23] Lues maligna may be especially aggressive, presenting with constitutional symptoms such as fever, malaise, and arthralgias, lymphadenopathy, mucosal and/or ocular involvement, and requiring hospitalization if incompletely treated.[23,24] Characteristic noduloulcerative lesions with rupioid crusts may be so grotesque in appearance and rapid in progression that is has been called malignant syphilis. The syphilitic endarteritis obliterans causes the papules and pustules to undergo central necrosis giving rise to "limpet-like" crusts resembling an "oyster shell." The discolored lesions, often on the central face are called "rupia" or rupioid crusts.[26] Other rare, but atypical, morphologies in the HIV-infected patient include vesiculo-necrotic lesions resembling congenital syphilis and disseminated herpetic infection and umbilicated papules and plaques.[23,24] The involvement of the palms and soles, so commonly found in other cases of secondary syphilis, is often absent in noduloulcerative syphilis. Most patients with malignant syphilis have high nontreponemal titers; however, negative or low positive titers (e.g., 1:8) that may serologically suggest latent infection have been reported in the setting of HIV-infected patients with malignant syphilis.[24]

Ocular syphilis can present at any stage of disease. In HIV infection, the severity of ocular syphilis does not correlate with immune status. Syphilis is the most common bacterial cause of uveitis in HIV-infected patients.[27] Acute, reversible, syphilitic blindness is a rare presentation of syphilis, but has been reported in HIV-infected patients.[28] Any HIV-positive patient with ocular syphilis should undergo a lumbar puncture for neurosyphilis.

Neurosyphilis, generally a hallmark of tertiary disease, may be precocious and present during early stages (primary or secondary syphilis) rather than after years of untreated infection.[29]

In addition, inability to fight infection in the HIV-positive patient may lead to the development of symptomatic neurosyphilis despite appropriate treatment for primary infection.[1] Neurosyphilis in HIV infection is asymptomatic in one-third of patients, but typically presents with "aseptic" meningitis, ocular involvement (uveitis, retinitis), and cranial nerve involvement.[1] The typical picture of aseptic meningitis of syphilis includes headache, lymphocytic pleocytosis, elevated cerebrospinal fluid (CSF) protein, and normal CSF glucose with manifestations of secondary syphilis. Cranial nerve II, followed by VIII, are the most commonly affected; but disease of cranial nerves III, IV, VI, and VII have also been reported.[1] The course of neurosyphilis of the meningovascular type represents syphilitic vasculitis of the vasa vasorum of the intracranial arteries (in the territory of the middle cerebral, basilar, or spinal arteries)[2] and is the prototypical late manifestation of neurosyphilis in HIV-infected patients. It may be so accelerated in an HIV-seropositive patient that the primary chancre may still be present at the time of the luetic stroke.[30] Stroke in a young HIV-positive patient – think syphilis. Other central nervous system (CNS) infections (herpes viruses, toxoplasmosis, cryptococcosis, progressive multifocal leukoencephalopathy, and other co-infections) may obscure the diagnosis of neurosyphilis in patients with AIDS.

Traditional serologic markers of both the nontreponemal tests (RPR or VDRL) and the treponemal tests (TPPA, *T. pallidum* particle hemagglutination assay; MHA-TP, microhemagglutination assay for antibodies to *T. pallidum*; and FTA-ABS, fluorescent treponemal antibody absorption test), which measure antibodies to *T. pallidum*, are generally reliable in the HIV-positive patient.[1] However titers may not correlate with the clinical presentation, making them difficult to interpret in the clinical setting. Higher than expected serologic titers are common in HIV. Delayed seroconversion may also occur. Occasionally, high nontreponemal titers in the HIV-positive patient may lead to the prozone phenomenon and subsequent false-negative nontreponemal tests.[1] In addition, in the HIV-positive patient, false-negative serologic tests for syphilis due to impaired humoral responses or false-positive serologic tests (11% of cases)[2] because of polyclonal B-cell activation inducing an increase in VDRL titers in the absence of reinfection in HIV-infected patients can make diagnosis difficult. Patients with HIV who are suspected of having syphilis but have a negative nontreponemal screen should be tested with a treponemal screen. In fact, specific treponemal tests are used by some laboratories to screen for syphilis.[1] Serologic response to therapy may also be hard to document in HIV-infected patients, as approximately 5% of HIV-infected patients are serofast.[4] Loss of treponemal-specific antibody titers has also been reported in HIV-infected patients.[4]

The unusual skin lesions of syphilis and potential for unreliable or difficult to interpret serologic studies in HIV-infected patients may make it necessary to obtain a skin biopsy to establish the diagnosis. The histopathology in HIV is the same as those in non-HIV infected patients. Some unusual variations have been reported in the HIV-infected population, however. Secondary syphilis histopathologically mimicking mycosis fungoides with atypical lymphoid infiltrates and epidermotropism,[31] lues maligna histopathologically misdiagnosed as "granulomatous mycosis fungoides,"[32] and secondary syphilis resembling leprosy with granulomatous infiltrates with epithelioid and giant multinucleated cells with multivacuolated cytoplasm[16] have been reported. *T. pallidum* has been detected in the hair follicle by immunohistochemical studies in an HIV-infected patient with alopecia syphilitica.[33] In noduloulcerative syphilis, skin biopsy may demonstrate necrotizing vasculitis, with spirochetes found on Warthin-Starry stain, although, more commonly, spirochetes are absent in malignant syphilis. The traditionally difficult detection of spirochetes in tissue sections using the silver stain, either the Steiner medication of the Dieterle technique or the Warthin-Starry technique, has been replaced with immunohistochemical staining using an anti-spirochete antibody. Polymerase chain reaction (PCR) can also be used to identify *T. pallidum* in skin biopsies.

In general, the treatment for syphilis in HIV-positive patients is the same as that for HIV-negative patients. However, the treatment of syphilis in HIV disease is complicated by the underlying immunodeficiency. Many authors believe that while *T. pallidum* is exquisitely sensitive to lysis by penicillin, complete eradication of the infection depends on the cooperation of an intact immune system. Cases of relapse or progression to (often precocious) tertiary syphilis have been documented despite adequate therapy.[18] In addition, the Jarisch-Herxheimer reaction may be more common in patients with HIV, especially those with malignant syphilis.[1]

The evaluation and treatment of neurosyphilis in HIV-infected patients is particularly controversial because, while CSF abnormalities may be present in primary syphilis and in patients infected with HIV, the prognostic significance of CSF abnormalities in primary or secondary syphilis in HIV disease is not known.[34] Therefore, it is currently a matter of active debate when the diagnosis of syphilis in HIV-infected individuals warrants a lumbar puncture with early treatment for neurosyphilis. The 2006 Centers for Disease Control (CDC) guidelines suggest that a lumbar puncture is indicated for any patient with signs or symptoms of neurosyphilis, ocular manifestations, active tertiary syphilis, or treatment failure and HIV-positive patients with any of the above or latent infection or infection of unknown duration.[34]

There are several cases reported of syphilis in the immunosuppressed, non-HIV-infected patient. Lues maligna has been reported in a chronic alcoholic.[35] Classic lesions of secondary syphilis with syphilitic hepatitis have been reported in several liver transplant patients.[36-38] One of these patients presented with a chancre, a maculopapular eruption, and meningitis two weeks after presenting with a transaminitis due to syphilitic hepatitis four years after liver transplant.[38] Syphilitic hepatitis[39] and secondary syphilis with a prozone phenomenon[40] have been reported after renal transplant. Secondary syphilis presenting with neurosyphilis and syphilitic hepatitis has also been reported in a cardiac transplant recipient.[41] Skin biopsy of a collarette of scale from a typical palm macule demonstrated an unusually large number of spirochetes with a Warthin-Starry stain, consistent with the patient's broad long term immunosuppression.

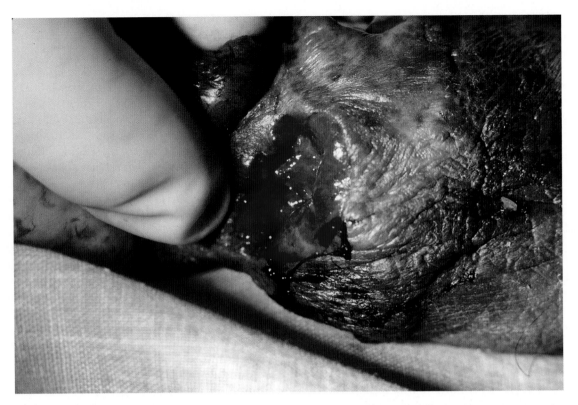

Figure 11.1.   Multiple syphilitic chancres on the penis of a 40-year-old human immunodeficiency virus (HIV)-positive man at the time of presentation with neurosyphilis of the meningovascular type. Nontender, clean-based ulcers with no undermining were present at the corona of the penis

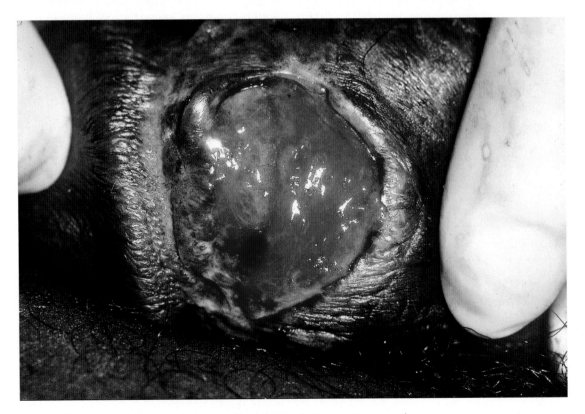

Figure 11.2.   The ulcerations were deep enough to expose the underlying bulbo spongiosus muscle

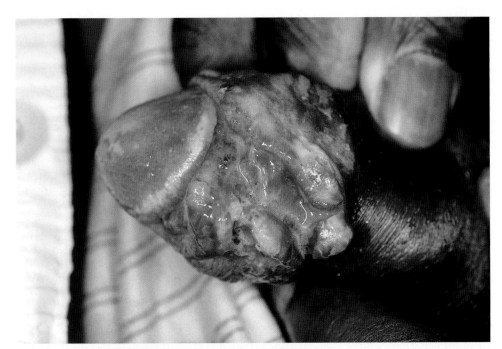

Figure 11.3. Large chancre of primary syphilis (biopsy proven) in an HIV-positive man who presented with conjunctivitis, arthritis, and positive fluorescent treponemal antibody (FTA) and venereal disease research laboratory (VDRL) test

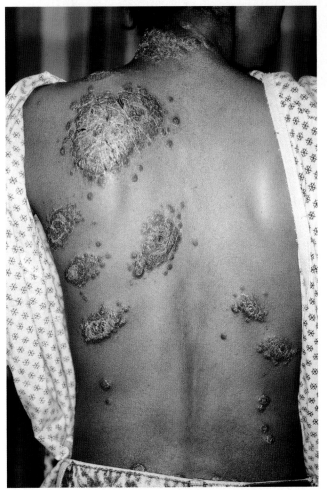

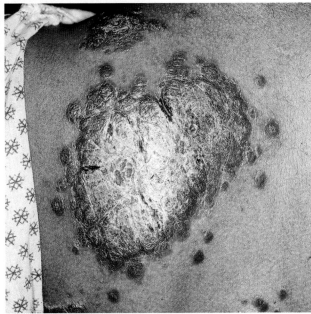

Figure 11.5. Close-up of corymbose secondary syphilis

Figure 11.4. Large psoriasiform plaques with satellite papules of corymbose secondary syphilis in an HIV-positive young woman. Skin biopsy demonstrated granulomatous inflammation with plasma cells. The VDRL was 1:512, FTA positive

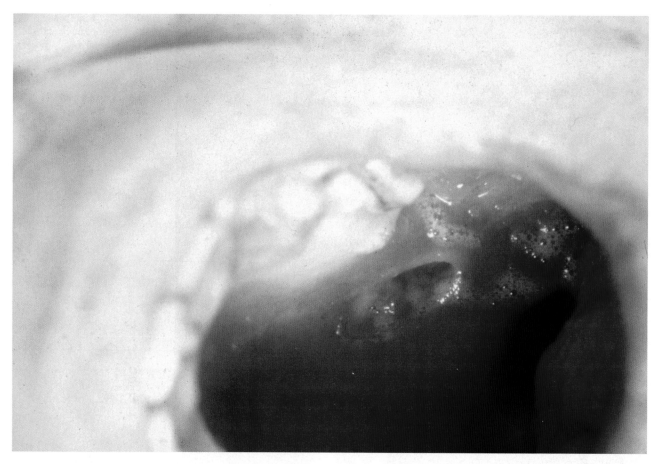

Figure 11.6.   Soft palate perforation clinically consistent with gummatous tertiary syphilis present at the same time as the skin rash of secondary syphilis in an HIV-positive homosexual with a rapid plasma regain (RPR) of 1:8192 (Courtesy of Mary Ruth Buchness, M.D., and Neal Gregory, M.D. From Gregory et al. [18])

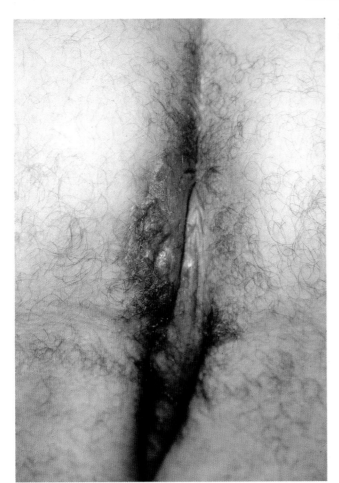

Figure 11.7. Multiple secondarily infected perianal chancres in an HIV-positive homosexual man

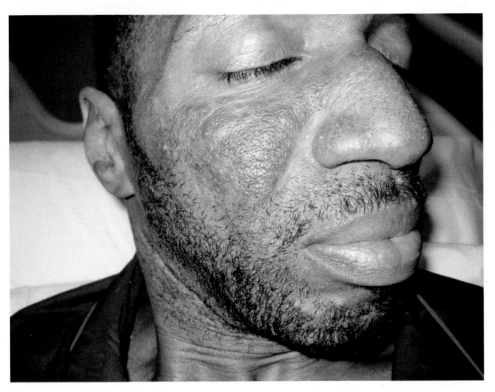

Figure 11.8. A 45-year-old man with newly diagnosed HIV/AIDS (acquired immune deficiency syndrome) and an 8-month history of a pruritic eruption involving his face, ears, hand, feet, and nails suggestive of acrokeratosis paraneoplastica. RPR was initially negative. After checking for a prozone phenomenon, his RPR was positive at 1:1. Cerebrospinal fluid venereal disease research disease laboratory (CSF VDRL) test was negative. Facial skin biopsy revealed a superficial and deep perivascular infiltrate of plasma cells. Spirochete immunoperoxidase stain was negative

References

1. Eaton M. Syphilis and HIV: old and new foes aligned against us. Curr Infect Dis Rep. 2009;11(2):157–62.
2. Lynn WA, Lightman S. Syphilis and HIV: a dangerous combination. Lancet Infect Dis. 2004;4(7):456–66.
3. Cusini M, Zerboni R, Muratori S, Monti M, Alessi E. Atypical early syphilis in an HIV-infected homosexual male. Dermatologica. 1988;177(5):300–4.
4. Stevenson J, Heath M. Syphilis and HIV infection: an update. Dermatol Clin. 2006;24(4):497–507, vi.
5. Ormond P, Mulcahy F. Sexually transmitted diseases in HIV-positive patients. Dermatol Clin. 1998;16(4):853–7, xvi.
6. Pleimes M, Hartschuh W, Kutzner H, Enk AH, Hartmann M. Malignant syphilis with ocular involvement and organism-depleted lesions. Clin Infect Dis. 2009;48(1):83–5.
7. Karp G, Schlaeffer F, Jotkowitz A, Riesenberg K. Syphilis and HIV co-infection. Eur J Intern Med. 2009;20(1):9–13.
8. Glover RA, Piaquadio DJ, Kern S, Cockerell CJ. An unusual presentation of secondary syphilis in a patient with human immunodeficiency virus infection. A case report and review of the literature. Arch Dermatol. 1992;128(4):530–4. Review.
9. Carbia SG, Lagodín C, Abbruzzese M, et al. Lichenoid secondary syphilis. Int J Dermatol. 1999;38(1):53–5.
10. Schröter R, Nher H, Petzoldt D. [Skin manifestations of syphilis maligna in HIV infection. Clinical observations in 3 cases]. Hautarzt. 1988;39(7):463–6. German.
11. Tosca A, Stavropoulos PG, Hatziolou E, et al. Malignant syphilis in HIV-infected patients. Int J Dermatol. 1990;29(8):575–8.
12. Trope BM, Lenzi ME. AIDS and HIV infections: uncommon presentations. Clin Dermatol. 2005;23(6):572–80.
13. Heller H, Fromowitz F, Fuhrer J. Luetic cervical adenitis in patients with human immunodeficiency virus type 1 infection. Arch Otolaryngol Head Neck Surg. 1992;118(7):757–8.
14. Radolf JD, Kaplan RP. Unusual manifestations of secondary syphilis and abnormal humoral immune response to Treponema pallidum antigens in a homosexual man with asymptomatic human immunodeficiency virus infection. J Am Acad Dermatol. 1988;18(2 Pt 2):423–8.
15. Kishimoto M, Lee MJ, Mor A, et al. Syphilis mimicking Reiter's syndrome in an HIV-positive patient. Am J Med Sci. 2006;332(2):90–2.
16. Fonseca E, García-Silva J, del Pozo J, et al. Syphilis in an HIV infected patient misdiagnosed as leprosy. J Cutan Pathol. 1999;26(1):51–4.
17. Kang SH, Lee D, Park JH, et al. Scrotal eczema-like lesion of secondary syphilis in an HIV-positive patient. Acta Derm Venereol. 2005;85(6):536–7.
18. Gregory N, Sanchez M, Buchness MR. The spectrum of syphilis in patients with human immunodeficiency virus infection. J Am Acad Dermatol. 1990;22(6 Pt 1):1061–7.
19. Cotterman C, Eckert L, Ackerman L. Syphilis mimicking tinea imbricata and erythema annulare centrifugum in an immunocompromised patient. J Am Acad Dermatol. 2009;61(1):165–7.
20. Shinkuma S, Abe R, Nishimura M, et al. Secondary syphilis mimicking warts in an HIV-positive patient. Sex Transm Infect. 2009;85(6):484.
21. Dalmau J, Alegre M, Sambeat MA, et al. Syphilitic nodules on the tongue. J Am Acad Dermatol. 2006;54(2 Suppl):S59–60.
22. Yébenes M, Toll A, Giménez-Arnau A, et al. Pseudotumoral primary syphilis on the tongue in an HIV positive patient. Clin Exp Dermatol. 2008;33(4):509–11.
23. Sands M, Markus A. Lues maligna, or ulceronodular syphilis, in a man infected with human immunodeficiency virus: case report and review. Clin Infect Dis. 1995;20(2):387–90.
24. Don PC, Rubinstein R, Christie S. Malignant syphilis (lues maligna) and concurrent infection with HIV. Int J Dermatol. 1995;34(6):403–7.
25. Tucker JD, Shah S, Jarell AD, et al. Lues maligna in early HIV infection case report and review of the literature. Sex Transm Dis. 2009;36(8):512–4.
26. Bhagwat PV, Tophakhane RS, Rathod RM, Shashikumar BM, Naidu V. Rupioid syphilis in an HIV patient. Indian J Dermatol Venereol Leprol. 2009;75(2):201–2.
27. Shalaby IA, Dunn JP, Semba RD, Jabs DA. Syphilitic uveitis in human immunodeficiency virus-infected patients. Arch Ophthalmol. 1997;115(4):469–73.
28. Oette M, Hemker J, Feldt T, et al. Acute syphilitic blindness in an HIV-positive patient. AIDS Patient Care STDS. 2005;19(4):209–11.
29. Bari MM, Shulkin DJ, Abell E. Ulcerative syphilis in acquired immunodeficiency syndrome: a case of precocious tertiary syphilis in a patient infected with human immunodeficiency virus. J Am Acad Dermatol. 1989;21(6):1310–2.
30. Held JL, Grossman ME. Syphilis associated with human immunodeficiency virus infection. J Am Acad Dermatol. 1989;20(2 Pt 1):295.
31. Liotta EA, Turiansky GW, Berberian BJ, Sulica VI, Tomaszewski MM. Unusual presentation of secondary syphilis in 2 HIV-1 positive patients. Cutis. 2000;66(5):383–6, 389.
32. D'Amico R, Zalusky R. A case of lues maligna in a patient with acquired immunodeficiency syndrome (AIDS). Scand J Infect Dis. 2005;37(9):697–700.
33. Nam-Cha SH, Guhl G, Fernández-Peña P, Fraga J. Alopecia syphilitica with detection of Treponema pallidum in the hair follicle. J Cutan Pathol. 2007;34 Suppl 1:37–40.
34. Centers for Disease Control and Prevention. Sexually transmitted diseases treatment guidelines, 2006. MMWR Morb Mortal Wkly Rep. 2006;55(RR-11):22–30.
35. Bayramgürler D, Bilen N, Yildiz K, Sikar A, Yavuz M. Lues maligna in a chronic alcoholic patient. J Dermatol. 2005;32(3):217–9.
36. Camara B, Kamar N, Bonafe JL, et al. Syphilis-related hepatitis in a liver transplant patient. Exp Clin Transplant. 2007;5(2):724–6.
37. Petersen LR, Mead RH, Perlroth MG. Unusual manifestations of secondary syphilis occurring after orthotopic liver transplantation. Am J Med. 1983;75(1):166–70.
38. Wolf SC, Kempf VA, Tannapfel A, et al. Secondary syphilis after liver transplantation: case report and review of the literature. Clin Transplant. 2006;20(5):644–9.
39. Johnson PC, Norris SJ, Miller GP, et al. Early syphilitic hepatitis after renal transplantation. J Infect Dis. 1988;158(1):236–8.
40. Taniguchi S, Osato K, Hamada T. The prozone phenomenon in secondary syphilis. Acta Derm Venereol. 1995;75(2):153–4.
41. Farr M, Rubin AI, Mangurian C, et al. Late syphilis in a cardiac transplant patient. J Heart Lung Transplant. 2006;25(3):358–61.

12

Gram-Positive Bacteria

BACILLUS SPECIES

Bacillus cereus, best known for causing mild food poisoning, has been recognized as a cause of life-threatening infection in the immunocompromised host.[1] It most commonly presents in a neutropenic patient as a single vesicle, pustule, or bulla on a digit or extremities with rapidly spreading cellulitis during the spring and summer.[2,3] The bulla may become necrotic and develop a black eschar. Lesions may mimic clostridial myonecrosis.[4] The lesion is usually painful and associated with high fever and negative blood cultures.[3] Gram stain of the aspirate smear or lesional biopsy shows large Gram-positive rods, which may be mistaken for *Clostridium* infection and treated with penicillin. *B. cereus* organisms are generally resistant to β-lactam antibiotics and most cephalosporins. The most useful drugs are vancomycin, carbapenems, and aminoglycosides.

Severe cases of *B. cereus* infection in immunosuppressed patients have been reported. Necrotizing fasciitis and brain abscesses developed in a 60-year-old neutropenic patient with myelodysplastic syndrome with *B. cereus* bacteremia.[5] The skin lesions and brain abscesses resolved when blood cultures became negative with antibiotic and hematopoietic growth factor therapy. A cirrhotic patient died of *B. cereus* bacterial peritonitis and necrotizing fasciitis.[6] *B. cereus* bacteremia presented as fever and a right thigh ulcer surrounded by a 5 × 5 cm area of "brawny, nontender erythema" that also cultured *B. cereus* in a patient with acute lymphoblastic leukemia undergoing chemotherapy.[7] The patient ultimately died of *B. cereus* mitral valve endocarditis, meningoencephalitis, and brain abscesses despite antibiotic therapy with penicillin, vancomycin, and ciprofloxacin.

Bacillus piliformis, which typically causes a disease in animals called Tyzzer's disease, is extremely rare in humans. However, *B. piliformis* has been reported to cause moderately painful, crusted, verrucous papules and nodules on the chest of a 32-year-old human immunodeficiency virus (HIV)-positive man with a CD-4 count of 80×10^9 cells/L.[8] The organism does not stain well with routine hematoxylin-and-eosin or Gram stains, but Silver and Warthin-Starry stains of a skin biopsy will demonstrate intracellular long, slender bacilli arranged in parallel bundles within keratinocytes.

M.E. Grossman et al., *Cutaneous Manifestations of Infection in the Immunocompromised Host*,
DOI 10.1007/978-1-4419-1578-8_12, © Springer Science+Business Media, LLC 2012

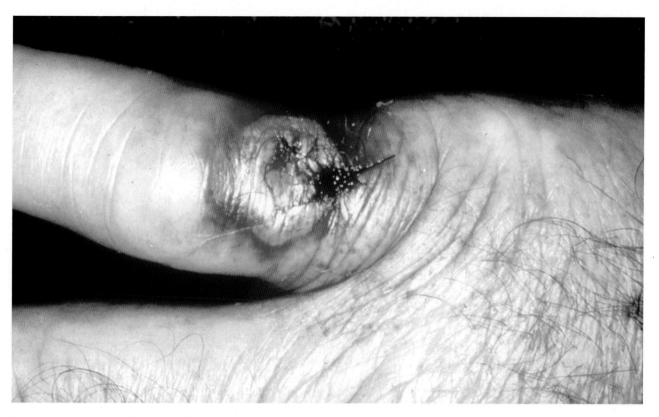

Figure 12.1.   Single, painful, flaccid bulla of *B. cereus* surrounded by purpura on the finger of a neutropenic patient with malignant lymphoma (Courtesy of Phillip Shapiro, M.D. From Khavari et al.[2], p. 543. Copyright 1991, American Medical Association)

CLOSTRIDIUM

Clostridia are Gram-positive, anaerobic, non-spore forming bacilli. Clostridial myonecrosis (gas gangrene) may be posttraumatic or spontaneous. Spontaneous or distant clostridial myonecrosis may be associated with immunosuppression, most commonly a silent colon carcinoma, an underlying hematologic tumor or neutrophil dysfunction. Almost all isolates from these infections have been *Clostridium perfringens* (60%) or the more virulent *Clostridium septicum* (30%). *Clostridium perfringens* is part of normal colonic flora while *C. septicum* is typically found in soil and animals, but is not a normal inhabitant of humans.[9] *C. septicum* may be more virulent because it is more aerotolerant and may survive dissemination and proliferate in a soft tissue site more easily than strict anaerobes such as *C. perfringens*.

Clostridial myonecrosis is clinically characterized by the sudden onset of severe pain in the involved site, rapid progression, and extreme toxicity.[10] Initially, the skin may be tense, edematous, and blanched. It then takes on a bronze discoloration and develops large hemorrhagic bullae. The serosanguinous fluid contains an abundance of Gram-positive rods and a paucity of inflammatory cells. Crepitus, although not prominent, can at times be detected by x-ray as gas about fascial planes and between muscle bundles. Involvement of underlying muscle is always more extensive than the evident skin involvement.

Nontraumatic clostridial myonecrosis with spreading cellulitis that appears spontaneously in an extremity due to *C. septicum* has a high frequency of association with colon carcinoma, especially carcinoma of the cecum.[9] An unusually aggressive and fatal infection with *C. septicum* presented as multifocal areas of cutaneous blue-purple mottling, bullae, and crepitus on the thigh, lateral chest, and left shoulder in a 64-year-old woman with chronic idiopathic neutropenia.[11] Fatal *C. perfringens* sepsis without skin lesions was reported in a patient with acute myeloid leukemia who received a pooled platelet transfusion where the same strain of *C. perfringens* was isolated from the venipuncture site of one of the donors.[12]

The diagnosis of clostridial myonecrosis requires a high index of suspicion, since the infection spreads rapidly and death may occur within 24–48 h. Gram stain of a bulla allows for a timely diagnosis. Cultures should be sent to determine future antibiotic use, but generally take too long to grow to be clinically helpful in the acute setting. Imaging with X-ray or computed tomography (CT) scan can demonstrate soft tissue gas (a late finding) and help determine the extent of infection.[13]

Most patients require a combination of surgical debridement and intravenous antibiotics. High-dose penicillin is the treatment of choice. In neutropenic patients, hematopoietic growth factors should be considered. The mortality rate of *C. perfringens* myonecrosis is 32%, while that of *C. septicum* is 79%.[13]

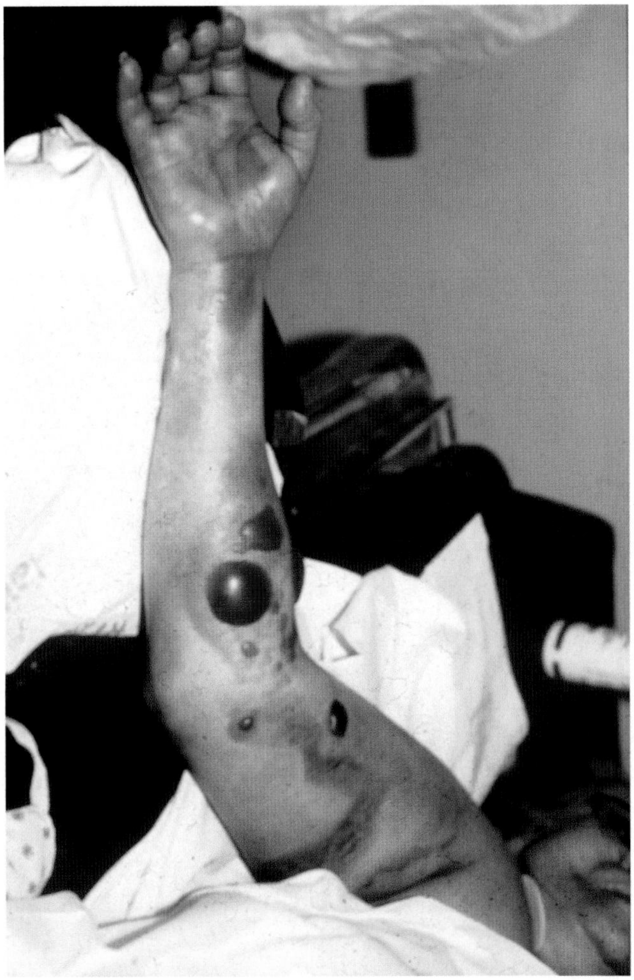

Figure 12.2. An 80-year-old woman with noninsulin-dependent diabetes presented to the emergency room febrile, toxic, and with a rapidly spreading cellulitis with hemorrhagic bullae. A Gram stain of the fluid showed Gram-positive rods. Surgery confirmed the myonecrosis, and a forequarter amputation was performed. *C. septicum* was cultured and carcinoma of the cecal colon was subsequently discovered

CORYNEBACTERIUM

Corynebacterium group JK, discovered by Johnson and Kaye in 1979, has been renamed *C. jeikeium*. Commonly referred to as diphtheroids or coryneforms, the organisms in this genus are small, pleomorphic, aerobic Gram-positive rods that are non-acid fast. Except for *C. diptheriae*, the other members of the genus *Corynebacterium* are part of the normal skin flora, rarely cause infection, and are susceptible to most antibiotics.

The most common sites of colonization by *C. jeikeium* are the perineum, rectal, and intertriginous (inguinal and axillary) areas. *C. jeikeium* colonization occurs most commonly in adult males over 16 or postmenopausal females with impaired mucocutaneous barriers to infection (particularly indwelling catheter placement), neutropenia, prolonged hospital stay, and/or previous treatment with broad-spectrum antibiotics.[14] The fact that colonization is most common in men over 16 and postmenopausal women may be related to increased cutaneous sebum which may promote the growth of lipophilic diphtheroids.[15] Although colonization leads to infection in a minority of patients, the risk factors for sepsis and colonization are the same. The strongest risk factors for infection are neutropenia and the presence of an indwelling catheter.

C. jeikeium causes sepsis in patients with hematologic malignancies, endocarditis after prosthetic heart valve placement, infection of ventricular cerebrospinal fluid (CSF) shunts, peritonitis in patients on peritoneal dialysis, and infection in patients status post major trauma.[14] In these groups, *C. jeikeium* is most aggressive in patients with hematologic malignancies, especially those undergoing chemotherapy or status post bone marrow transplantation. This is also the group that almost exclusively develops skin lesions with *C. jeikeium* infection. The most common sites of infection in patients with hematologic malignancies with *C. jeikeium* sepsis are the skin (48% of patients) and the lungs (36% of patients).[14]

Primary cutaneous infection with *C. jeikeium* occurs at breaks in the skin barrier due to bone marrow biopsy, intravascular catheter insertion, or fissures (especially perirectal) which serve as a portal of entry into the bloodstream, leading to septicemia.[16] Primary skin lesions typically present as cellulitis or infection at sites of trauma or nosocomial inoculation.[17] Chronic osteomyelitis of the metatarsal sesamoid with a plantar ulcer with surrounding erythema and a draining fistula occurred in a patient with rheumatoid arthritis treated with prednisone and methotrexate.[18]

Secondary skin and soft tissue infections with *C. jeikeium* develop in the course of septicemia at previously normal sites distant from the original access point of the organism. Skin lesions of hematogenously disseminated infection may present as single to multiple, nontender, noninflamed 2 × 2 cm subcutaneous nodules that do not spontaneously drain but are purulent upon surgical drainage[14]; bright red, non-blanching papules with satellite petechiae and central necrosis or pustulation on the trunk and/or extremities[17]; erythematous macules and papules[19]; or multiple erythematous to purpuric papules on the face, trunk, and extremities, resolving with hyperpigmentation.[19] Histopathology in several cases revealed a dermal inflammatory infiltrate surrounding an amorphous, basophilic, granular mass made up of an eosinophilic matrix of basophilic rods mimicking botryomycosis.[19]

Vancomycin is the treatment of choice for *C. jeikeium* and should be continued through recovery of the bone marrow. Linezolid is also effective. The mortality of *C. jeikeium* septicemia in patients with hematologic malignancies approaches 34%, but is only 5% in patients whose bone marrow recovers.[14] Therefore, hematopoietic growth factors should be considered.

Figure 12.3. Acute cellulitis of the right first toe due to *C. jeikeium* in a patient with acute myelocytic leukemia. The infection began as a paronychia that spread proximally (From Dreizen S, et al. Unusual mucocutaneous infections in immunosuppressed patients with leukemia – expansion of an earlier study. Postgrad Med 1986;79(4): 287–294)

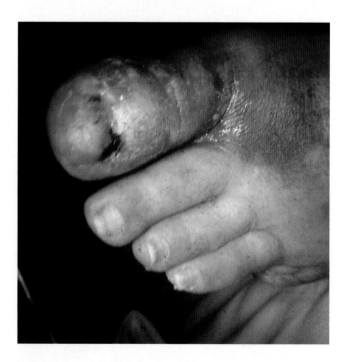

Nocardia

Nocardia is an aerobic, branching, beaded, filamentous bacteria found in soil, dust, and decaying organic matter (rotting vegetation). *Nocardia* is not part of the normal human flora and any isolate must be carefully evaluated.[20] Infections in humans are most commonly due to *N. asteroides* but infections with *N. brasiliensis*, *N. otitidiscaviarum (caviae)*, *N. nova*, *N. farcinica*, *N. cyriacigeorgica*, and *N. transvalensis* have been reported. *N. niigatensis* and *N. asiatica* infections are rare. Infection typically occurs via the respiratory route. The lungs are the most frequently involved organs, followed by the skin and central nervous system. While most *Nocardia* species respond to the combination of trimethoprim-sulfamethoxasole, *N. farcinica* has a high degree of antibiotic resistance.

The presentation of nocardiosis in immunocompetent and immunosuppressed patients is similar. Cutaneous nocardial infections in the normal or immunocompromised host may be due to primary inoculation or secondary dissemination. Primary cutaneous nocardiosis occurs as (a) mycetoma; (b) sporotrichoid or lymphocutaneous infection[21]; and (c) superficial skin infections such as abscesses,[22] ulcers,[23] "cold" or warm nodules which may become crusted or ulcerate, cellulitis, and granulomas. Secondary cutaneous involvement due to hematogenous spread from the lung may occur as abscesses, pustules, and "cold" or warm nodules, which may ulcerate. Secondary involvement due to hematogenous spread may be indistinguishable from primary cutaneous nocardiosis. All patients presenting with cutaneous lesions should be evaluated by imaging for lung and central nervous system involvement, as the skin may be the sign of disseminated infection[24] and disseminated disease may be asymptomatic. In the immunosuppressed patient, late dissemination to the skin and other organs, especially the central nervous system, can occur during appropriate therapy for a previously diagnosed pulmonary nocardial infection. Dissemination from the primary cutaneous disease to other organs is rare.

Nocardiosis in immunosuppressed patients may arise in the setting of hematologic malignancy, organ transplantation, iatrogenic immunosuppressive therapy, or HIV disease. Patients on tumor necrosis factor-alpha (TNF-alpha) inhibitors have also been reported to develop nocardiosis.[25,26] Infection due to the primary immunodeficiency associated with Down syndrome and chronic variable immunodeficiency have been reported. Iatrogenic immunosuppression for bullous pemphigoid, connective tissue diseases, sarcoidosis, idiopathic thrombocytopenic purpura, pemphigus vulgaris, and rheumatoid arthritis has been associated with nocardiosis. In patients with HIV infection, *Nocardia* usually presents with CD4 counts ≤ 100 cells/mm³ and often occurs simultaneously with an acquired immune deficiency syndrome (AIDS) defining infection.[27] Uncommonly, it is the presenting sign of HIV disease.[27] In HIV-positive patients, the clinical picture of pulmonary nocardiosis with or without dissemination may be very similar to tuberculosis leading to delay in diagnosis and poor outcome.

Nocardiosis is more common after solid organ transplantation than bone marrow transplantation. In the organ transplant patient, *N. nova* is the most common cause of disseminated infection.[28] Independent risk factors for *Nocardia* infection in organ transplant recipients include high-dose steroid therapy, prior infection with cytomegalovirus, and high calcineurin inhibitor serum levels in the 30 days prior to infection.[28] While some experts note that prophylactic use of trimethoprim-sulfamethoxasole to prevent Pneumocystis pneumonia in immunosuppressed patients helps prevent nocardial infections, nocardiosis is frequently reported in patients compliant with their prophylactic regimen.[28] This suggests that there is a difference between prophylactic and treatment doses of trimethoprim-sulfamethoxasole in the prevention and treatment of *Nocardia*.

Primary cutaneous nocardiosis in immunosuppressed patients has presented in myriad ways. A tender, erythematous, edematous subcutaneous nodule due to *N. asteroides* developed on the plantar surface of the right hallux in a 13-year-old boy status post bone marrow transplantation for aplastic anemia.[29] *N. asteroides* cervical lymph node abscess, presenting as an inflamed and enlarged right cervical mass, presented concomitantly with cryptococcal meningitis as the initial sign of HIV in a 35-year-old man.[27] A 30-year-old Algerian woman with systemic scleroderma and polymyositis overlap treated with prednisone and cyclosporine developed a firm, painful, forearm nodule without lymphadenopathy due to *N. farcinica*.[30] *N. asteroides* mycetoma involving the bone developed at the site of a prior burn injury on the dorsal foot in an 81-year-old woman with myelodysplastic syndrome.[31] *N. asteroides* gluteal muscle abscess presenting as severe pain without overlying edema or erythema was reported in a patient with systemic lupus erythematosus on prednisolone and monthly cyclophosphamide.[32] A similar case of an adductor muscle abscess due to *N. asteroides*, this time presenting as a warm swelling, was reported in a cardiac transplant recipient.[33] Tender subcutaneous cystic nodules, without overlying erythema or edema, upon incision and drainage, drained a yellow-white discharge that grew *N. asteroides* in a patient with pulmonary sarcoidosis on chronic prednisolone therapy.[34] *N. asteroides* caused a dorsal foot cellulitis with an overlying hemorrhagic bulla in a patient with systemic lupus erythematosus on prednisone.[35] A patient with psoriatic arthritis treated with intra-articular steroid injections into the right hand developed fluctuating, erythematous, scaling nodules and scattered papulopustules on the dorsal right hand due to *N. brasiliensis*.[36] Although the patient liked to garden, traumatic inoculation could not be confirmed. *N. farcinica* sialoadenitis and submandibular abscess disseminated from the submandibular triangle to the axilla, arm, scapula, chest, abdomen, and legs in a patient with nephrotic syndrome on chronic prednisolone.[37] A 45-year-old man with Crohn's disease treated with chronic prednisone developed multiple erythematous papulopustules on the leg 6 weeks after beginning infliximab infusions.[26] Although cultures never grew, *Nocardia* was confirmed by polymerase chain reaction (PCR) on skin biopsy. An HIV-positive gardener with a CD4 count of 189 cells/μl presented with thigh and retroauricular ulcers due to *N. asiatica*.[38] Concomitant cutaneous phaeohyphomycosis and nocardiosis have been reported. Infection with *Exophiala spinifera* and *N. asteroides* developed on the hand of an 85-year-old farmer with idiopathic thrombocytopenic purpura on prednisolone and azathioprine.[39] A country worker status post liver transplantation presented with sporotrichoid cold nodules on the leg due to *N. brasiliensis* and *Exophiala jeanselmei*.[40] Lymphocutaneous *Nocardia* is often misdiagnosed as sporotrichosis because of its appearance, a history of trauma or gardening, and because both organisms live in the soil. A renal transplant patient developed fungating masses on the left knee and shin due to *N. niigatensis* after sustaining a laceration to the left knee.[41]

Disseminated infection is usually associated with *Nocardia asteroides* in immunocompromised hosts, although cases due to other *Nocardia* species have been reported, especially in solid organ transplant recipients. Pustules of the face and trunk in a renal transplant patient with a cavitary lung lesion were caused by *Nocardia asteroides*[42] and by *N. caviae* in a similar case.[43] In a man with metastatic renal carcinoma on high-dose systemic steroids, *N. caviae* disseminated from pulmonary abscesses to the skin, with pustules scattered over his body.[44] *N. asteroides* chest wall abscess developed in an HIV-positive patient with pulmonary and cerebral nocardiosis.[27] Nocardiosis was the presenting sign of HIV infection in this patient. Widespread hemorrhagic ulceronodules of disseminated *N. brasiliensis* developed in a steroid-dependent asthmatic patient.[45] A cardiac transplant patient presented with a pulmonary nodule due to *N. transvalensis* that was initially sensitive to treatment with trimethoprim-sulfamethoxazole.[46] Several months later, the patient developed cerebral abscesses and subcutaneous nodules on the hip and popliteal fossa that were both culture positive for the same strain of *N. transvalensis* that had developed resistance to sulfas.[46] *N. farcinica* presented as subcutaneous and muscle abscesses in the lower abdomen, adrenal glands, and lungs, cerebral nodules, and subcutaneous nodules on the legs in a 69-year-old liver transplant recipient.[47] Spontaneously draining scalp nodules with occipital and cervical lymphadenopathy, a 3-cm erythematous nonfluctuant soft tissue mass on the back, and a cavitary lung lesion and pulmonary nodules with cultures from both the blood and a scalp lesion demonstrating *N. farcinica* presented in a 76-year-old man with Churg-Strauss syndrome on corticosteroids and methotrexate.[48] An 85-year-old female with polymyalgia rheumatica on chronic prednisolone presented with pulmonary consolidation, an iliac fossa draining sinus and fluctuant swelling on the flank followed by fluctuant abscesses of the forearm, thigh, and chest due to *N. cyriacigeorgica*.[49] An echocardiogram demonstrated endocarditis and the patient died 2 days later.

Several cases of nocardiosis in Behcet's disease, sometimes mimicking a flare of the disease, with cutaneous, neurologic, pulmonary, and ocular involvement, have been reported. Patients with Behcet's disease who present with what appears to be a flare of the disease despite immunosuppressive treatment should be evaluated for an opportunistic infection. A patient with Behcet's disease treated with prednisone and monthly intravenous pulses of cyclophosphamide developed neurologic symptoms, vision loss, folliculitis, and painful inflammatory nodules on the chest mimicking a flare of Behcet's disease.[50] The patient was found to have *N. asteroides* pulmonary abscess by culture and the neurologic abscesses and cutaneous lesions resolved with treatment of *Nocardia*. A 29-year-old man with Behcet's disease treated with corticosteroids and azathioprine developed cavitary lung lesions and uveitis, followed by fluctuant nodules on the back, abdomen, and perianal area, scleral perforation, and a brain abscess.[51] *N. asteroides* was cultured from both the skin and ocular tissue. A 24-year-old man with Behcet's disease on methylprednisolone, azathioprine, and cyclosporine presented with fever, cough, hemoptysis, and suppurative cutaneous nodules, followed by brain abscesses.[51] Sputum and skin cultures grew *N. farcinica*. A *N. cyriacigeorgica* culture positive 10 × 7 cm abscess on the left clavicle along with pulmonary disease thought to be due to the same organism developed in a patient with Behcet's disease on corticosteroids, azathioprine, and cyclosporine.[52]

The diagnosis of nocardiosis can be challenging. Skin lesions of *Nocardia* infection may be overlooked and underestimated because of the resemblance to pyogenic bacterial infections, because the infections may be treated empirically without culture, or the cultures are discarded before *Nocardia* species have time to grow. *Nocardia* species are Gram-positive, variably acid-fast, and are not seen on routine hematoxylin and eosin preparations or on sections stained with periodic acid-Schiff for fungi. Gomori methenamine silver or Brown-Brenn stains are needed. Blood cultures are rarely positive. Cultures of tissue or fluid may take 2–4 weeks to grow; so, unless the laboratory is alerted to the clinician's suspicion of *Nocardia*, cultures may be discarded prematurely. In addition, serial smears and cultures are often required to make the diagnosis. Clues to the diagnosis of nocardial infection include: (a) history of traumatic inoculation; (b) occupational exposure (farmer, gardener); (c) tendency for cutaneous infection to recur; (d) worsening of infection despite standard antibiotics; (e) chronic suppurative or posttraumatic cutaneous infections with negative cultures; and (f) the presence of acid-fast organisms, which may represent *Nocardia* species.[53] *Nocardia* should be suspected in any immunosuppressed patient presenting with lung nodules and cutaneous lesions. Pleural and pericardial involvement in the compromised patient are particularly suggestive of nocardiosis.[24]

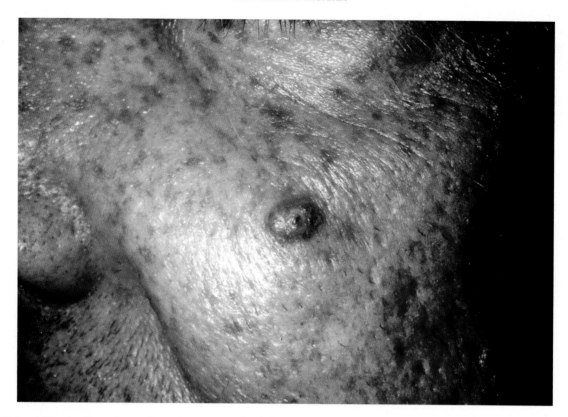

Figure 12.4. A 47-year-old renal transplant patient presented with fever, a cavitating pulmonary nodule, and a sparse number of pustules on his trunk and face

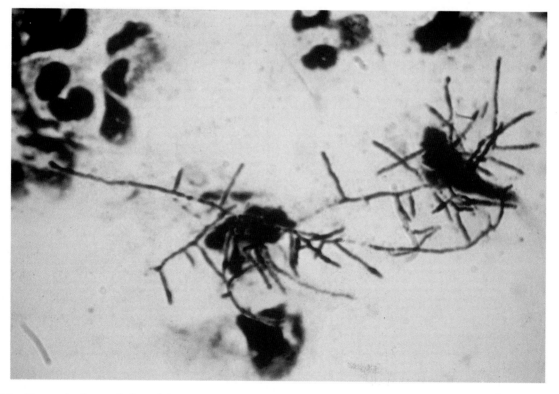

Figure 12.5. Gram stain of a pustule showed characteristic Gram-positive, delicately branching filaments of *Nocardia asteroides* cultured from his skin and lung

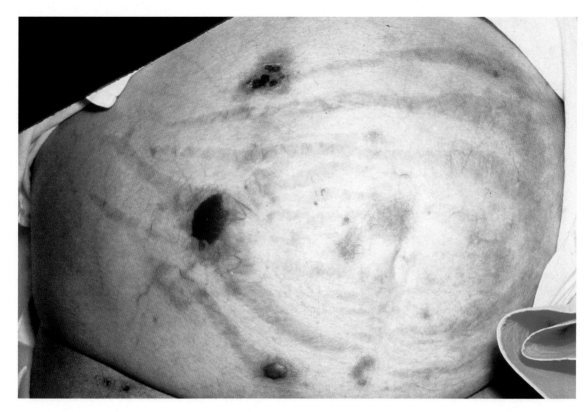

Figure 12.6. Hemorrhagic ulceronodules due to *N. brasiliensis* in the abdominal striae of a steroid-dependent asthmatic patient (Courtesy of Joseph L. Jorizzo, M.D. From Schreiner et al.[45] p. 1186. Copyright 1986, American Medical Association)

Figure 12.7. An 83-year-old male renal transplant recipient presented with a 3-month history of non-healing ulcerated nodules near the site of a previous in situ squamous cell carcinoma excision site on the left preauricular cheek. Biopsy and tissue culture revealed the presence of primary cutaneous nocardiosis

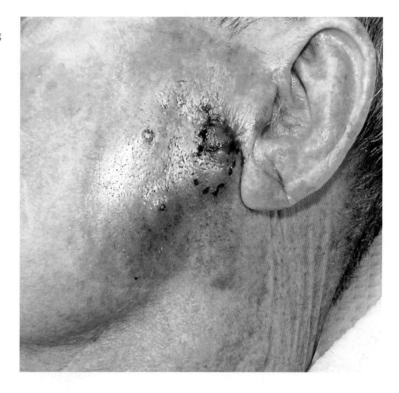

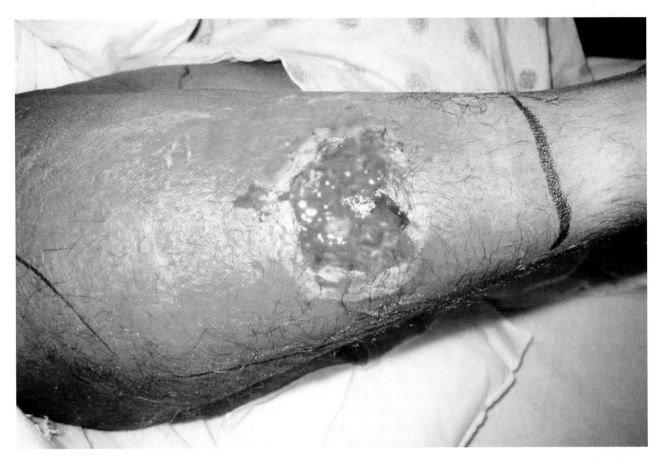

Figure 12.8. A 53-year-old physician with idiopathic chronic neutropenia presented with fever, night sweats, chills, and a left arm ulceration with surrounding "cellulitis" not responsive to antibiotics. The lesion began as an enlarging pustule 3 weeks after gardening and fixing a drip system in Arizona and 2 weeks after gardening in Merced, California. Ipsilateral axillary lymphadenopathy was present. Wound culture and skin biopsy culture grew *Nocardia brasiliensis* (Courtesy of Kanade Shinkai, M.D., Ph.D., and Tiffany Scharschmidt, M.D.)

STAPHYLOCOCCUS

Staphylococci are frequent colonizers of normal skin but commonly infect certain compromised individuals including: diabetics; children with chronic granulomatous disease; patients with cancer (particularly hematologic malignancies), including cutaneous T cell lymphoma[54]; those receiving interleukin-2-based immunotherapy; patients with leukopenia, granulocytic chemotactic defects, or hyperimmunoglobulinemia E syndrome; and those with AIDS. The increase in staphylococcal infections, particularly those due to S. epidermidis, may be related to the use of permanent indwelling central venous catheters.

While community acquired methicillin-resistant S. aureus (CA-MRSA) can be observed in immunosuppressed patients, it is more common in young and healthy patients who live in crowded conditions or have close physical contact with others.[55] However, MRSA carriage and infection rates have been shown to be higher in HIV-infected men who have sex with men (MSM) without evidence of immune suppression than in healthy MSM controls.[56] The USA 300 strain with the staphylococcal cassette chromosome (SCCmec IV) is closely associated with HIV infection. Patients with HIV disease develop MRSA infections due to the same strain with which they are colonized. In one study, the risk factor for colonization in HIV-positive patients was only prior antibiotic use[56] while in another study, the risk factors for colonization or infection with MRSA in HIV-positive patients included prior antibiotic use, a central venous catheter, presence of a dermatologic disease, and total number of days in the hospital.[57] Another study noted that CA-MRSA infections in HIV-positive MSM were associated with high risk sex and drug-using behaviors and environmental exposures, but not with immune status.[58]

The literature on MRSA infections in solid organ transplant recipients is sparse. In liver transplant recipients, MRSA occurs in the first 3 months after transplantation with infections occurring in the blood, wounds, abdomen, and lower respiratory tract.[59] A 32-year-old renal transplant recipient suffered for several months with recurrent MRSA furunculosis and cellulitis treated with appropriate antibiotics, incision and drainage, and nasal mupirocin.[59] Despite this treatment, 7 months later, he developed a MRSA iliopsoas abscess and osteomyelitis of the L5 vertebral body and left transverse process. Necrotizing fasciitis due to S. aureus is uncommon. Necrotizing fasciitis due to MRSA as the single pathogen has been reported in 2 renal transplant recipients[59,60] and a previously undiagnosed AIDS patient.[61]

Staphylococcal scalded skin syndrome (SSSS) is a distinctive form of toxin mediated erythema caused by infection most often with S. aureus type 71, phage group 2. The Staphylococcus produce epidermolytic toxins (exfoliating toxin-A and exfoliating toxin-B) that are not excreted in either infants or adults with impaired renal function. SSSS can occur in adults immunosuppressed because of systemic steroids or malignancy, status-post transplantation,[62] or infected with HIV.[63] SSSS in adults differs from SSSS in children because of the much greater incidence of positive blood cultures for S. aureus and the higher

mortality rate.[64] Another staphylococcal toxin was responsible for a toxic shock-like illness in five AIDS patients with a prolonged desquamative erythroderma[65] and mucosal infection lasting for several weeks. This is distinguished from classic toxic shock syndrome by its subactue and recalcitrant course and by less frequent multi-organ failure.

Blistering distal dactylitis, tender tense bullae most often affecting the fingertip fat pad, was historically caused by group A beta-hemolytic Streptococcus, but there are increasing reports of blistering distal dactylitis due to S. aureus. S. aureus -induced blistering dactylitis was reported in an adult with Crohn's disease on high dose systemic steroids.[66] Two HIV-positive patients presented with S. aureus blistering distal dactylitis on the dorsal fingers, one with bulla that rapidly evolved into erosions on two fingers of the same hand, and the other presented with an enlarging bulla on the dorsal thumb.[67] Multiple bullae may be a predictor that S. aureus is the causative agent.[68] A lymphocutaneous syndrome (nodules in a sporotrichoid pattern) due to S. aureus occurred in a patient with Wegener's granulomatosis treated with cyclophosphamide, prednisone, and hemodialysis. Blastomycosis-like pyoderma (verrucous plaques with multiple pustules, an elevated border and pseudoepitheliomatous hyperplasia with multiple abscesses on biopsy) due to S. aureus was observed in a case of chronic myeloid leukemia.[69]

A group of renal transplant patients with recurrent staphylococcal cellulitis of the elbow was described by Wolfson et al.[70] All four patients had a similar clinical problem they termed "transplant elbow." These patients all had the adverse effects of chronic corticosteroid therapy: marked atrophy and poor wound healing of the skin with increased susceptibility to trauma and a steroid-induced proximal myopathy of their legs so that they could not rise from a seated position without pushing off with their elbows and traumatizing them. The recurrent episodes of cellulitis continued until adequate protection was provided to the elbows.

Cutaneous staphylococcal infections are frequent in HIV-infected patients with the incidence increasing with the degree of immunodeficiency. Bullous impetigo of the intertriginous areas, facial or truncal folliculitis, furunculosis, or ecthyma develops. HIV infection is also a risk factor for pyomyositis due to S. aureus.[71] Secondary staphylococcal infection frequently develops in AIDS patients with underlying dermatoses. Patients may continue to develop new lesions even while receiving appropriate therapy based on the antibiotic sensitivity of the cultured strain.[72]

Superficial bacterial infections in HIV-positive patients may have unusual clinical pictures. Molluscum contagiosum-like dermal abscesses due to S. aureus occurred in a patient with multiple infections and AIDS.[73] Duvic reported cases of intertriginous or axillary staphylococcal infection that clinically resembled candidiasis.[74] Violaceous plaques up to 10 cm in diameter with superficial pustules and crusts, culture-positive for S. aureus, were observed in HIV-infected patients.[75] The atypical plaque-like staphylococcal folliculitis required prolonged oral and topical antibiotic treatment. Botryomycosis, a rare chronic suppurative infection most commonly due to *S. aureus* and characterized by granules in tissue, has been described in patients with AIDS and with hyper-IgE syndrome (Job syndrome).[76,77] One HIV-positive patient presented with an index finger ulcer with grey vesicles at the margin, keratotic papules in a sporotrichoid pattern on the arm and painful ulcerations on the buttocks and toes.[77] An atypical presentation of botryomycosis in AIDS includes pruritic pink granulomatous papules and pustules on the posterior neck, oral commissures, upper trunk, and antecubital fossae, some with umbilicated centers and some with overlying crust.[78]

Cancer patients who develop cutaneous toxicities after treatment with the epidermal growth factor receptor inhibitors have a high rate (38%) of bacterial infection at the site of the cutaneous toxicity, most commonly due to methicillin-sensitive *Staphylococcus aureus* (MSSA), followed by MRSA.[79] Leukopenic patients were found to be at greatest risk for infection.

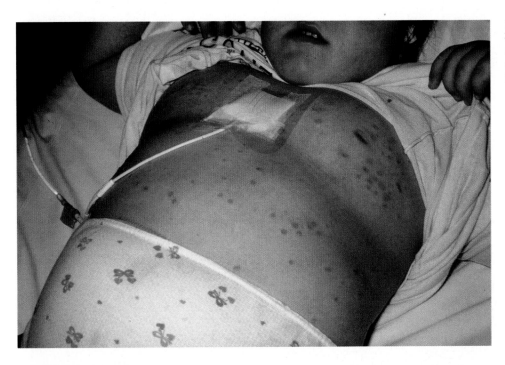

Figure 12.9. A monomorphous bullous eruption due to *S. aureus* developed in a 12-year-old during chemotherapy for acute lymphocytic leukemia

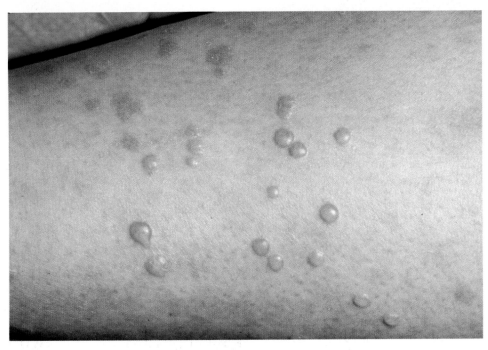

Figure 12.10. Tense nonumbilicated vesicles and bullae contained a pure culture of *S. aureus* and readily resolved with antibiotics

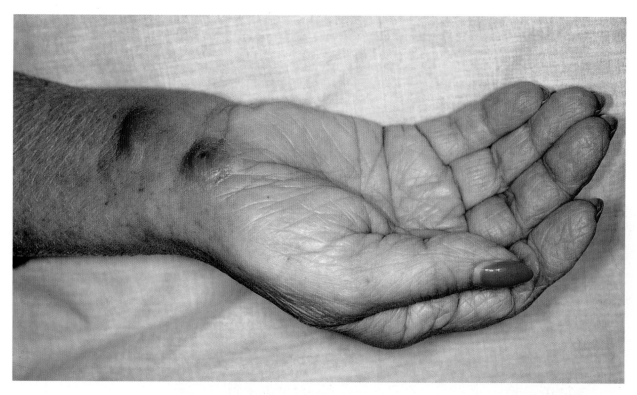

Figure 12.11. Sporotrichoid tender erythematous nodules of *S. aureus* developed in a 65-year-old woman on chronic corticosteroid therapy

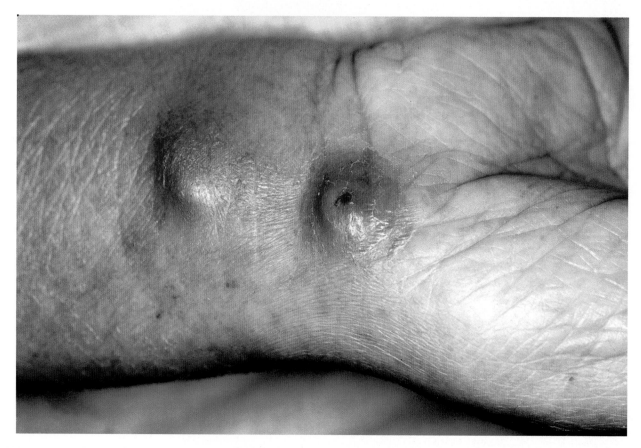

Figure 12.12. Close-up of the wrist nodules. Skin biopsy and culture demonstrated *S. aureus*

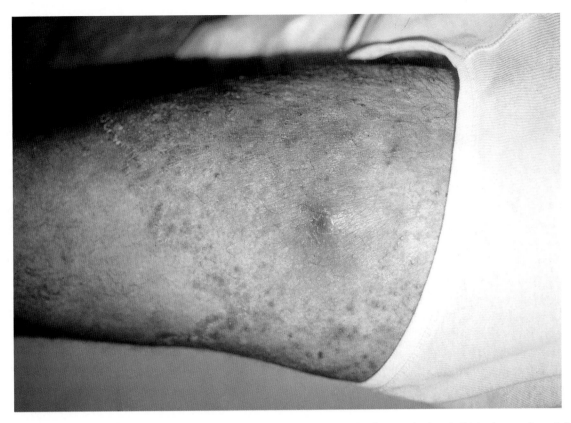

Figure 12.13.   Recurrent bacterial abscesses due to *S. aureus* developed in the broken skin barrier of a chronic *Trichophyton rubrum* infection in a heart transplant patient

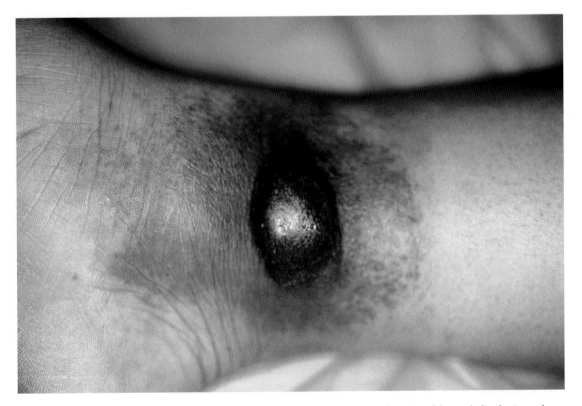

Figure 12.14.   *Staphylococcus aureus* hemorrhagic bulla of the ankle was the presenting manifestation of the myelodysplastic syndrome

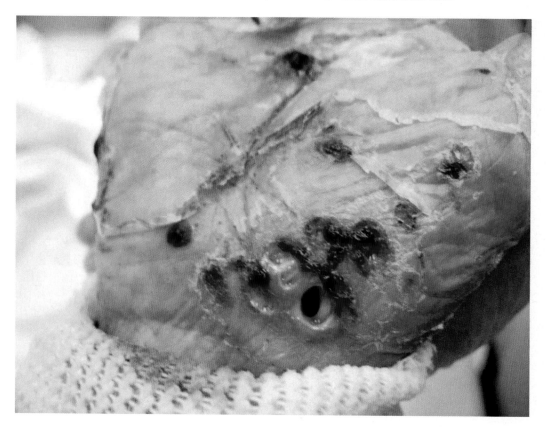

Figure 12.15. A 75-year-old man with a history of dilantin hypersensitivity syndrome was treated with systemic steroids and developed methicillin-resistant *S. aureus* (MRSA) botryomycosis of the palm and persistent bacteremia

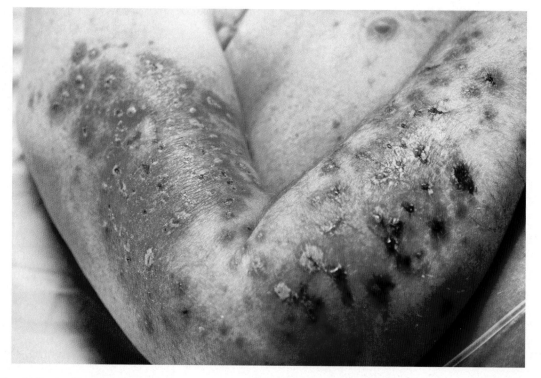

Figure 12.16. A 74-year-old man with neutropenia secondary to newly diagnosed follicular lymphoma had *S. aureus* and group B *Streptococcus* ecthyma seen on the arm

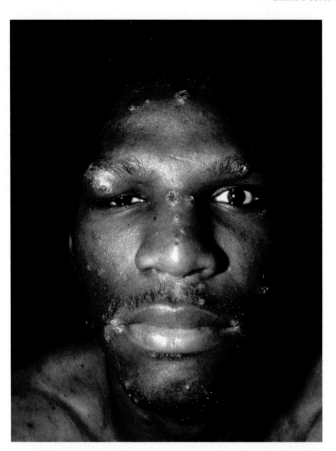

Figure 12.17. A 30-year-old human immunodeficiency virus (HIV)-positive African-American man developed crusted papules and nodules, some with central ulceration on his face, scalp, neck, chest, and arms. Skin biopsy and culture demonstrated *S. aureus* botryomycosis (Courtesy of Ed Milano, M.D.)

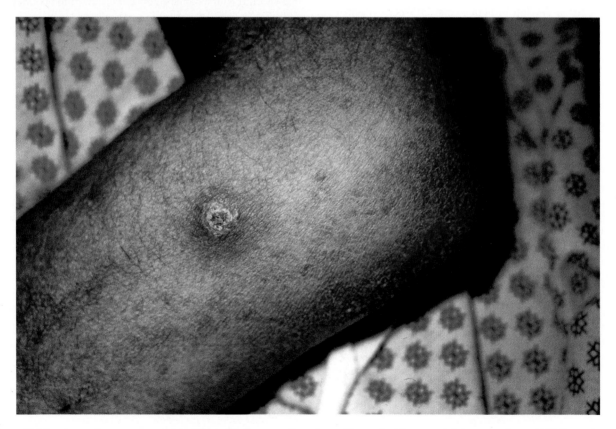

Figure 12.18. An erythematous crusted nodule on the forearm of a patient with acquired immune deficiency syndrome (AIDS) was due to a complex infection by more than one pathogen: *S. aureus* and *Histoplasma*

Streptococcus

Streptococcal infections in the immunocompromised host may be clinically atypical. In addition, organisms that have been historically limited to certain patient populations are increasingly reported in immunosuppressed patients.

Streptococcus pyogenes (group A β-hemolytic Streptococcus)

Ecthyma due to *Streptococcus pyogenes* (group A β-hemolytic *Streptococcus*), was remarkable for extensive, bilaterally symmetrical skin involvement and bacteremia in a homosexual man with AIDS.[80]

Facial erysipelas due to group A β-hemolytic *Streptococcus* (*Streptococcus pyogenes*) was atypical in two patients with hypereosinophilic syndrome on long-term systemic steroids: the facial lesion followed the onset of fever by 48 h in one; in the other, there was a striking absence of erythema of the facial lesions and there was the presence of bacteremia, which is rare in uncomplicated facial erysipelas.[81]

Streptococcal cellulitis-adenitis is typically caused by group B streptococci (*Streptococcus agalactiae*) and presents in infants less than 2 months of age. However, streptococcal cellulitis-adenitis caused by group A β-hemolytic streptococci also occurs in homosexual men with AIDS. Typically, rapidly enlarging inguinal nodes with fever, leukocytosis, and no obvious genital or skin lesion develop in homosexual HIV-positive men. An unusual case of group A streptococcal cellulitis-adenitis in a homosexual HIV-positive man was complicated by a scarlatiniform eruption and a streptococcal toxic shock-like syndrome.[82] Streptococcal toxic shock syndrome in a 68-year-old with rheumatoid arthritis on systemic steroids, hydroxychloroquine and leflunomide presented with multiple hemorrhagic bullae and advancing erythema on the right upper forequarter.[83]

Group B Streptococcus (Streptococcus agalactiae)

Invasive infections with Group B *Streptococcus* are most common in neonates and pregnant women. However, immunodeficiency and malignancies, as well as older age and diabetes mellitus, are emerging risk factors for skin and soft-tissue infections with this organism.[84] Co-infection with *Staphylococcus aureus* is not uncommon. Cutaneous manifestations include erysipelas/cellulitis (25%), infections of wounds or ulcers, myositis, necrotizing fasciitis, and toxic shock syndrome.[84]

Streptococcus pneumoniae

Streptococcus pneumoniae is an uncommon cause of soft tissue infections, but the incidence may be rising due to increasing numbers of immunosuppressed patients.[85] As opposed to patients with diabetes mellitus and substance abuse who present with *S. pneumoniae* cellulitis of the limbs, adult patients with hematologic disease (multiple myeloma or macroglobulinemia), systemic lupus erythematosus, or nephrotic syndrome and pediatric patients with hypogammaglobulinemia tend to present with facial and neck cellulitis.[86] Patients with pneumococcal cellulitis commonly present with bulla formation and violaceous or brownish skin discoloration. A disproportionate number of cases of pneumococcal cellulitis have been reported among patients with systemic lupus erythematosus (SLE). Alcoholism and asplenia (functional or anatomical) may be considered an additional risk factor for pneumococcal cellulitis.[87]

Necrotizing fasciitis caused by *S. pneumonia* is exceedingly rare, but has been reported in patients with cirrhosis, systemic lupus erythematosus, diabetes mellitus, rheumatoid arthritis, mixed connective tissue disease, idiopathic thrombocytopenic purpura, and status-post renal transplantation.[88] Cutaneous involvement most commonly presents on the lower extremities, followed by the upper extremities and trunk.

Acute infectious purpura fulminans occurring the setting of disseminated intravascular coagulation due to streptococcal infection was reported in 5 immunosuppressed patients (AIDS, rheumatoid arthritis on systemic steroids, idiopathic thrombocytopenia on systemic steroids, metastatic renal cell carcinoma, and non-Hodgkin's lymphoma).[89] Four of the patients had asplenia or functional hyposplenia. Blood cultures were positive for *Streptococcus pneumonia* in 4 cases and group A β-hemolytic *Streptococcus* in one case. Group A streptococcus is a rare cause of purpura fulminans. Patients presented with symmetric acral purpura, with striking involvement of the nose that evolved into gangrene, consistent with the diagnosis of peripheral symmetric gangrene.

Group G Streptococcus

Erysipelas was atypical in a patient with cured Hodgkin's disease who presented with patchy, macular erythema involving the buttocks and both thighs (more resembling a drug eruption than erysipelas) due to group G *Streptococcus*.[90]

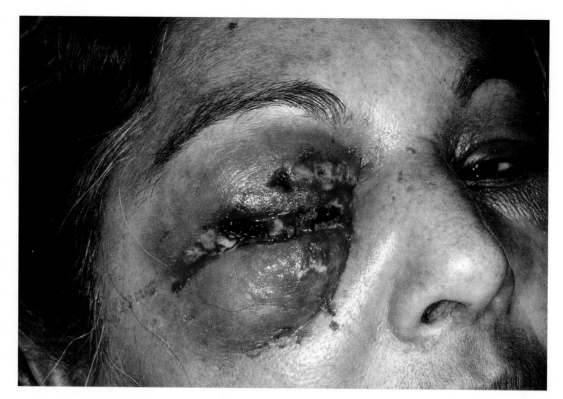

Figure 12.19. A 28-year-old woman with systemic lupus erythematosus (SLE) on prednisone, mycophenolic acid and hydroxychloroquine developed fever, swelling of her left eye, nausea, and vomiting. Magnetic resonance imaging (MRI) showed periorbital cellulitis and inflammatory changes in the masseter and temporalis muscles. Total hemolytic complement 8 (60–144 nL), C3 48 (83–177 nL), C4 7 (16–47 nL). *Streptococcus* group A cellulitis/gangrene resolved with antibiotics and no surgical debridement

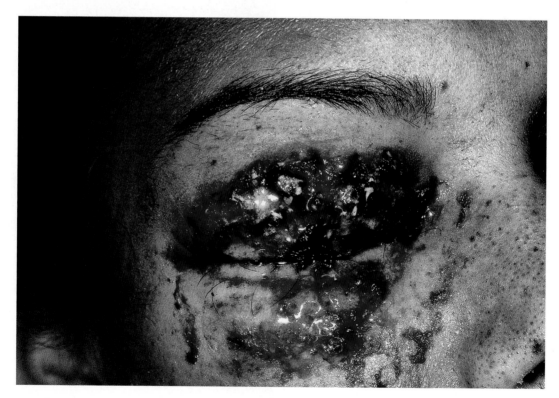

Figure 12.20. Follow-up appearance approximately 48 h after inception of intravenous (IV) antibiotics

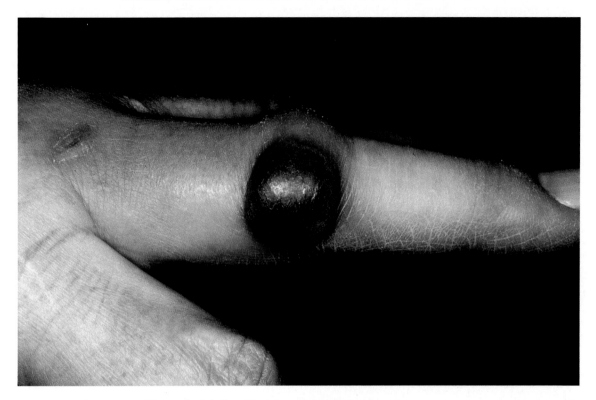

Figure 12.21.   Group A streptococcal hemorrhagic bulla and lymphangitis in refractory anemia

Figure 12.22.   Woman with a history of metastatic non-small cell lung cancer who recently completed a cycle of chemotherapy 2 weeks prior to the development of Group G *Streptococcus* bacteremia and perineal bullous cellulitis. Skin tissue and bulla fluid cultures were positive for Group G *Streptococcus*

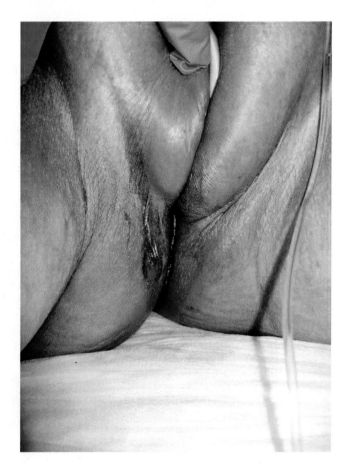

References

Bacillus Species

1. Jaruratanasirikul S, Kalnauwakul S, Lekhakula A. Traumatic wound infection due to *Bacillus cereus* in an immunocompromised patient: a case report. Southeast Asian J Trop Med Public Health. 1987;18(1):112–4.

2. Khavari PA, Bolognia JL, Eisen R, et al. Periodic acid-Schiff-positive organisms in primary cutaneous *Bacillus cereus* infection. Case report and an investigation of the periodic acid-Schiff staining properties of bacteria. Arch Dermatol. 1991;127(4):543–6.

3. Henrickson KJ, Shenep JL, Flynn PM, Pui CH. Primary cutaneous *Bacillus cereus* infection in neutropenic children. Lancet. 1989;1(8638):601–3.

4. Meredith FT, Fowler VG, Gautier M, Corey GR, Reller LB. *Bacillus cereus* necrotizing cellulitis mimicking clostridial myonecrosis: case report and review of the literature. Scand J Infect Dis. 1997;29(5):528–9.

5. Mori T, Tokuhira M, Takae Y, et al. Successful non-surgical treatment of brain abscess and necrotizing fasciitis caused by *Bacillus cereus*. Intern Med. 2002;41(8):671–3.

6. Lee YL, Shih SD, Weng YJ, Chen C, Liu CE. Fatal spontaneous bacterial peritonitis and necrotizing fasciitis with bacteraemia caused by *Bacillus cereus* in a patient with cirrhosis. J Med Microbiol. 2010;59 (Pt 2):242–4.

7. Cone LA, Dreisbach L, Potts BE, Comess BE, Burleigh WA. Fatal *Bacillus cereus* endocarditis masquerading as an anthrax-like infection in a patient with acute lymphoblastic leukemia: case report. J Heart Valve Dis. 2005;14(1):37–9.

8. Smith KJ, Skelton HG, Hilyard EJ, et al. *Bacillus piliformis* infection (Tyzzer's disease) in a patient infected with HIV-1: confirmation with 16S ribosomal RNA sequence analysis. J Am Acad Dermatol. 1996;34(2 Pt 2):343–8.

Clostridium

9. Burke MP, Opeskin K. Nontraumatic clostridial myonecrosis. Am J Forensic Med Pathol. 1999;20(2):158–62.

10. Dellinger EP. Severe necrotizing soft-tissue infections. Multiple disease entities requiring a common approach. JAMA. 1981;246(15):1717–21.

11. Tehrani H, Gillespie PH, Cormack GC. Fatal multifocal metastasis of *Clostridium septicum*: a case report. Br J Plast Surg. 2004;57(7):673–5.

12. McDonald CP, Hartley S, Orchard K, et al. Fatal *Clostridium perfringens* sepsis from a pooled platelet transfusion. Transfus Med. 1998;8(1):19–22.

13. Smith-Slatas CL, Bourque M, Salazar JC. *Clostridium septicum* infections in children: a case report and review of the literature. Pediatrics. 2006;117(4):e796–805.

Corynebacterium

14. van der Lelie H, Leverstein-Van Hall M, Mertens M, et al. Corynebacterium CDC group JK (*Corynebacterium jeikeium*) sepsis in haematological patients: a report of three cases and a systematic literature review. Scand J Infect Dis. 1995;27(6):581–4.

15. Jerdan MS, Shapiro RS, Smith NB, Virshup DM, Hood AF. Cutaneous manifestations of Corynebacterium group JK sepsis. J Am Acad Dermatol. 1987;16(2 Pt 2):444–7.

16. Guarino MJ, Qazi R, Woll JE, Rubins J. Septicemia, rash, and pulmonary infiltrates secondary to Corynebacterium group JK infection. Am J Med. 1987;82(1):132–4.

17. Olson JM, Nguyen VQ, Yoo J, Kuechle MK. Cutaneous manifestations of *Corynebacterium jeikeium* sepsis. Int J Dermatol. 2009;48(8):886–8.

18. Ordóñez-Palau S, Boquet D, Gil-Garcia M, Pardina-Solano M. Chronic osteomyelitis of the metatarsal sesamoid due to *Corynebacterium jeikeium* in a patient with rheumatoid arthritis. Joint Bone Spine. 2007;74(5):516–7.

19. Jucglà A, Sais G, Carratala J, et al. A papular eruption secondary to infection with *Corynebacterium jeikeium*, with histopathological features mimicking botryomycosis. Br J Dermatol. 1995;133(5):801–4.

Nocardia

20. Ambrosioni J, Lew D, Garbino J. Nocardiosis: updated clinical review and experience at a tertiary center. Infection. 2010;38(2):89–97.

21. Moeller CA, Burton III CS. Primary lymphocutaneous *Nocardia brasiliensis* infection. Arch Dermatol. 1986;122(10):1180–2.

22. Nishimoto K, Ohno M. Subcutaneous abscesses caused by *Nocardia brasiliensis* complicated by malignant lymphoma. A survey of cutaneous nocardiosis reported in Japan. Int J Dermatol. 1985;24(7):437–40.

23. Boixeda P, España A, Suarez J, Buzon L, Ledo A. Cutaneous nocardiosis and human immunodeficiency virus infection. Int J Dermatol. 1991;30(11):804–5.

24. [No authors listed]. Case records of the Massachusetts General Hospital. Weekly clinicopathological exercises. Case 29-2000. A 69-year-old renal transplant recipient with low grade fever and multiple pulmonary nodules. N Engl J Med. 2000;343(12):870–7.

25. Fabre S, Gibert C, Lechiche C, Jorgensen C, Sany J. Primary cutaneous *Nocardia otitidiscaviarum* infection in a patient with rheumatoid arthritis treated with infliximab. J Rheumatol. 2005;32(12):2432–3.

26. Singh SM, Rau NV, Cohen LB, Harris H. Cutaneous nocardiosis complicating management of Crohn's disease with infliximab and prednisone. CMAJ. 2004;171(9):1063–4.

27. Lee CC, Loo LW, Lam MS. Case reports of nocardiosis in patients with human immunodeficiency virus (HIV) infection. Ann Acad Med Singapore. 2000;29(1):119–26.

28. Peleg AY, Husain S, Qureshi ZA, et al. Risk factors, clinical characteristics, and outcome of Nocardia infection in organ transplant recipients: a matched case-control study. Clin Infect Dis. 2007;44(10):1307–14.

29. Freites V, Sumoza A, Bisotti R, et al. Subcutaneous *Nocardia asteroides* abscess in a bone marrow transplant recipient. Bone Marrow Transplant. 1995;15(1):135–6.

30. Auzary C, Mouthon L, Soilleux M, et al. Localized subcutaneous *Nocardia farcinica* abscess in a woman with overlap syndrome between systemic scleroderma and polymyositis. Ann Med Interne (Paris). 1999;150(7):582–4.

31. Furumoto H, Sasaki T, Tatebayashi K, Shimizu T, Mikami Y. Profound skin infection with bone involvement due to *Nocardia asteroides* in a patient with myelodysplastic syndrome. J Dermatol. 2001;28(10):582–3.

32. Balbir-Gurman A, Schapira D, Nahir AM. Primary subcutaneous nocardial infection in a SLE patient. Lupus. 1999;8(2):164–7.

33. Stamenkovic SA, Madden BP. *Nocardia asteroides* abscess after heart transplantation. J Heart Lung Transplant. 2001;20(7):789–91.

34. Hashimoto Y, Hiruma M, Hisamichi K, et al. Primary cutaneous nocardiosis with multiple, subcutaneous abscesses in a patient with sarcoidosis. J Dermatolog Treat. 2002;13(4):201–3.

35. Lopes JO, Silva CB, Kmohan C, et al. Acute primary cutaneous *Nocardia asteroides* infection in a patient with systemic lupus erythematosus. Case report. Rev Inst Med Trop Sao Paulo. 1995;37(6):547–50.

36. Aydingöz IE, Candan I, Dervent B, Hitit G. Primary cutaneous nocardiosis associated with intra-articular corticosteroid injection. Int J Dermatol. 2001;40(3):196–8.

37. Shimizu T, Furumoto H, Asagami C, et al. Disseminated subcutaneous *Nocardia farcinica* abscesses in a nephrotic syndrome patient. J Am Acad Dermatol. 1998;38(5 Pt 2):874–6.

38. Iona E, Giannoni F, Brunori L, et al. Isolation of *Nocardia asiatica* from cutaneous ulcers of a human immunodeficiency virus-infected patient in Italy. J Clin Microbiol. 2007;45(6):2088–9.

39. Takahara M, Imafuku S, Matsuda T, et al. Concurrent double infections of the skin: phaeohyphomycosis and nocardiosis in a patient with idiopathic thrombocytopenic purpura. J Am Acad Dermatol. 2005;53(5 Suppl 1):S277–80.

40. Parra IH, Galimberti R, Galimberti G, Guanella B, Kowalczuk A. Lymphocutaneous nocardiosis and cutaneous pheohyphomycosis in a liver transplant recipient. Int J Dermatol. 2008;47(6):571–4.

41. Park I, Lee W, Cho J, et al. *Nocardia niigatensis* infection in a kidney transplant recipient. Transpl Int. 2009;22(5):583–5.

42. Shapiro PE, Grossman ME. Disseminated *Nocardia asteroides* with pustules. J Am Acad Dermatol. 1989;20(5 Pt 2):889–92.

43. Christoph I. Pulmonary *Cryptococcus neoformans* and disseminated *Nocardia brasiliensis* in an immunocompromised host. Case report. N C Med J. 1990;51(5):219–20.

44. Arroyo JC, Nichols S, Carroll GF. Disseminated *Nocardia caviae* infection. Am J Med. 1977;62(3):409–12.

45. Schreiner DT, de Castro P, Jorizzo JL, Solomon AR, Holder WR. Disseminated *Nocardia brasiliensis* infection following cryptococcal disease. Arch Dermatol. 1986;122(10):1186–90.

46. Lopez FA, Johnson F, Novosad DM, Beaman BL, Holodniy M. Successful management of disseminated *Nocardia transvalensis* infection in a heart transplant recipient after development of sulfonamide resistance: case report and review. J Heart Lung Transplant. 2003;22(4):492–7.

47. Jimenez-Galanes Marchan S, Meneu Díaz JC, Caso Maestro O, et al. Disseminated nocardiosis: a rare infectious complication following non-heart-beating donor liver transplantation. Transplant Proc. 2009;41(6):2495–7.

48. Smilack JD. Images in clinical medicine. Pulmonary and disseminated nocardiosis. N Engl J Med. 1999;34(12):885.

49. Cargill JS, Boyd GJ, Weightman NC. *Nocardia cyriacigeorgica*: a case of endocarditis with disseminated soft-tissue infection. J Med Microbiol. 2010;59(Pt 2):224–30.

50. Auzary C, Du Boutin LT, Wechsler B, Chollet P, Piette JC. Disseminated nocardiosis presenting as a flare of Behçet's disease. Rheumatology (Oxford). 2001;40(8):949–52.

51. Korkmaz C, Aydinli A, Erol N, et al. Widespread nocardiosis in two patients with Behçet's disease. Clin Exp Rheumatol. 2001;19(4):459–62.

52. Arslan U, Tuncer I, Uysal EB, Inci R. Pleuropulmonary and soft tissue *Nocardia cyriacigeorgici* infection in a patient with Behçet's disease. Saudi Med J. 2007;28(9):1435–7.

53. Kalb RE, Kaplan MH, Grossman ME. Cutaneous nocardiosis. Case reports and review. J Am Acad Dermatol. 1985;13(1):125–33.

Staphylococcus

54. Nguyen V, Huggins RH, Lertsburapa T, et al. Cutaneous T-cell lymphoma and *Staphylococcus aureus* colonization. J Am Acad Dermatol. 2008;59(6):949–52.

55. Elston DM. Community-acquired methicillin-resistant *Staphylococcus aureus*. J Am Acad Dermatol. 2007;56(1):1–16.

56. Shet A, Mathema B, Mediavilla JR, et al. Colonization and subsequent skin and soft tissue infection due to methicillin-resistant *Staphylococcus aureus* in a cohort of otherwise healthy adults infected with HIV type 1. J Infect Dis. 2009;200(1):88–93.

57. Onorato M, Borucki MJ, Baillargeon G, et al. Risk factors for colonization or infection due to methicillin-resistant *Staphylococcus aureus* in HIV-positive patients: a retrospective case-control study. Infect Control Hosp Epidemiol. 1999;20(1):26–30.

58. Lee NE, Taylor MM, Bancroft E, et al. Risk factors for community-associated methicillin-resistant *Staphylococcus aureus* skin infections among HIV-positive men who have sex with men. Clin Infect Dis. 2005;40(10):1529–34. Epub 2005 Apr 13.

59. Adeyemi OA, Qi C, Zembower TR, et al. Invasive infections with community-associated methicillin-resistant *Staphylococcus aureus* after kidney transplantation. J Clin Microbiol. 2008;46(8):2809–13. Epub 2008 Jun 4.

60. Audard V, Pardon A, Claude O, et al. Necrotizing fasciitis during de novo minimal change nephrotic syndrome in a kidney transplant recipient. Transpl Infect Dis. 2005;7(2):89–92.

61. Olsen RJ, Burns KM, Chen L, Kreiswirth BN, Musser JM. Severe necrotizing fasciitis in a human immunodeficiency virus-positive patient caused by methicillin-resistant *Staphylococcus aureus*. J Clin Microbiol. 2008;46(3):1144–7.

62. Strauss G, Mogensen AM, Rasmussen A, Kirkegaard P. Staphylococcal scalded skin syndrome in a liver transplant patient. Liver Transpl Surg. 1997;3(4):435–6.

63. Farrell AM, Ross JS, Umasankar S, Bunker CB. Staphylococcal scalded skin syndrome in an HIV-1 seropositive man. Br J Dermatol. 1996;134(5):962–5.

64. Ito Y, Funabashi Yoh M, Toda K, et al. Staphylococcal scalded-skin syndrome in an adult due to methicillin-resistant *Staphylococcus aureus*. J Infect Chemother. 2002;8(3):256–61.

65. Cone LA, Woodard DR, Byrd RG, et al. A recalcitrant, erythematous, desquamating disorder associated with toxin-producing staphylococci in patients with AIDS. J Infect Dis. 1992;165(4):638–43.

66. Zemtsov A, Veitschegger M. *Staphylococcus aureus*-induced blistering distal dactylitis in an adult immunosuppressed patient. J Am Acad Dermatol. 1992;26(5 Pt 1):784–5.

67. Scheinfeld N. A review and report of blistering distal dactylitis due to *Staphylococcus aureus* in two HIV-positive men. Dermatol Online J. 2007;13(2):8.

68. Norcross Jr MC, Mitchell DF. Blistering distal dactylitis caused by *Staphylococcus aureus*. Cutis. 1993;51:353–4.

69. Dutta TK, James J, Baruah MC, Ratnakar C. Blastomycosis-like pyoderma in a case of chronic myeloid leukaemia. Postgrad Med J. 1992;68(799):363–5.

70. Wolfson JS, Sober AJ, Rubin RH. Dermatologic manifestations of infection in the compromised host. Annu Rev Med. 1983;34:205–17.

71. Fox LP, Geyer AS, Grossman ME. Pyomyositis. J Am Acad Dermatol. 2004;51(2):308–14.

72. Crum-Cianflone NF. Recurrent neck infection in a person with HIV/AIDS. AIDS Read. 2006;16(3):129–32.

73. Boudreau S, Hines HC, Hood AF. Dermal abscesses with *Staphylococcus aureus*, cytomegalovirus and acid-fast bacilli in a patient with acquired immunodeficiency syndrome (AIDS). J Cutan Pathol. 1988;15(1):53–7.

74. Duvic M. Staphylococcal infections and the pruritus of AIDS-related complex. Arch Dermatol. 1987;123(12):1599.

75. Becker BA, Frieden IJ, Odom RB, Berger TG. Atypical plaquelike staphylococcal folliculitis in human immunodeficiency virus-infected persons. J Am Acad Dermatol. 1989;21(5 Pt 1):1024–6.

76. Patterson JW, Kitces EN, Neafie RC. Cutaneous botryomycosis in a patient with acquired immunodeficiency syndrome. J Am Acad Dermatol. 1987;16(1 Pt 2):238–42.

77. de Vries HJ, van Noesel CJ, Hoekzema R, Hulsebosch HJ. Botryomycosis in an HIV-positive subject. J Eur Acad Dermatol Venereol. 2003;17(1):87–90.

78. Templet JT, Straub R, Ko C. Botryomycosis presenting as pruritic papules in a human immunodeficiency virus-positive patient. Cutis. 2007;80(1):45–7.

79. Eilers Jr RE, Gandhi M, Patel JD, et al. Dermatologic infections in cancer patients treated with epidermal growth factor receptor inhibitor therapy. J Natl Cancer Inst. 2010;102(1):47–53.

Streptococcus

80. Hewitt WD, Farrar WE. Bacteremia and ecthyma caused by *Streptococcus pyogenes* in a patient with acquired immunodeficiency syndrome. Am J Med Sci. 1988;295(1):52–4.
81. Cupps TR, Cotton DJ, Schooley RT, Fauci AS. Facial erysipelas in the immunocompromised host. Report of two cases. Arch Dermatol. 1981;117(1):47–9.
82. Janssen F, Zelinsky-Gurung A, Caumes E, Decazes JM. Group A streptococcal cellulitis-adenitis in a patient with acquired immunodeficiency syndrome. J Am Acad Dermatol. 1991;24(2 Pt 2):363–5.
83. Chikkamuniyappa S. Streptococcal toxic shock syndrome and sepsis manifesting in a patient with chronic rheumatoid arthritis. Derm Online J. 2004;10(1):7.
84. Sendi P, Johansson L, Norrby-Teglund A. Invasive group B Streptococcal disease in non-pregnant adults: a review with emphasis on skin and soft-tissue infections. Infection. 2008;36(2):100–11.
85. DiNubile MJ, Albornoz MA, Stumacher RJ, et al. Pneumococcal soft-tissue infections: possible association with connective tissue diseases. J Infect Dis. 1991;163(4):897–900.
86. Parada JP, Maslow JN. Clinical syndromes associated with adult pneumococcal cellulitis. Scand J Infect Dis. 2000;32(2):133–6. Review.
87. Lawlor MT, Crowe HM, Quintiliani R. Cellulitis due to *Streptococcus pneumoniae*: case report and review. Clin Infect Dis. 1992;14(1):247–50.
88. Yamashiro E, Asato Y, Taira K, et al. Necrotizing fasciitis caused by *Streptococcus pneumoniae*. J Dermatol. 2009;36(5):298–305.
89. Ward KM, Celebi JT, Gmyrek R, Grossman ME. Acute infectious purpura fulminans associated with asplenism or hyposplenism. J Am Acad Dermatol. 2002;47(4):493–6.
90. Shama S, Calandra GB. Atypical erysipelas caused by group G streptococci in a patient with cured Hodgkin's disease. Arch Dermatol. 1982;118(11):934–6.

13

Gram-Negative Bacteria

AEROMONAS

Aeromonas species are gram-negative anaerobic rods found in fresh water lakes and streams. They have also been recovered from chlorinated tap water, including hospital water supplies. *Aeromonas* infections of freshwater traumatic wounds cause a characteristic clinical picture indistinguishable from group A streptococcal infection in normal hosts. Rapidly progressive cellulitis develops within 8–48 h after trauma with freshwater exposure, followed by suppuration and necrosis around the wound, often requiring surgical debridement. Fasciitis, myonecrosis, and osteomyelitis may develop. *Aeromonas hydrophilia* is the species that causes most soft tissue infections and bacteremias. Other species isolated include *A. veronii* subtype sobria and *A. caviae*.[1]

In immunosuppressed patients, *Aeromonas* can cause various infections that are likely to be fatal including severe cellulitis, fulminant necrotizing infections, and ecthyma gangrenosum.[2,3] Myonecrosis and gas production have occurred with *Aeromonas* and can simulate clostridial gas gangrene.[4]

Aeromonas septicemia in immunocompromised patients with various types of leukemia, solid neoplasms, and hepatic cirrhosis occurs without an obvious portal of entry. The infection may be nosocomially acquired or spread from the gastrointestinal tract. Most patients with *Aeromonas* sepsis do not present with diarrhea. Since the organism can be found in fish, turtles, and other marine animals, eating contaminated freshwater seafood may be a source of human infection. In *Aeromonas* sepsis, characteristically multiple hemorrhagic bullae occur on the trunk or extremity and rapidly evolve to extensive necrotizing fasciitis and profound shock.[1]

Other skin and soft tissue infections that may be seen with a history of water contact and should be differentiated from *Aeromonas* infections include: (a) *Vibrio* species after contact with salt water; (b) *Erysipelothrix rhusiopathiae* (erysipeloid), after contact with fish; (c) *Mycobacterium marinum*, also known as swimming pool granuloma; (d) *Burkholderia pseudomallei*, formerly *Pseudomonas pseudomallei* (Whitmore's disease or melioidosis) in Southeast Asia; (e) *Pseudomonas aeruginosa* in hot tubs; (f) *Chromobacterium* species with recreational water contact; (g) *Prototheca wickerhamii*; and (h) *Legionella* species.

M.E. Grossman et al., *Cutaneous Manifestations of Infection in the Immunocompromised Host*,
DOI 10.1007/978-1-4419-1578-8_13, © Springer Science+Business Media, LLC 2012

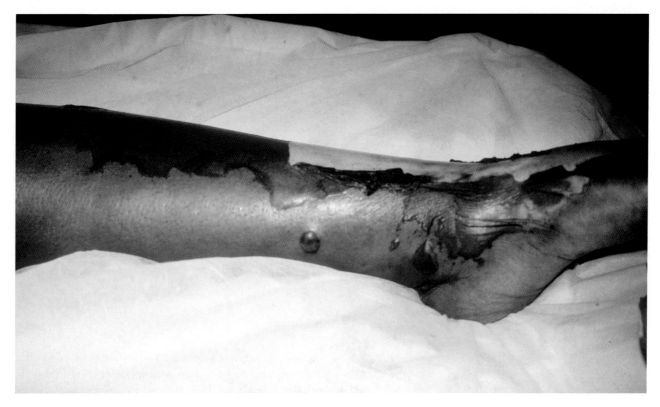

Figure 13.1. Necrotizing hemorrhagic bullae of a human immunodeficiency virus (HIV)-negative, intravenous drug abuser with cirrhosis who developed septic shock and multiorgan failure and then died. *Aeromonas* species was cultured from the blood and bullae

BARTONELLA

Bartonella (formerly *Rochalimaea*) species are small pleomorphic fastidious gram-negative bacilli that belong to the alpha-2 subdivision of Proteobacteria, a group that includes the genera *Rickettsia, Ehrlichia, Brucella,* and the plant pathogen *Agrobacterium tumefaciens*.[5] They require blood-enriched media and environments with high carbon dioxide levels in order to grow and are rarely cultured in the microbiology laboratory. The genus *Bartonella* has expanded to 20 currently identified species. At least 8 of these are responsible for human disease. The number of recognized species of *Bartonella* and human diseases caused by them will probably increase in the future.

The first member of the *Bartonella* genus, *B. bacilliformis*, was identified in the Andes Mountain region of Peru by Alberto Barton in the early 1900s. Prior to this discovery, the self-experimenting medical student, Daniel Carrion, had linked the development of the chronic form of infection, verruga peruana, to the acute form of disease, known as Oroya fever. Oroya fever, or Carrion's disease, is a febrile hemolytic anemia transmitted by the female sandfly, *Lutzomyia verrucarum*. Verruga peruana (Peruvian wart) is an eruptive angiomatosis of the skin, which appears as "red warts." *Bartonella henselae*, which is transmitted among cats by fleas and to humans by cat contact, cat scratches, or tick bites, is the pathogenic agent of cat scratch disease. The disease typically presents with lymphadenopathy and skin or visceral lesions. *Bartonella quintana* is the pathogenic agent of Trench fever transmitted by the body louse. Described during World War I and rarely thereafter, the disease now primarily occurs in human immunodeficiency virus (HIV) seronegative homeless men with chronic alcoholism living in urban areas. The disease follows a cyclic clinical evolution of relapsing fever, malaise, chills, anorexia, sweating, headache, conjunctival injection, myalgias, arthralgias, and crops of truncal erythematous macules or papules.

Bacillary angiomatosis (BA) was first reported in an acquired immune deficiency syndrome (AIDS) patient in 1983[6] followed by multiple reports by dermatologists.[7-9] The etiologic agents for BA were originally designated as new species in the genus *Rochalimaea*. However, the agents of bacillary angiomatosis have been reclassified as *Bartonella henselae* and *Bartonella quintana*. Though bacillary angiomatosis is not a manifestation of cat scratch disease, it is considered that a scratch, bite, or contact with a cat can be a risk factor since the cat is the main source of *Bartonella henselae*. AIDS-associated BA was most frequently seen in patients with a CD4 count less than 100 cells/mm.[3] BA occurs less often in other immunocompromised hosts, including cardiac, hepatic, renal, and bone marrow transplant recipients, patients undergoing chemotherapy for hematologic malignancies (acute and chronic leukemia, lymphoma, especially chronic lymphocytic leukemia [CLL]), and rarely in immunocompetent individuals.[10] The incidence of BA has dropped dramatically since the introduction of highly active antiretroviral treatment (HAART) regimens and prophylactic antibiotics.

BA often presents with constitutional signs and symptoms such as fever, chills, malaise, headache, and anorexia with or without weight loss. *Bartonella* infections can be the cause of fever of unknown origin in HIV-infected patients with disseminated disease. Because of the difficulty of culturing the organism and the nonspecific clinical presentation, the diagnosis is often neglected in the absence of skin lesions.

Various organs can be affected by BA, including the liver, spleen, bone marrow, lymph nodes, skeletal muscle,[11,12] conjunctiva, brain, mucosal surfaces of the gastrointestinal and respiratory tracts, and skin. The skin lesions are the most frequent clinical manifestation of BA.[13,14] The head is the most common site, but lesions may occur on the trunk and the extremities, particularly when the lesions are numerous. The characteristic cutaneous lesion present in 55–90% of BA is a single or multiple asymptomatic bright red to purple papules, which may be disseminated over the entire surface of the body, sometimes numbering more than 1,000. The reddish-purple papule is firm, from 1 mm to 1 cm, and may be smooth, verrucous, or pedunculated. Clinically these lesions look like the verruga peruana of Carrion's disease due to *Bartonella bacilliformis*. Although the skin lesions appear vascular, they rarely ulcerate or bleed like pyogenic granulomas or Kaposi's sarcoma, the major clinical differential diagnoses. Subcutaneous nodules, the second common morphology of BA, are smooth surfaced and skin colored. These nodules can be associated with underlying bony defects or coexist with the generalized red papules. Individual nodules may be up to several centimeters in size. A third type of lesion is an indurated hyperpigmented and hyperkeratotic plaque with indistinct borders or a cellulitic plaque typically found on the extremities which may overlie deeper osseous involvement.[15] In one case, BA produced a large ($10 \times 10 \times 2$ cm) fungating mass with central ulceration, purulence, and necrosis on the ankle of an HIV-positive man,[16] and another case demonstrated a friable, ulcerating, and fungating mass affecting the entire left side of the face of a 46-year-old HIV-positive man.[17] Anal, conjunctival,[18,19] nasal,[20] and gastrointestinal mucosal[21] involvement have been reported.

Oral lesions of BA are usually described as bluish purplish macules and papules. The sites of highest frequency are the palate and gingiva, followed by the buccal and labial mucosa and tongue. Some cases are ulcerated, nodular, granulomatous, exophytic,[22] or fungating masses.[23]

Histologically, the most characteristic features of BA are lobular vascular proliferations consisting of plump endothelial cells lining vessels and protruding into vascular lumina. Neutrophils and leukocytoclastic debris are characteristically found throughout the lesions. Purplish granular material representing clumps of bacilli is seen on hematoxylin and eosin staining. Warthin-Starry, Steiner, or Dieterle silver stains best reveal that these aggregates represent bacteria individually or more commonly in clumps and tangled masses.[24]

Bone involvement of BA produces isolated painful or painless lytic lesions, most commonly affecting the distal extremities, including the radius or tibia, and sometimes with overlying skin changes or soft tissue mass. Involvement of the ribs and vertebra has been reported. Radiographically osteolytic bone lesions or osteomyelitis with aggressive periosteal reaction is seen on plain films, and bone scans are always positive.[25]

Peliosis hepatis, a peculiar form of BA affecting the liver, was first described in 1990. It may present as an isolated condition or it may develop concomitantly with cutaneous and extracutaneous BA. Prior to the AIDS pandemic, peliosis hepatis (PH) was a rarity associated with chronic infection, malignant tumors, immunosuppressive agents such as azathioprine and cyclosporin, and the use of anabolic and androgenic steroids. PH presents with weight loss, fever, abdominal pain, and hepatosplenomegaly.

Elevated alkaline phosphatase with a normal or slightly elevated bilirubin and aminotransferase level are typical. Severe anemia may result as a consequence of sequestration of blood in the multiple dilated capillaries and blood filled cavernous spaces in the liver. Most cases of bacillary PH occur in HIV patients with AIDS, whereas granulomatous hepatitis is more common in immunocompetent patients. Both types of liver involvement have been reported in transplant patients.[26]

Bartonella infections in HIV-infected patients with bone lesions and subcutaneous masses are more often caused by *B. quintana*. Peliosis hepatis and lymph node lesions in HIV-infected patients are usually caused by *Bartonella henselae*.[27]

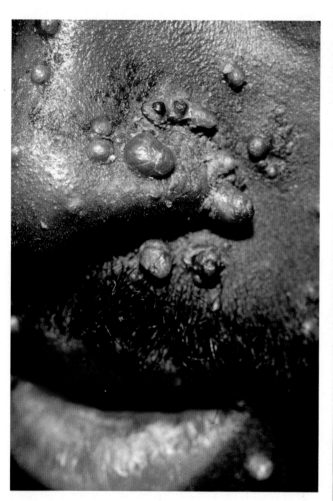

Figure 13.2. A 24-year-old homeless, HIV-positive man with pulmonary tuberculosis developed more than 100 asymptomatic 2–4 mm red-purple papules over his face and trunk of bacillary angiomatosis

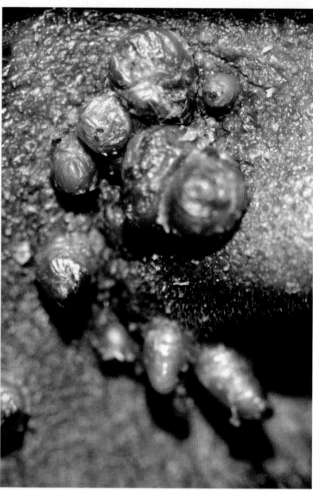

Figure 13.3. Close-up of the red accuminate and filiform papules on the alae nasi

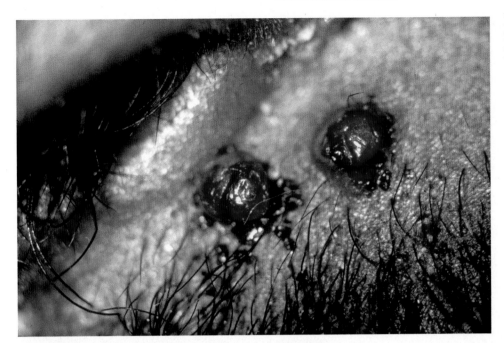

Figure 13.4. Two of the pyogenic granuloma-like papules of bacillary angiomatosis oozing because of their friability

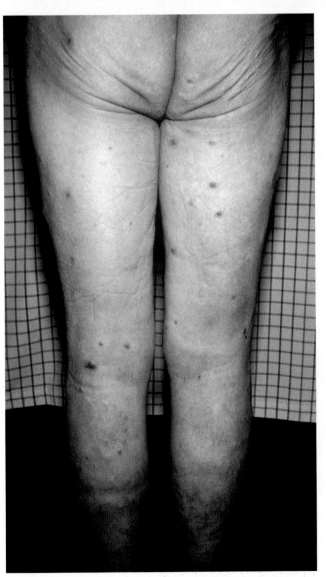

Figure 13.5. A 46-year-old HIV-positive man with multiple 3–4 mm red-purple papules over his buttocks, thighs, and legs of bacillary angiomatosis

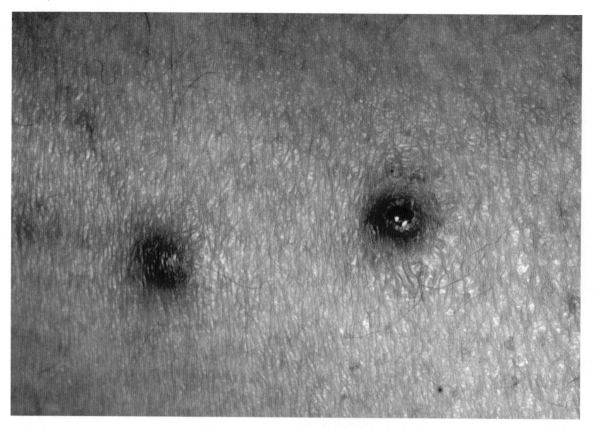

Figure 13.6.   Close-up demonstrates a bright red papule with a collarette of epidermis

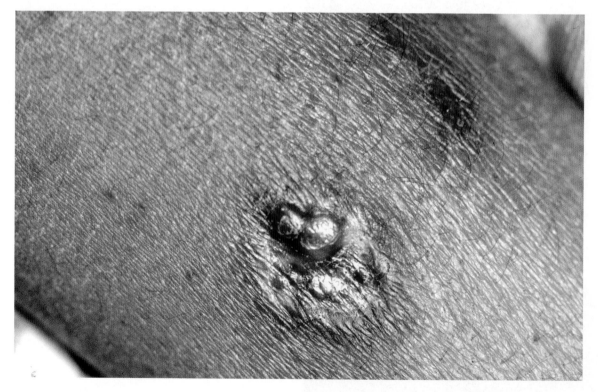

Figure 13.7.   A 37-year-old HIV-positive intravenous drug abuser suddenly developed 0.5–1 cm red-purple papules at "skin popping" scars as well as on normal skin scattered over the body

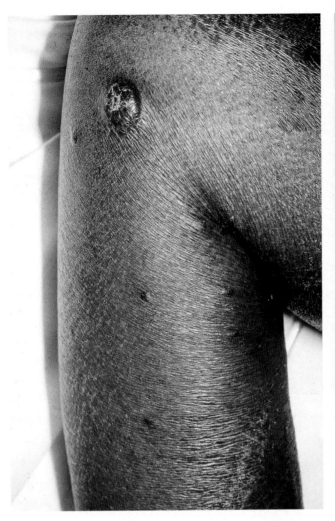

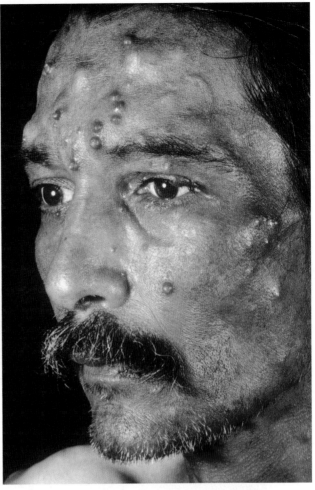

Figure 13.8. A 2-cm red nodule of bacillary angiomatosis on the extremity with smaller surrounding papules

Figure 13.9. All of the characteristic lesions of bacillary angiomatosis are seen on the face of this patient with AIDS: pyogenic granuloma-like papules, hyperpigmented indurated plaques, and subcutaneous nodules (Courtesy of Mary Ruth Buchness, M.D.)

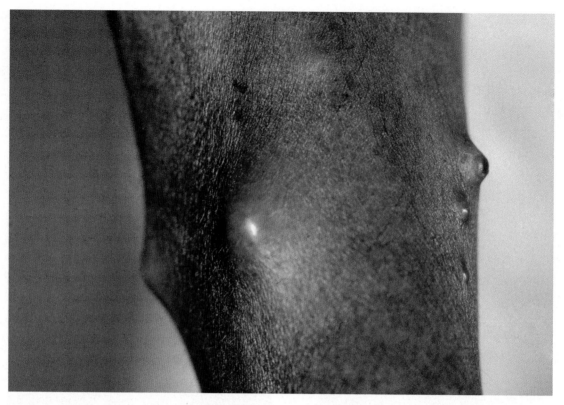

Figure 13.10. Subcutaneous dome-shaped nodules of bacillary angiomatosis on the forearm of an AIDS patient (Courtesy of Mary Ruth Buchness, M.D.)

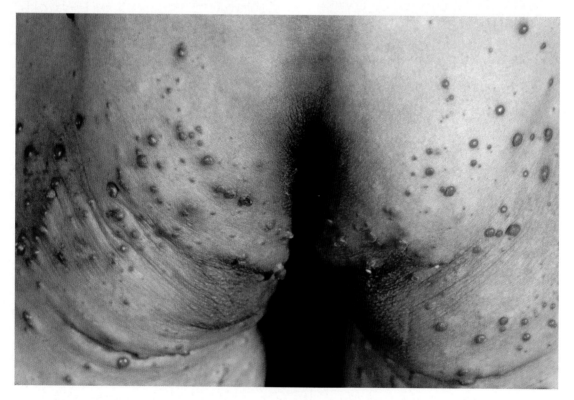

Figure 13.11. Multiple bright red, berrylike, and pedunculated papules and nodules of bacillary angiomatosis on the buttocks of an AIDS patient. The surrounding skin is normal. Several lesions have coagulated blood on their surface (Courtesy of Mary Ruth Buchness, M.D.)

CHROMOBACTERIUM VIOLACEUM

Chromobacterium violaceum is a rare but frequently fatal infection due to a morphologically and geographically distinct human pathogen. It is a common saprophytic, catalase-producing anaerobic gram-negative rod that is commonly found in soil and water in tropical and sub-tropical climates between latitudes 35° north and 35° south. Cutaneous infection is rare and usually occurs with exposure of broken or injured skin to contaminated muddy or stagnant water or soil in patients with neutrophil dysfunction or HIV infection. The presence of this frequently fatal infection has led to the new diagnosis of immunodeficiency in patients, especially young children with chronic granulomatous disease. Certain pathogenic *C. violaceum* endotoxin-producing strains are able to withstand phagocytosis by the host immune response.

Infection in the skin tends to present with cellulitis, pustules, ulcers, or abscesses accompanied by severe systemic symptoms including fevers, myalgias, and abdominal pain. A 13-year-old patient presented with violaceous plaques studded with vesicles on the forearm and scalp that grew *Chromobacterium* on tissue culture. Biopsy revealed a necrotizing leukocytoclastic vasculitis. Gram stain was negative but culture on tryptophan-enhanced media was positive with water insoluble violet pigment characteristic of *C. violaceum*. The patient was subsequently diagnosed with chronic granulomatous disease.[28] *Chromobacterium* infection can progress with the development of multiple metastatic visceral abscesses involving the liver, lung, and spleen and fulminant septic shock.

CITROBACTER

The genus *Citrobacter* belongs to the family of Enterobacteriaceae and comprises 11 species of anaerobic, motile, gram-negative bacilli. The majority of infections are associated with *C. freundii* and *C. koseri* (formerly named *C. diversus*). *Citrobacter* species traditionally considered harmless contaminants or bacteria with low virulence are now being increasingly recognized as human pathogens. The incidence of infections with *Citrobacter* is increasing in the immunocompromised population. *Citrobacter* is commonly found in water, soil, food, and occasionally as a colonizer of the human gastrointestinal tract, a location that can serve as a reservoir of infection.

Atypical cellulitis during anti-CD20 monoclonal antibody treatment of B cell-chronic lymphocytic leukemia due to *Citrobacter koseri* was reported in a febrile 60-year-old woman with "bilateral inflammatory erysipelas predominating on the right leg." The culture of the skin biopsy but not the blood was positive for *C. koseri*.[29] Typical cellulitis due to *C. braakii* in a diabetic renal transplant recipient[30] and due to *C. diversus* in a patient with multiple myeloma[31] have been reported.

Ecthyma gangrenosum-like lesions were described in an 8-month old with acute myelogenous leukemia as a 1 × 3 cm punched out ulcer on the inferior buttock. Gram stain of the skin biopsy demonstrated numerous gram-negative rods around the blood vessels. Tissue and blood cultures grew *C. freundii*.[32] A febrile neutropenic 18-year-old with acute lymphocytic leukemia developed a 7 × 10 cm hemorrhagic ulcer with central bullae and ascending lymphangitis on the right leg with a hemorrhagic pustule on the same leg and Janeway lesions on the palm. *C. freundii* was cultured from the blood and an aspirate of the right leg ulcer.[33] An 8 × 10 cm tender ecchymosis on the right shoulder of a febrile neutropenic 55-year-old woman with acute myelomonocytic leukemia developed a purple necrotic center and an erythematous indurated circumference. *Citrobacter* was cultured from the blood and an aspirate of the lesion.[34]

Enterobacter

Enterobacter cloacae, a gram-negative bacterium, can cause hemorrhagic bullae in the immunocompromised host.[35] *Enterobacter* species are found in low numbers in the gastrointestinal tract. *Enterobacter*, particularly *E. cloacae*, can cause nosocomial sepsis. Although endogenous flora may be the source of infection,

E. cloacae sepsis has been traced to contaminated medicinal, intravenous, and other hospital products. *Enterobacter* bacteremia typically occurs in debilitated or immunocompromised patients and often in the setting of an intensive care unit, systemic steroid therapy, and broad-spectrum antibiotics. The use of third-generation cephalosporins in particular has been associated with the emergence of resistant *Enterobacter* strains.

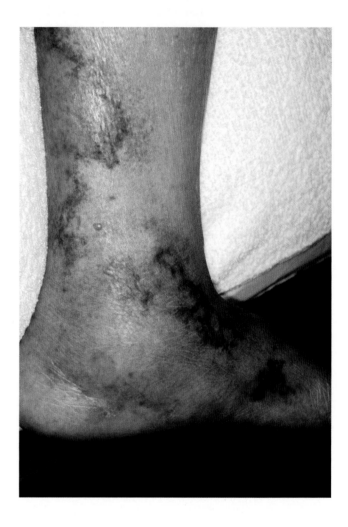

Figure 13.12.   Hemorrhagic bullae on the foot and leg of a 75-year-old patient with diverticulosis and inactive bullous pemphigoid on systemic steroids. *E. cloacae* was cultured from the bullae and blood. Diverticulosis was the likely source of the *Enterobacter* organisms

ESCHERICHIA COLI

Escherichia coli is a gram-negative aerobic non-spore forming rod. It is a normal inhabitant of the gastrointestinal tract, from where it can spread if normal anatomic barriers are interrupted as with chemotherapy for acute leukemia. *E. coli* infections of the urinary tract with or without obstruction are more common than infection of the hepatobiliary tree. *E. coli* may produce abscesses anywhere in the body. Subcutaneous infections may be found at the site of insulin injections in diabetics, in extremities with ischemic gangrene, or in surgical wounds. Perirectal phlegmon are not uncommon in leukemic patients. Ecthyma gangrenosum, considered pathognomonic for *Pseudomonas aeruginosa*, has also been described with multiple other gram-negative organisms including *E. coli*. The most common sites for ecthyma gangrenosum are the gluteal, axillary, perineal regions, and the extremities. *E. coli* ecthyma gangrenosum has been reported in patients with lung cancer undergoing chemotherapy, in a patient with multiple myeloma who developed a lesion on the lower extremity secondary to an *E. coli* urinary tract infection, and on the upper arm of a neutropenic man with acute myelogenous leukemia.[36]

Acral hemorrhagic bullae may be an early sign of *E. coli* septicemia. The bullae may be serous or hemorrhagic, on normal appearing skin or overlying a cellulitis. Fisher et al. described tense subepidermal bullae from urosepsis in a 71-year-old woman with multiple myeloma receiving chemotherapy.[37] Cultures of the urine, blood, and bullae grew *E. coli*. Hemorrhagic cellulitis on the left upper chest, shoulder, and left upper extremity developed at the site of a recently placed dialysis catheter and arteriovenous fistula with hemorrhagic bullae on the left hand in a 66-year-old with steroid dependent rheumatoid arthritis and anti-neutrophilic cytoplasmic antibody associated vasculitis. Cultures of the blood and bullae grew *E. coli*.[38] Chapman et al. described a neutropenic woman with acute granulocytic leukemia with *E. coli* urosepsis and two painful subcutaneous nodules on each leg which enlarged to 7 by 7 and 10 by 10 cm each. Over 24 h the erythema spread, became purpuric, and developed bullous centers containing *E. coli*.[39]

E. coli cellulitis in the immunocompromised host is rare and impossible to distinguish from streptococcal cellulitis. The risk factors for gram-negative cellulitis include neutropenia, diabetes mellitus, corticosteroid treatment, renal or hepatocellular insufficiency, and chronic alcohol consumption.[40,41] Rapidly progressive upper limb cellulitis in a 21-year-old with acute lymphoblastic leukemia and neutropenia from chemotherapy was stopped by amputation proximal to the infection.[42] Dreizen et al. reported a digital ulcerative cellulitis caused by *E. coli* following an accidental skin puncture in a patient with acute myelocytic leukemia.[43] Spontaneous *E. coli* cellulitis of the thigh with fever, pain, and redness developed 8 days post liver transplantation for end-stage liver disease due to hepatitis C. Numerous bullae developed at the site of the infection. Spontaneous gram-negative cellulitis has been well described in patients with hepatic cirrhosis and nephrotic syndrome that all share similar features: significant hypoalbumenemia, peripheral edema, and immunosuppression.[44]

Malakoplakia is a rare granulomatous disease most frequently seen in immunocompromised patients, many as a result of renal transplantation. It has rarely been associated with AIDS.[45] The pathogenesis of malakoplakia is unknown, but thought to represent defective bacterial killing by macrophages of common pathogens. The most common bacteria cultured from malakoplakia are gram-negative rods (*E. coli*, *Klebsiella* species and *Enterobacter* species) and gram-positive cocci (*Staphylococcus aureus* and several varieties of *Streptococcus* and *Enterococcus* species).[46] Cutaneous involvement is rare and typically perianal.[47] Cutaneous malakoplakia may present as abscesses, masses, draining sinuses, papules, nodules, or ulcerations. The diagnosis can only be made by skin biopsy that demonstrates numerous large Hansemann macrophages (packed with eosinophilic granules diastase resistant and periodic acid Schiff positive) that contain Michaelis-Gutmann bodies (MG bodies). MG bodies are intracytoplasmic basophilic ring-shaped spherules that have a targetoid center and are positive on von Kossa staining. Electron microscopic examination reveals hydroxyapatite crystals arranged in a concentric fashion. Rod-shaped bacilli can be seen on Warthin-Starry silver stain.

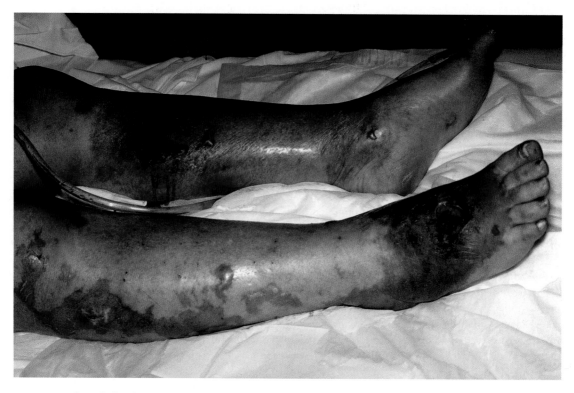

Figure 13.13.   Hemorrhagic bullae due to *Escherichia coli* from urosepsis in a 71-year-old woman with an ischemic right leg

Figure 13.14.   Patient with end-stage acquired immune deficiency syndrome (AIDS) developed purpura fulminans in the setting of *Escherichia coli* sepsis. Skin tissue culture was also positive for *E. coli*

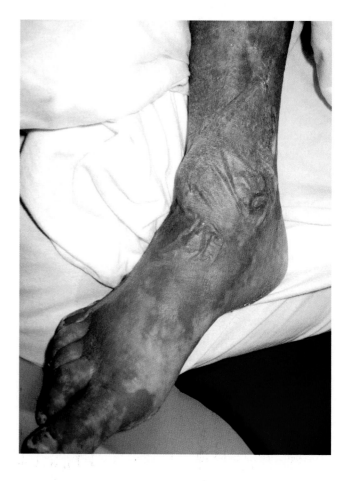

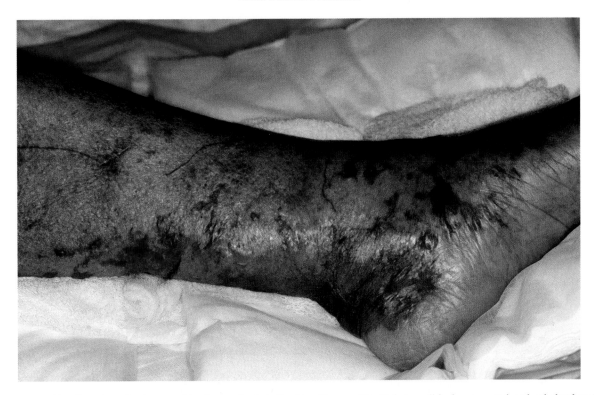

Figure 13.15. *E. coli* sepsis and culture positive hemorrhagic bullae in a 94-year-old with hairy cell leukemia, antiphosphopholipid antibody syndrome, splenomegaly, and transfusion dependent cold aggutinin hemolytic anemia despite rituximab

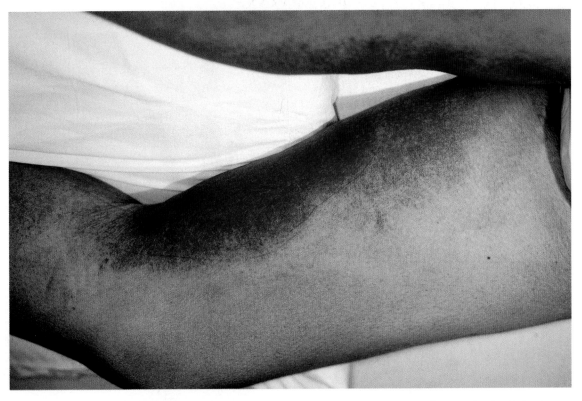

Figure 13.16. A 52-year-old with systemic lupus erythematosus and nephritis on high-dose systemic steroids, pancytopenia, and fever developed a tender purpuric thigh cellulitis. Surgical consultation and biopsy excluded necrotizing fasciitis. Blood and skin biopsy cultures grew *E. coli* before she died

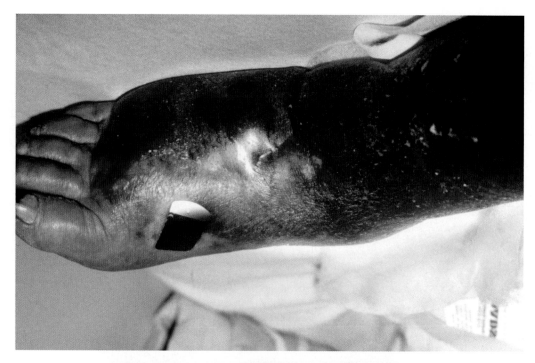

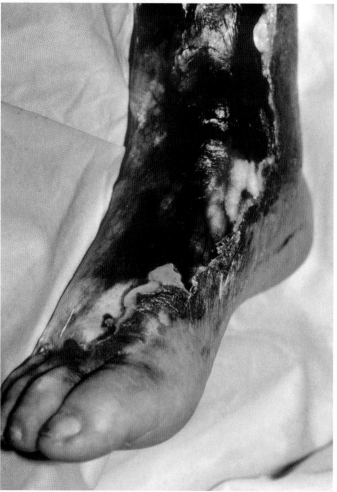

Figure 13.17. and 13.18. A 74-year-old status post orthotopic heart transplant for ischemic cardiomyopathy (status post left leg vein harvested for coronary artery bypass graft [CABG]) developed *E. coli* necrotizing bullous cellulitis of the left foot and lower leg requiring multiple debridements and skin graft procedures

HELICOBACTER CINAEDI

Helicobacter cinaedi (formerly named *Campylobacter cinaedi*) is a fastidious gram-negative spiral bacillus. It inhabits the intestinal tract of various animals including rats, hamsters, dogs, cats, foxes, wild birds, and monkeys. Hamsters in particular are known to be a common natural reservoir. Microbiologic diagnosis is difficult because *H. cinaedi* rarely grows on traditional media. The median time to detection of *H. cinaedi* on culture is 6 days and up to 10 days in some cases as opposed to 2 days for most other bacterial species. Some microbiology laboratories may not hold specimens for a sufficient period of time to allow for growth. The organism is not routinely observed on gram stain but can be detected by dark field or acridine orange staining. Together with the culturing difficulty, this may lead to under diagnosis of *H. cinaedi* infections.

Helicobacter cinaedi is an unusual opportunistic pathogen found predominantly in severely immunocompromised patients with AIDS, malignancy, or post-transplantation. The more immunocompromised the patient, the more severe the symptoms. Even though *H. cinaedi* lives in the intestinal tract, the clinical symptoms of infection include fever, rash, arthritis, leg pain, and other systemic or local symptoms rather than abdominal pain, diarrhea, and other gastrointestinal complaints.[48]

Nonspecific cutaneous manifestations of *H. cinaedi* have been reported without histopathologic examination. A recurrent diffuse erythematous macular and patchy eruption occurred in a 53-year-old with B-cell lymphoma. Each episode of fever and rash (with diarrhea the second time) was accompanied by positive blood cultures for *H. cinaedi*.[49] Tender, well-demarcated, hyperpigmented macules occurred in an afebrile patient with X-linked agammaglobulinemia and recurrent *H. cinaedi* bacteremia.[50]

The common dermatologic manifestations of *H. cinaedi* bacteremia are large, multifocal plaques of cellulitis involving the extremities with monoarticular large joint arthritis adjacent to the area of cellulitis.[51,52] In a young HIV-positive male, the presence of bilateral cellulitis (especially in the absence of chronic venous stasis dermatitis) is a rare clinical presentation and should alert the clinician to consider *H. cinaedi* infection. An area resembling superficial thrombophlebitis may be present with *H. cinaedi* bacteremia.[53] It has been suggested that endovascular infection may be a feature of *H. cinaedi* bacteremia.[54]

Immunocompromised patients with *H. cinaedi* usually require prolonged or multiple courses of antibiotics for the relapsing bacteremia. Recurrent bacteremia may be associated with recurrent skin lesions, cellulitis, or localized leg pain.[54] In cases of HIV-infected men who present with cellulitis, recurrent cellulitis, or multifocal cellulitis, especially if initial blood culture reports are negative, *H. cinaedi* infection should be considered, because of the slow growth of this organism in blood cultures.

KLEBSIELLA

Klebsiella pneumoniae are encapsulated gram-negative bacilli found among the normal flora of the mouth and intestinal tract. *Klebsiella*, a virulent respiratory pathogen, is closely related to the genera *Enterobacter* and *Serratia*. Many clinical isolates of *Klebsiella* are found in patients with complicated and obstructive urinary tract disease. In a study of hospital acquired (nosocomial) gram-negative infections, the most frequently isolated organism was *Klebsiella pneumoniae* followed by *Escherichia coli* and *Pseudomonas aeruginosa*.[55]

Klebsiella may present with acral hemorrhagic bullae in the compromised host. Pubic cellulitis with numerous ulcerations (called ecthyma gangrenosum by the authors), culture positive for *Klebsiella* in the vulvar and perianal area, developed post chemotherapy for metastatic nasopharyngeal carcinoma in a 54-year-old woman.[56] Cellulitis of the leg became increasingly painful with the appearance of bullae and progressed to necrotizing fasciitis in a 66-year-old diabetic on prednisolone and methotrexate for ankylosing spondylitis. Early surgical debridement was limb saving.[57] Nonclostridial crepitant cellulitis due to *Klebsiella* on the extremities in patients with diabetes has been reported. DiGioia et al. described fatal crepitant cellulitis with underlying myonecrosis in an alcoholic.[58] The infection was presumably metastatic from a *Klebsiella* osteomyelitis months earlier. A similar presentation of nonclostridial crepitant cellulitis due to *Klebsiella* in a diabetic following a closed fracture of the femur was described by Napgezek and Hall.[59]

Impetigo-like vegetating nasal lesions caused by *Klebsiella* developed in a 56-year-old diabetic post chemotherapy for metastatic breast cancer.[60] Noma-like gangrenous cheilitis due to *Klebsiella* in a child with cyclic neutropenia and hereditary myeloperoxidase deficiency was reported.[61]

Figure 13.19. The forearms of a 34-year-old woman with a 2-year history of metastatic malignant thymoma. She had been on systemic steroids when the skin lesions developed

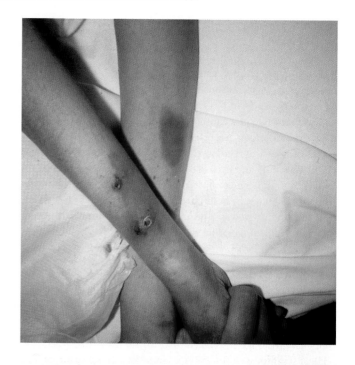

Figure 13.20. An erythematous plaque with a central hemorrhagic necrotic bullae was biopsied. Skin biopsy demonstrated vascular thrombosis with a diffuse neutrophilic infiltrate

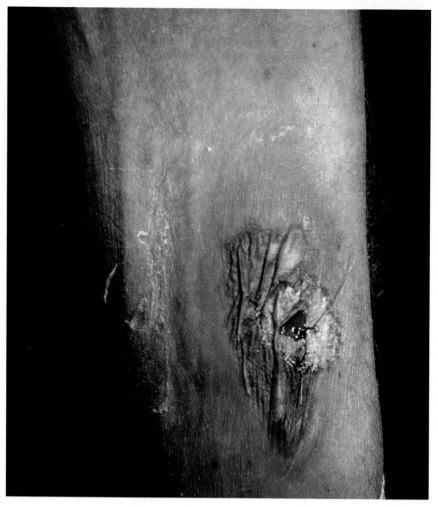

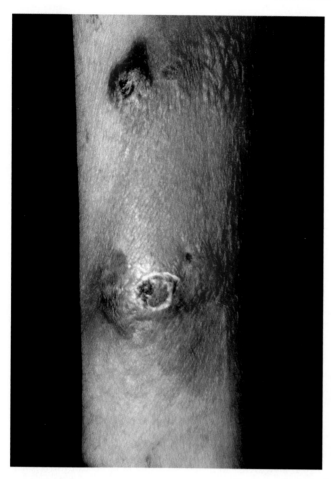

Figure 13.21. Similar hemorrhagic necrotic bullae developed on the other forearm. Blood and wound cultures grew *K. pneumoniae*. The patient died 4 days later

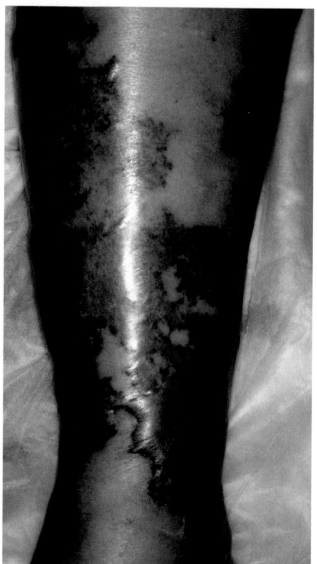

Figure 13.23. A 52-year-old on thalidomide for multiple myeloma received pulse dexamethasone. She developed diarrhea and abdominal pain due to *Strongyloides stercoralis* followed by pulmonary infiltrates, septic shock, and hemorrhagic bullae of her legs due to *Klebsiella*

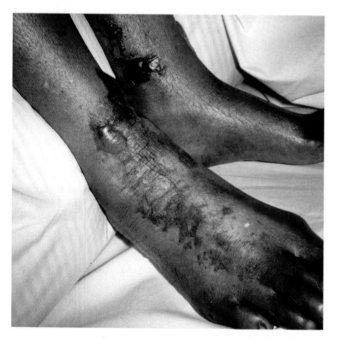

Figure 13.22. Hemorrhagic bullae on the feet of a neutropenic alcoholic due to *Klebsiella* sepsis

Legionella

Infections due to *Legionella* species have been described in numerous outbreaks and case reports since the first isolation of the gram-negative bacterium following an outbreak at a convention of veterans in Philadelphia, Pennsylvania in 1976. *Legionella* is primarily considered a pulmonary pathogen of immunocompromised patients and a rare cause of cellulitis and soft tissue infection in the compromised host. *Legionella* should be considered in the etiology of cellulitis in cases: (1) that are refractory to conventional antibiotics routinely administered for skin and soft tissue infections; (2) when routine cultures for bacteria, fungi, and mycobacteria are negative; (3) when gram stain of the purulent material demonstrates neutrophils with no organisms; or (4) when the infection relapses after weeks of antibiotic treatment. *Legionella* pneumonia is often not present with the skin infection.

There are more than 50 species of *Legionella* with multiple serogroups. The first case of *Legionella pneumophilia* cellulitis in a 66-year-old man with advanced follicular lymphoma was reported in 1993.[62] He had a rapidly spreading necrotizing cellulitis which started near the site of a thoracentesis and spread down to his thigh. He required surgical debridement. *L. pneumophilia* was cultured from the surgical specimen and confirmed by direct immunoflourescence with a monoclonal antibody to *L. pneumophilia*. A second case of *L. pneumophilia* cellulitis in a 65-year-old woman on high-dose systemic steroids for interstitial lung disease and idiopathic thrombocytopenia purpura presented on her right posterior thigh and gluteal fold.[63] A skin biopsy was culture positive and the cellulitis relapsed on her right lower extremity 2 weeks after completing a successful course of antibiotic therapy. The skin biopsy culture on buffered charcoal yeast extract agar (BCYE, the preferred growth media for clinical isolation of *Legionella*), direct immunofluorescence and a blood culture were all positive for *L. pneumophilia*. This case illustrates that relapsing *Legionella* infection can occur in the immunocompromised patient even after prolonged therapy with antimicrobials that are ordinarily curative after shorter durations of therapy.

Other *Legionella* species have been reported to cause skin and soft tissue infections in immunocompromised patients. *L. micdadei* produced cellulitis of the right calf followed by a soft tissue abscess at the right lateral malleolus in a 62-year-old woman on prednisone and cyclophosphamide for necrotizing vasculitis of the kidney.[64] A renal transplant recipient developed necrotizing cellulitis of the hand and arm due to *L. micdadei* necessitating amputation of the limb.[65] Tissue smears obtained at amputation showed acid-fast organisms confirmed by direct and indirect fluorescent antibody staining to be *L. micdadei*. *L. micdadei* is the only *Legionella* species reported to be acid-fast in tissue sections but is not acid-fast when grown in culture. *L. maceachernii* produced multiple tender fluctuant red nodules on the forearm and face with a swollen tender fifth finger in a 68-year-old woman with polymyalgia rheumatica on prednisone and methotrexate.[66] Routine cultures from the frank pus of a nodule were negative and the biopsy of the nodules demonstrated dermal

suppurative neutrophilic and granulomatous inflammation. The organism was grown on BYCE medium and confirmed to be *Legionella* by direct fluorescent antibody. Prolonged courses of antibiotics (i.e., 8 weeks) may be required to eradicate the *Legionella* soft tissue infection. A 73-year-old woman with nephrotic syndrome and IgA gammopathy of undetermined etiology had recurrent soft tissue abscesses due to *L. cinnatiensis*.[67] She subsequently developed a disseminated diffuse large B-cell lymphoma to explain the gammopathy and her susceptibility to this unusual cause of multiple routine culture negative skin abscesses. Among the scarce reports of extrapulmonary *Legionella* infection was a 66-year-old woman with chronic lymphocytic leukemia and a cellulitis with a central skin abscess due to *L. feeleii*.[68]

The source of *Legionella* species in all of these immunocompromised patients with skin and soft tissue infection was not reported. *Legionella* are found in a large variety of aquatic habitats (lakes, streams, coastal oceans), particularly warm man-made waters (water heaters, air-conditioning and cooling towers, baths, hot water plumbing systems, and recirculating water systems).

Morganella

The genera *Proteus*, *Providencia*, and *Morganella* are related members of the family Enterobacteriaceae. *Morganella morganii* (formerly *Proteus morganii*) is a gram-negative bacillus ubiquitous in the environment, found in soil, water, sewage, and as part of the normal fecal flora.

M. morganii is an infrequent cause of opportunistic nosocomial infection. Reports of *Morganella* infection in immunocompromised hosts are infrequent but include pyomyositis in a patient with AIDS and hepatic cirrhosis with positive serology for hepatitis B and C.[69] *Morganella* is a rare cause of acral hemorrhagic bullae. In the case reported by Bagel and Grossman, multiple factors predisposed the patient to *Morganella* sepsis including malignant lymphoma, chemotherapy, neutropenia, systemic steroids, multiple hospitalizations, and multiple courses of broad-spectrum antibiotics.[70] The authors observed a fatal case of cellulitis with hemorrhagic bullae due to *M. morganii* in an 81-year-old man on high-dose prednisone and chlorambucil. He had a history of myelodysplastic syndrome, refractory anemia, and a malignant lymphoma. A 60-year-old woman with poorly controlled diabetes and metastatic adenocarcinoma of the colon developed a heel ulcer followed by cellulitis of the calf. She developed hemorrhagic bullae in the swollen red leg and gas within the fascial planes of the muscles on computerized tomography followed by positive blood cultures for *Morganella morganii* and septic shock. *Morganella*, part of the normal flora of the colon in this patient with inoperable colon cancer, may have been the source of the bacteremia. *Morganella* ferments glucose with the production of gas, which in the tissues of this diabetic is the source of the non-clostridial gas gangrene.[71]

Ecthyma gangrenosum like lesions were reported in an 84-year-old with drug induced neutropenia. Skin biopsy cultures were positive and blood cultures were negative for *Morganella*.[72]

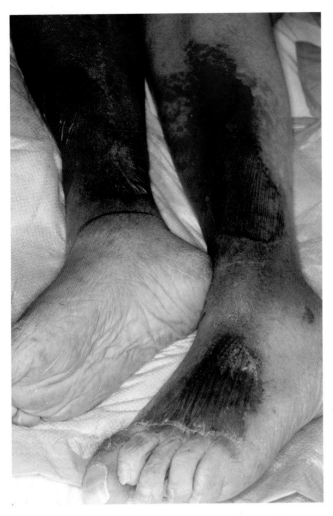

Figure 13.24. Hemorrhagic bullae on the dorsum of the left foot and on the lower legs. Gram stain of the bullae aspirate revealed gramnegative rods, and cultures from the bullae and blood grew *Morganella morganii*

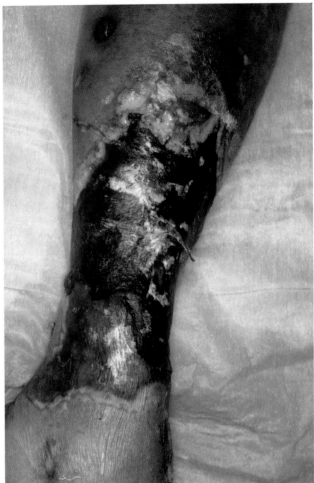

Figure 13.25. The bullae enlarged, ruptured, and developed eschars with deepening necrosis requiring debridement of both calves down to muscle. The patient died before skin grafting or amputation could be performed

PSEUDOMONAS

Pseudomonas aeruginosa is a gram-negative rod primarily encountered as a nosocomial pathogen. *Pseudomonas aeruginosa* septicemia is a common cause of bacteremia in immunocompromised patients, most often in neutropenic leukemics during chemotherapy, burn victims, and those with solid malignancies. The risk factors associated with *P. aeruginosa* infections include granulocytopenia, intravascular catheterization, intravenous drug use, cystic fibrosis, chronic ambulatory peritoneal dialysis, corticosteroid administration, hospitalization, previous antimicrobial treatment, chemotherapy, and immunosuppression associated with organ transplantation. The site of origin of the *Pseudomonas* is most commonly the respiratory or genitourinary tract. *P. aeruginosa* infection can also be acquired from any of the moist reservoirs patients come in contact with including showers, sinks, and flower vases.

The dermatologic manifestations of *Pseudomonas* sepsis include ecthyma gangrenosum, hemorrhagic bullae, gangrenous or bullous cellulitis, small papules on the trunk resembling rose spots of typhoid fever, grouped petechiae, erysipelas-like lesions with hyperesthesia,[73] erythematous or violaceous subcutaneous nodules, and necrotizing or malignant external otitis.

Ecthyma gangrenosum (EG) has classically been considered a pathognomonic sign of *Pseudomonas aeruginosa* septicemia. Multiple other gram-negative bacterial, fungal, and viral infections have been reported to cause ecthyma gangrenosum or EG-like lesions in the immunocompromised host. Most cases of ecthyma gangrenosum have been associated with septicemia, but it has also rarely been reported without bacteremia due to *Pseudomonas*.[74] Most often ecthyma gangrenosum occurs as a life-threatening septicemic infection in neutropenic leukemics. It also occurs in any kind of immunodeficiency associated with severe neutropenia, AIDS, burn patients, underlying malignancies, and in organ transplant recipients. Ecthyma gangrenosum occurs predominantly in the anogenital area, axillae, and legs as single or multiple lesions. It begins as vesicles or erythematous or purpuric macules that become edematous and evolve into necrotic vesicles or hemorrhagic bullae up to several centimeters in diameter in a matter of hours. They subsequently become painless ulcers with central gray black eschars with surrounding erythema or a red halo. The necrosis may extend as deep as muscle. Pus is minimal. Lesions at various stages of development may be present at different sites in the same patient.[75]

Pathologically, there is perivascular cuffing of organisms with infiltration of the outer layers of arterial and venous walls, relative intimal sparing, and a lack of inflammatory response. The gram-negative bacilli invade the adventitial and medial layers of the small vessel walls. This differs from other forms of bacterial vasculitis in which septic intraluminal thrombi attach to bacteria and invade the endothelium.

Ecthyma gangrenosum, usually considered a bacteremic form of *Pseudomonas* sepsis, can also be the result of primary or localized infection in the absence of bacteremia in the immunocompromised host. In contrast to the bacteremic cases of ecthyma gangrenosum, the non-bacteremic patients were more often female, had a better prognosis,[76-78] and the source may be inoculation at the site of minor trauma.

Gangrenous or necrotizing cellulitis is a progressive cellulitis in the neutropenic patient.[79,80] It begins with a tense, erythematous patch of skin without clear areas of demarcation. The area is tender. The skin becomes bullous, purpuric, or cyanotic and then develops blackened areas of necrosis and gangrene with accompanying systemic toxicity. Progressive cellulitis or the development of necrosis while the patient is on antibiotic therapy is an indication for surgical debridement. Surgery at the time when it would be maximally beneficial is often delayed because of thrombocytopenia, concern for the resultant cosmetic defect and the need for reconstruction, and the uncertainty about the extent of the soft tissue infection. The course is often fulminant, and surgical intervention is often delayed until it is too late and overwhelming sepsis occurs. When clinical improvement occurs, it is associated with increasing neutrophil counts or a change in the status of the malignancy.

Pseudomonas can also cause necrotizing gangrene in neutropenic leukemics in the absence of septicemia. Progression from edema, erythema, and hemorrhagic bullae to finally necrosis of the nose, paranasal area, and vulva with tissue loss has occurred in acute leukemia.[81] Cutaneous nasal necrosis with palatal ulceration can develop in *Pseudomonas* bacteremia in immunologically and nutritionally compromised infants. Massive facial necrosis with systemic *Pseudomonas* infection has been reported with concomitant systemic lupus erythematosus.

Subcutaneous nodules are encountered less frequently than bullae in *Pseudomonas* bacteremia. The subcutaneous nodules may be the only manifestation of *Pseudomonas* septicemia or may be accompanied by characteristic lesions of *Pseudomonas* including ecthyma gangrenosum and hemorrhagic bullae. Unlike ecthyma gangrenosum, which occurs most frequently in the anogenital and axillary regions, bullae and subcutaneous nodules are distributed widely over the skin. A solitary subcutaneous nodule as a manifestation of *Pseudomonas* sepsis was described in a heart transplant recipient with *P. aeruginosa* maxillary sinusitis.[82] Clinically, the lesions are tender, erythematous, fluctuant or nonfluctuant nodules.[83] The absence of fluctuation may be due to the lack of pus seen with chemotherapy-induced neutropenia, but more often is due to the deep location of the abscess. Some nodules resolve with appropriate intravenous antibiotic therapy alone. Other nodules require incision and drainage. Surgical intervention is indicated when fever, toxicity, or subcutaneous nodules persist despite antibiotic therapy.[84] Deep persistence of viable organisms in the subcutaneous pseudomonal nodules of a neutropenic patient or the patient who becomes neutropenic again with another course of chemotherapy may require a prolonged course of antibiotics to eradicate the infection.

Malignant or invasive otitis externa which occurs predominantly in elderly diabetics has been reported in patients with HIV disease.[85]

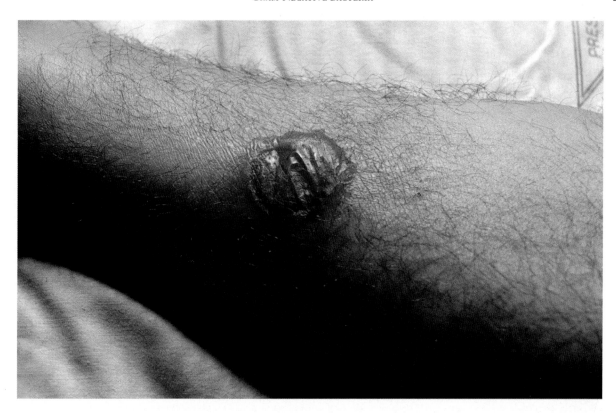

Figure 13.26. *Pseudomonas* ecthyma gangrenosum

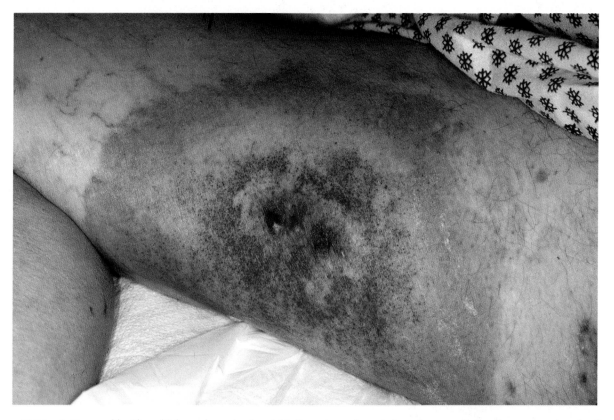

Figure 13.27. A 69-year-old with multiple myeloma developed febrile neutropenia post chemotherapy with *Pseudomonas* sepsis and ecthyma gangrenosum on the medial thigh. Blood and skin cultures grew *Pseudomonas*

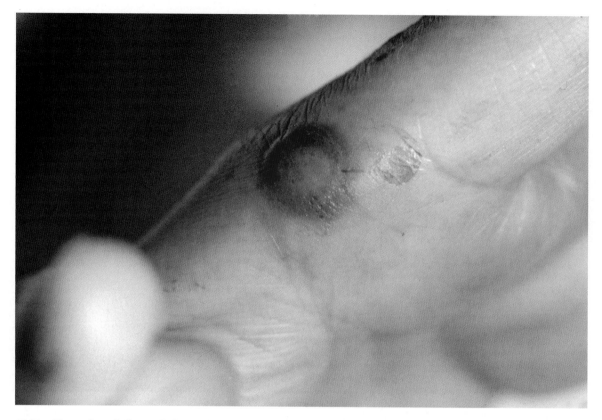

Figure 13.28.   Hemorrhagic bullae on the hand of woman with *Pseudomonas* sepsis and cancer

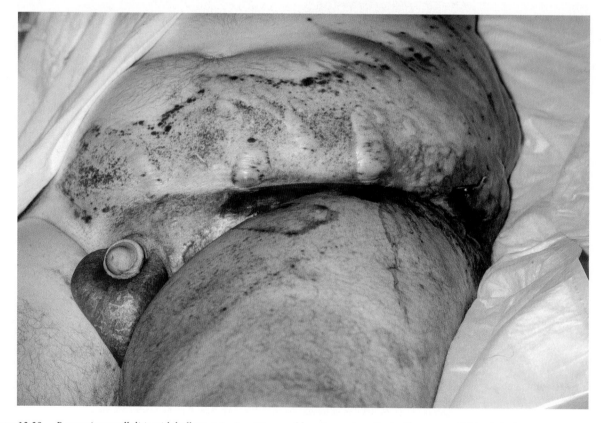

Figure 13.29.   *P. aeruginosa* cellulitis with bullous striae in a 17-year-old neutropenic patient with acute myeloblastic leukemia

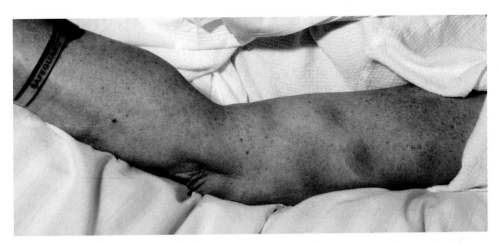

Figure 13.30.–13.32. Approximately 60 nontender, nonfluctuant, red-hot, subcutaneous nodules on the proximal arms, legs, and face of a febrile 56-year-old woman with ovarian adenocarcinoma during chemotherapy. *P. aeruginosa* was cultured from blood, urine, and skin biopsy (suppurative panniculitis)

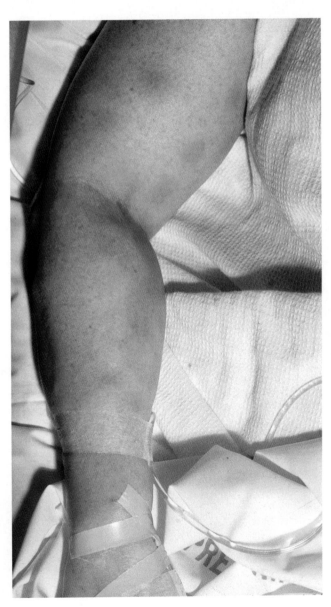

Figure 13.31.

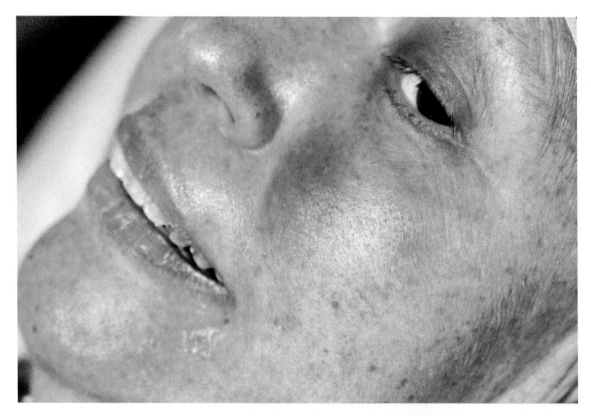

Figure 13.32.

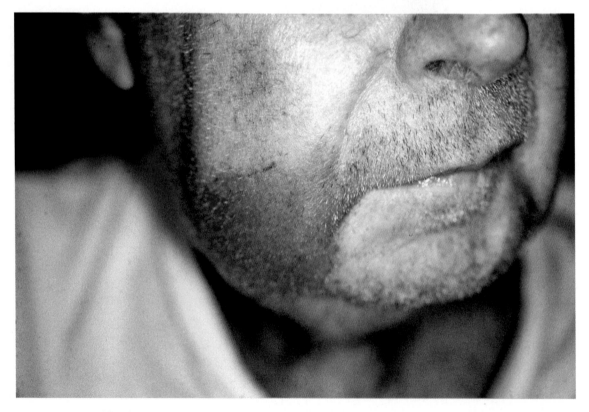

Figure 13.33. A 73-year-old with acute myelogenous leukemia (AML) developed febrile neutropenia post chemotherapy with *Pseudomonas aeruginosa* bacteremia and facial cellulitis. Computed axial tomography (CAT) scan of the face, head, and neck was normal

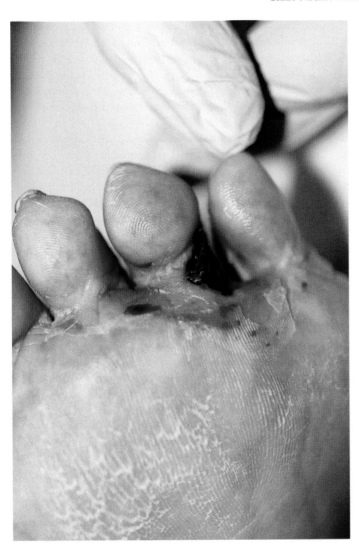

Figure 13.34. A 75-year-old woman with a history of high-grade myelodysplastic syndrome versus evolving AML who developed hemorrhagic bullae which ulcerated with necrotic eschars on her feet and axillae following chemotherapy. Cultures of the ulcerations were positive for *Pseudomonas aeruginosa* (Courtesy of Alexis Young, M.D.)

Salmonella

Salmonella species are gram-negative bacilli belonging to the family Enterobacteriaceae. Non-typhoidal *Salmonella* is increasingly recognized as an invasive pathogen in the immunocompromised host. Patients with hematological malignancy, advanced or disseminated solid cancer, renal transplantation, HIV infection, systemic lupus erythematosus, chronic granulomatous disease, and those receiving long-term corticosteroids, immunosuppressive medication, and tumor necrosis factor inhibitors are at greatest risk of invasive *Salmonella* infection.[86] Extra-intestinal infections such as bacteremia, infectious endarteritis (mycotic abdominal aortic aneurysm), subcutaneous abscess, hemorrhagic cellulitis, or necrotizing fasciitis develop mainly in the immunocompromised host.[87] *Salmonella* bacteremia in the absence of gastrointestinal infection or diarrhea is a useful marker for underlying immunosuppression and high mortality.[88]

Cutaneous manifestations of *Salmonella* infection in the immunocompromised host are rare. Zoonotic transmission of *Salmonella* from reptiles or amphibians (including turtles, iguanas, lizards, and snakes) represents a risk factor to the immunocompromised patient as it did for a 12-year-old receiving chemotherapy for an unresectable glioma. He developed a soft tissue infection, without gastroenteritis, from his pet turtle.[89] Necrotizing fasciitis due to *Salmonella* has been rarely reported. Necrotizing fasciitis developed after a diarrheal illness in a 57-year-old woman status post peripheral blood stem cell transplantation for multiple myeloma on high doses of thalidomide and dexamethasone[90] and in a patient with multiple myeloma after receiving bortezomib.[91] Both cases cultured *S. enteritidis*. A 19-year-old Arab woman with systemic lupus erythematosus on chronic corticosteroids living in Israel presented with painful swelling of both legs due to multiple gas-forming *Salmonella enteritidis* leg abscesses and osteomyelitis mimicking deep vein thrombosis.[92] Hemorrhagic bullae and bacteremia due to *Salmonella enteritidis typhimurium* developed in a 16-year-old girl on chronic corticosteroids for systemic lupus erythematosus. The bullae progressed to necrosis and abscess formation which did not heal by the time she died 2 weeks later of cryptococcal pneumonia.[93]

Serratia

Serratia marcescens is an aerobic gram-negative bacillus closely related to *Enterobacter* and *Klebsiella*. The organism is widespread in the environment. The organism can survive under harsh conditions and is often a contaminant in a variety of disinfectants, cleansing and irrigating solutions, respirators, and catheters, some of which have been the sources of outbreaks. It colonizes the respiratory tracts and urinary tracts of hospitalized patients. *Serratia* can cause a variety of nosocomial infections. Multi-drug resistant strains are reported with increasing frequency in hospitals.

Serratia is recognized as an opportunistic pathogen in the immunocompromised host. It has a particular association with injection drug users. Multiple cases of *Serratia* cellulitis have been reported. The infection typically begins in a benign fashion with ill-defined erythema, edema, warmth, and tenderness but rapidly progresses with toxicity, bullae, necrosis, and sometimes crepitance.[94] Bullous cellulitis progressed to necrotizing fasciitis in a 40-year-old with systemic lupus erythematosus on systemic steroids and peritoneal dialysis. The *Serratia* cellulitis started from a skin biopsy of leukocytoclastic vasculitis involving the lower legs and feet.[95] Necrotizing fasciitis due to *Serratia marcescens* has also been reported in a 49-year-old diabetic with metastatic small cell lung cancer following chemotherapy[96] and in a 73-year-old with minimal change nephropathy on systemic steroids.[95] Sudden appearing painful nodules and abscesses on the lower extremities with multiple violet bordered ulcers due to *Serratia* occurred in a 73-year-old with chronic obstructive pulmonary disease in the setting of chronic steroid use and venous insufficiency.[97]

Serratia is a significant cause of infection in older children and adults with chronic granulomatous disease (CGD).[98] The infections have a different pattern than infants. Skin infections form large poorly healing ulcers and frequently occur with metastatic spread of infection to multiple sites. In four cases of neutropenic leukemics with *Serratia* sepsis, cutaneous findings included a metastatic thigh abscess in one patient and diffuse edematous facial swelling in three patients.[99] Rapid onset facial swelling with a necrotizing forehead ulceration, culture positive for *Serratia marcescens*, developed in a healthy 31-year-old who developed drug induced agranulocytosis.[100]

In an HIV-infected 33-year-old, asymptomatic, disseminated skin-colored papules, more prevalent on the trunk with scarce pustules, were reported. Skin biopsies and cultures confirmed *Serratia marcescens* perifolliculitis.[101]

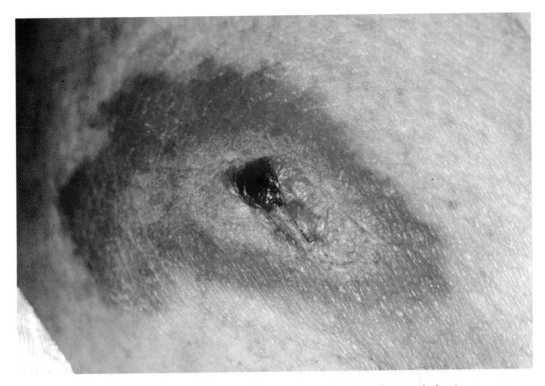

Figure 13.35. Ecthyma gangrenosum due to *Serratia* near the axilla in a patient with acute myelogenous leukemia

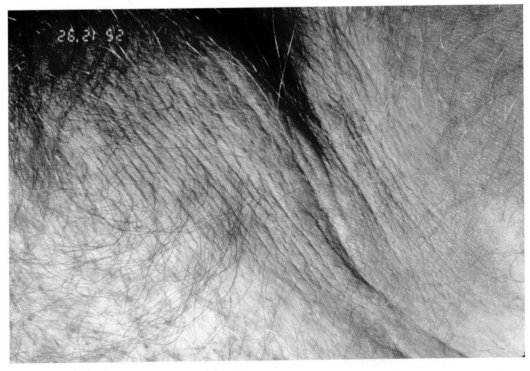

Figure 13.36.–13.38. A 53-year-old with acute myelogenous leukemia developed fever, neutropenia, and a tender axillary rash after induction chemotherapy. Figure 13.36 shows an 8×15 cm edematous, erythematous, exquisitely tender plaque in the right axilla. Figure 13.37 shows several firm subcutaneous nodules that were present within the area of cellulitis and in the opposite axilla. Skin biopsies demonstrated cellulitis with extensive eccrine gland necrosis without surrounding neutrophilic infiltrate. Tissue culture revealed *S. marcescens* resistant to multiple antibiotics. Figure 13.38 shows that, despite antibiotics and a rising white blood cell count, the patient developed extensive cutaneous necrosis of the entire right axilla. It healed by secondary intention (Courtesy of FC Fehl, III, M.D.)

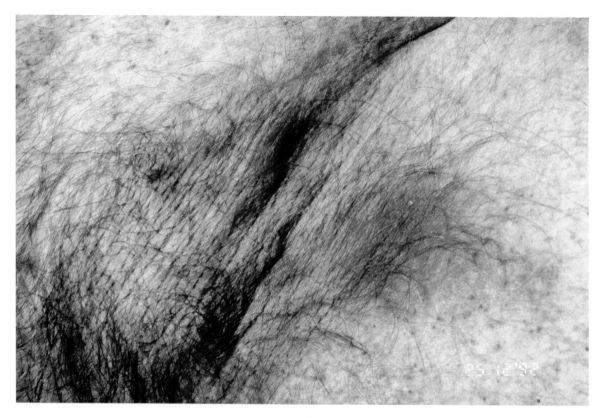

Figure 13.37.

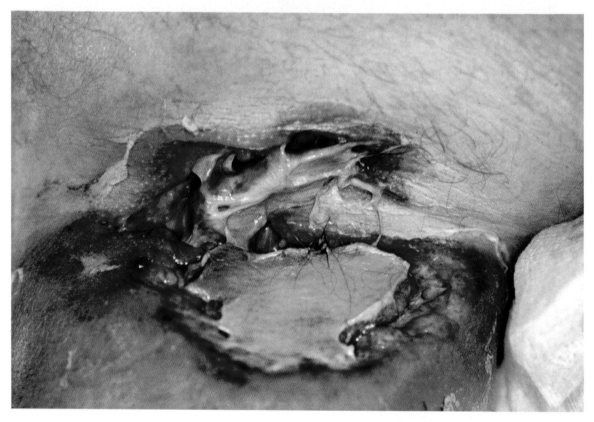

Figure 13.38.

STENOTROPHOMONAS

Stenotrophomonas maltophilia (SM) is the only recognized species in this new genus, originally included in the genus *Pseudomonas* and then *Xanthomonas*. SM is a nosocomial gram-negative bacillus found in aquatic environments, with a significant mortality rate in the immunocompromised host. It frequently colonizes fluids used in the hospital setting including nebulizers, water baths, intravenous fluids, tap water faucets,[102] oxygen humidifier water reservoirs, and dialysis machines. The majority of infections occur in patients with malignancy after prolonged hospitalizations particularly in the intensive care unit, following mechanical ventilation or in patients with tracheostomies, and after exposure to broad-spectrum antimicrobial agents (particularly beta-lactams, carbapenems, and fluoroquinolones) due to the organisms' intrinsic resistance to these agents which results in overgrowth and facilitates superinfection with SM.[103] Other risk factors for infection with this emerging opportunistic pathogen include leukemia, lymphoma, prolonged neutropenia, mucositis due to chemotherapy, radiation or graft versus host disease, diarrhea,[103] or a central venous catheter.

Mucocutaneous and soft tissue infections due to SM are becoming recognized more frequently. Skin manifestations include primary cellulitis, metastatic nodules or cellulitis, gangrenous cellulitis, soft tissue necrosis, ecthyma gangrenosum, and infected mucocutaneous ulcers.[104]

SM can cause metastatic nodules that mimic disseminated fungal infection. The lesions are warm, firm, nonfluctuant tender, well-demarcated or poorly delineated skin or subcutaneous nodules with overlying redness or violaceous erythema.[105-108] They involve the extremities, scalp, back, and abdomen. The lesions increase in size and number over days.[109] The nodules may have surrounding cellulitis or tender areas of cellulitis in areas distant from the nodules. Two cases with central black necrosis and two cases of ulceration of the nodules have been reported.[109] Skin biopsy of a nodule usually demonstrates the gram-negative rods and is culture positive for SM.

Vartivarian reported five cases of cellulitis associated with catheter use. All had tender cellulitis without clear demarcation of the borders. None had leukemia and none had received prior antibiotics.[109] One patient had cellulitis surrounding a neck mass (lymphoma) and the other four patients had exudative lesions at the catheter insertion sites.[109] SM cellulitis of the left arm developed in a febrile 47-year-old with relapsed acute myelogenous leukemia (AML), neutropenic from chemotherapy on broad-spectrum antibiotics. Cultures of blood and skin biopsy grew SM and the cellulitis resolved with trimethoprim-sulfamethoxazole.[110]

The mucocutaneous lesions of SM are infected ulcers of the gingiva, lip, and buccal mucosa. Son reported rapid, progressive, severe edematous, erythematous necrotic plaques with bulla formation around the lips in a 47-year-old with AML as ecthyma gangrenosum.[111] Blood and tissue cultures revealed SM, resistant to the antibiotics he had been treated with before his demise.

Ecthyma gangrenosum may be a rare cutaneous complication of SM bacteremia.[112] Fatal gangrenous cellulitis started as tender erythema around a Hickman type central venous catheter on the chest wall of a neutropenic 29-year-old with aplastic anemia. The skin and soft tissue infection of the chest wall spread despite removal of the catheter. SM was traced to the tap water faucets in the patient's room.[102] Perineal gangrenous cellulitis with bullae developed in a 31-year-old neutropenic leukemic following chemotherapy. SM was cultured from the bullae and the blood.[113]

Figure 13.39. A 65-year-old man with stage III-A Hodgkin's disease, febrile, pancytopenic from chemotherapy, on broad-spectrum antibiotics, developed a 10-cm erythematous nonfluctuant deep plaque on the hip. Blood and skin biopsy of the phlegmon cultured *Stenotrophomonas maltophilia*

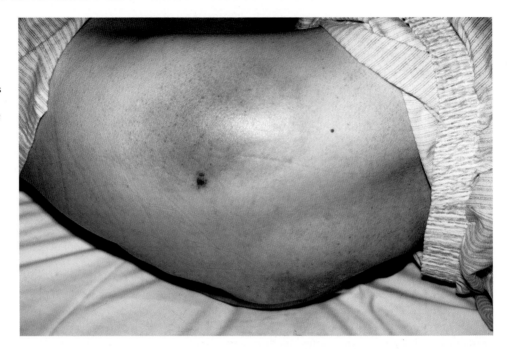

Figure 13.40. A 31-year-old woman febrile and pancytopenic after chemotherapy for acute myelogenous leukemia developed a rapidly spreading cellulitis on the right flank, buttocks, and perineum after 12 days of broad-spectrum antibiotics. Two bullae developed at the center of the lesion. Culture of the blister fluid and blood yielded *Stenotrophomonas maltophilia*. Necrotic lesions developed at the sites of the bullae (Courtesy of Selim Aractingi, M.D. From Phalm et al.[113] Copyright 1992, American Medical Association)

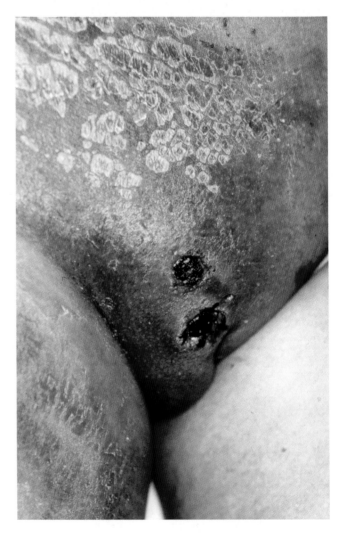

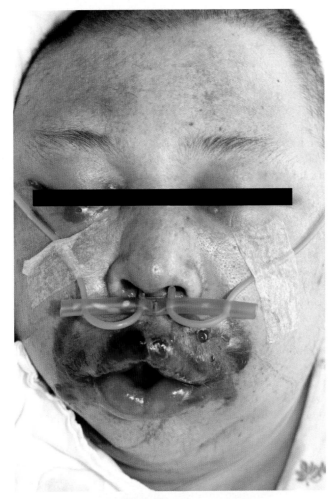

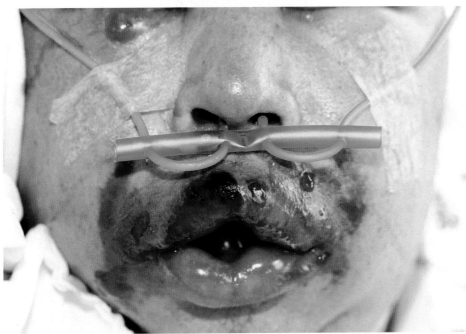

Figure 13.41. and 13.42. A 47-year-old man with acute myelogenous leukemia 10 days status post allogeneic bone marrow transplant developed erythematous, necrotic, hemorrhagic bullae around the lips and below the eye. Blood and tissue cultures grew *Stenotrophomonas maltophilia* (Courtesy of Joo Young Roh, M.D.)

Vibrio

Vibrio vulnificus is a gram-negative halophilic (salt-loving or salt-requiring) bacillus found in sea water worldwide, especially warm brackish seas in summer months. *V. vulnificus*, an opportunistic pathogen that causes serious life threatening infection, is classified into a primary septicemia (more common) and a wound infection (less common) type. Vulnificus, Latin for "wounding" is an appropriate name for this vibrio which may cause extensive soft tissue destruction.

Other marine halophilic vibrios (including *V. alginolyticus*, *V. damsela* [*Photobacterium damsela*], and *V. parahaemolyticus*)[114] can cause similar soft tissue infections or septicemias. *V. vulnificus* is the most common of these species involved.

V. vulnificus is capable of causing severe wound infection by direct penetration or injury in a marine environment or from exposure of pre-existing wounds to sea water or during seafood handling (fins of tilapia, St. Peter's fish). The wound infections begin within 4 h to 4 days after contact with sea water. Most patients develop edema, cellulitis, and bullae at the wound site followed by fever, chills, hypotension, and necrotizing fasciitis requiring debridement. Infections can mimic gas gangrene in their rapidity and destructiveness.

The primary septicemic type occurs in immunocompromised patients with underlying liver disease (including hemochromatosis and other syndromes involving chronic iron overload, alcoholic, and other causes of cirrhosis), hematologic disease, and other disorders associated with immunosuppression (AIDS,[115] immunosuppressive medications, long-term steroid use, organ transplantation,[116] malignancy, and lymphoma[117]). These compromised patients acquire the organism through the gastrointestinal tract, without causing gastrointestinal symptoms, after recent consumption of raw seafood (particularly oysters, mussels, clams, and whole scallops, filter feeders in which the organism is concentrated; crabs, eels, mullet, and sea bass) or inadequately cooked shellfish from seawater close to estuaries. Bacteremia in the susceptible immunocompromised host occurs during the summer months following the ingestion of raw molluscan shellfish. The clinical course of infection is characterized by abrupt onset of fever and chills without any apparent source of sepsis, bullous skin lesions, hypotension, and shock. The skin lesions are distinctive and rapidly progressive. They start as edematous, erythematous, or ecchymotic areas that evolve to vesicles or large hemorrhagic bullae on the extremities or trunk. Necrotic ulcers develop that extend to fascia and cause extensive soft tissue destruction and gangrene. New lesions may develop while the patient is on antibiotics.[118] Other metastatic or secondary cutaneous lesions from *Vibrio* bacteremia include cellulitis, edema, hemorrhagic bullae, and severe pain associated with purpura but without inflammatory signs of erythema or heat.[119]

The prognosis for *V. vulnificus* septicemia is very poor with a mortality greater than 50%. Therefore early diagnosis and urgent aggressive treatment are important. The differential diagnosis includes other cutaneous and soft tissue infections such as necrotizing fasciitis due to group A streptococci. High serum creatine phosphokinase (CPK) levels are useful in the diagnosis of these two bacterial infections.[120] These infections can have a fulminant course resulting in death within 24–48 h after hospital admission. Some *Vibrio* infections progressed rapidly to death, before clinicians could initiate surgical interventions.[121]

REFERENCES

Aeromonas

1. Ko WC, Chuang YC. Aeromonas bacteremia: review of 59 episodes. Clin Infect Dis. 1995;20(5):1298–304.
2. Francis YF, Richman S, Hussain S, Schwartz J. Aeromonas hydrophila infection: ecthyma gangrenosum with aplastic anemia. N Y State J Med. 1982;82(10):1461–4.
3. Wolff RL, Wiseman SL, Kitchens CS. Aeromonas hydrophila bacteremia in ambulatory immunocompromised hosts. Am J Med. 1980;68(2):238–42.
4. Cui H, Hao S, Arous E. A distinct cause of necrotizing fasciitis: Aeromonas veronii biovar sobria. Surg Infect (Larchmt). 2007;8(5):523–8.

Bartonella

5. Maguiña C, Guerra H, Ventosilla P. Bartonellosis. Clin Dermatol. 2009;27(3):271–80.
6. Stoler MH, Bonfiglio TA, Steigbigel RT, Pereira M. An atypical subcutaneous infection associated with acquired immune deficiency syndrome. Am J Clin Pathol. 1983;80(5):714–8.
7. Cockerell CJ, Whitlow MA, Webster GF, Friedman-Kien AE. Epithelioid angiomatosis: a distinct vascular disorder in patients with the acquired immunodeficiency syndrome or AIDS-related complex. Lancet. 1987;2(8560):654–6.
8. LeBoit PH, Berger TG, Egbert BM, et al. Epithelioid haemangioma-like vascular proliferation in AIDS manifestation of cat scratch disease bacillus infection. Lancet. 1988;1(8592):960–3.
9. Knobler EH, Silvers DN, Fine KC, Lefkowitch JH, Grossman ME. Unique vascular skin lesions associated with human immunodeficiency virus. JAMA. 1988;260(4):524–7.
10. Petersen K, Earhart KC, Wallace MR. Bacillary angiomatosis in a patient with chronic lymphocytic leukemia. Infection. 2008;36:480–4.
11. Whitfeld MJ, Kaveh S, Koehler JE, Mead P, Berger TG. Bacillary angiomatosis associated with myositis in a patient infected with human immunodeficiency virus. Clin Infect Dis. 1997;24(4):562–4.
12. Husain S, Singh N. Pyomyositis associated with bacillary angiomatosis in a patient with HIV infection. Infection. 2002;30:50–3.
13. Chian CA, Arrese JE, Piérard GE. Skin manifestations of Bartonella infections. Int J Dermatol. 2002;41(8):461–6.
14. Spach DH. Bacillary angiomatosis. Int J Dermatol. 1992;31(1):19–24.
15. Manders SM. Bacillary angiomatosis. Clin Dermatol. 1996;14:295–9.
16. Fagan WA, DeCamp NC, Kraus EW, Pulitzer DR. Widespread cutaneous bacillary angiomatosis and a large fungating mass in an HIV-positive man. J Am Acad Dermatol. 1996;35:285–7.
17. Kiss A, Moodley M, Sheldon J, Tun M. Misdiagnosed bacillary angiomatosis. S Afr Med J. 2007;97:1050.
18. Edmonson BC, Morris WR, Osborn FD. Bacillary angiomatosis with cytomegaloviral and mycobacterial infections of the palpebral conjunctiva in a patient with AIDS. Ophthal Plast Reconstr Surg. 2004;20(2):168–70.
19. Tsai PS, DeAngelis DD, Spencer WH, Seiff SR. Bacillary angiomatosis of the anterior orbit, eyelid and conjunctiva. Am J Ophthal. 2002;134:433–5.
20. Vickery CL, Dempewolf S, Porubsky ES, Faulk CT. Bacillary angiomatosis presenting as a nasal mass epistaxis. Otolaryngol Head Neck Surg. 1996;114:443–6.
21. Chang AD, Drachenberg CI, James SP. Bacillary angiomatosis associated with extensive esophageal polyposis: a new mucocutaneous manifestation of acquired immunodeficiency disease (AIDS). Am J Gastroenterol. 1996;91(10):2220–3.
22. López de Blanc S, Sambuelli R, Femopase F, et al. Bacillary angiomatosis affecting the oral cavity. Report of two cases and review. J Oral Pathol Med. 2000;29(2):91–6.
23. Julian RS, Dierks EJ, McMunn III W. Fungating mass of the anterior maxilla. J Oral Maxillofac Surg. 1999;57:1449–54.
24. Karem KL, Paddock CD, Regnery RL. Bartonella henselae, B. quintana, and B. bacilliformis: historical pathogens of emerging significance. Microbes Infect. 2000;2(10):1193–205.
25. Bruckert F, de Kerviler E, Zagdanski AM, et al. Sternal abscess due to Bartonella (Rochalimaea) henselae in a renal transplant patient. Skeletal Radiol. 1997;26(7):431–3.
26. Bonatti H, Mendez J, Guerrero I, et al. Disseminated Bartonella infection following liver transplantation. Transplant Int. 2006;19(8):683–7.
27. Koehler JE, Sanchez MA, Garrido CS, et al. Molecular epidemiology of Bartonella infection sin patients with bacillary angimatosis-peliosis. N Engl J Med. 1997;337(26):1876–83.

Chromobacterium violaceum

28. Brown KL, Stein A, Morrell DS. Ecthyma gangrenosum and septic shock syndrome secondary to Chromobacterium violaceum. J Am Acad Dermatol. 2006;54(5 Suppl):S224–8.

Citrobacter

29. Kluger N, Cartron G, Bessis D, Guillot B, Girard C. Citrobacter koseri cellulitis during anti-CD20 monoclonal antibody (ofatumumab) treatment for B-cell chronic lymphocytic leukaemia. Acta Derm Venereol. 2010;90(1):99–100.
30. Gupta R, Rauf SJ, Singh S, Smith J, Agraharkar ML. Sepsis in a renal transplant recipient due to Citrobacter braakii. South Med J. 2003;96(8):796–8.
31. Bishara J, Gabay B, Samra Z, Hodak E, Pitlik S. Cellulitis caused by Citrobacter diversus in a patient with multiple myeloma. Cutis. 1998;61(3):158–9.
32. Reich HL, Williams Fadeyi D, Naik NS, Honig PJ, Yan AC. Nonpseudomonal ecthyma gangrenosum. J Am Acad Dermatol. 2004;50(5 Suppl):S114–7.
33. Schlossberg D, Ricci JA, Fugate JS. Dermatologic manifestations of citrobacter septicemia. J Am Acad Dermatol. 1981;5(5):613–5.
34. Grant MD, Horowitz HI, Lorian V. Gangrenous ulcer and septicemia due to citrobacter. N Engl J Med. 1969;280(23):1286–7.

Enterobacter

35. Livingston W, Grossman ME, Garvey G. Hemorrhagic bullae in association with Enterobacter cloacae septicemia. J Am Acad Dermatol. 1992;27:637–8.

Escherichia coli

36. Patel JK, Perez OA, Viera MH, Halem M, Berman B. Ecthyma gangrenosum caused by Escherichia coli bacteremia: a case report and review of the literature. Cutis. 2009;84(5):261–7.
37. Fisher K, Berger BW, Keusch GT. Subepidermal bullae secondary to Escherichia coli septicemia. Arch Dermatol. 1974;110(1):105–6.
38. Hansen EA, Cunha BA. Escherichia coli chest-wall hemorrhagic cellulitis associated with central-line placement. Heart Lung. 2000;29(6):450–2.
39. Chapman RA, Van Slyck EJ, Madhavan T. Skin lesions associated with E. coli sepsis in a patient with acute leukemia. Henry Ford Hosp Med J. 1980;28(1):47–8.
40. Castanet J, Lacour JP, Perrin C, et al. Escherichia coli cellulitis: two cases. Acta Derm Venereol. 1992;72(4):310–1.
41. Yoon TY, Jung SK, Chang SH. Cellulitis due to Escherichia coli in three immunocompromised subjects. Br J Dermatol. 1998;139(5):885–8.
42. Brzozowski D, Ross DC. Upper limb Escherichia coli cellulitis in the immunocompromised. J Hand Surg Br. 1997;22(5):679–80.
43. Dreizen S, McCredie KB, Bodey GP, Keating MJ. Unusual mucocutaneous infections in immunosuppressed patients with leukemia–expansion of an earlier study. Postgrad Med. 1986;79(4):287–94.

44. Paterson DL, Gruttadauria S, Lauro A, Scott V, Marino IR. Spontaneous gram-negative cellulitis in a liver transplant recipient. Infection. 2001;29(6):345–7.

45. Barnard M, Chalvardjian A. Cutaneous malakoplakia in a patient with acquired immunodeficiency syndrome (AIDS). Am J Dermatopathol. 1998;20(2):185–8.

46. Wittenberg PG, Douglass MC, Azam M, et al. Cutaneous malacoplakia in a patient with the acquired immunodeficiency syndrome. Arch Dermatol. 1998;134(2):244–5.

47. Palou J, Torras H, Baradad M, et al. Cutaneous malakoplakia. Report of a case. Dermatologica. 1988;176(6):288–92.

Helicobacter cinaedi

48. Minauchi K, Takahashi S, Sakai T, et al. The nosocomial transmission of Helicobacter cinaedi infections in immunocompromised patients. Intern Med. 2010;49(16):1733–9. Epub 2010 Aug 13.

49. Uçkay I, Garbino J, Dietrich PY, et al. Recurrent bacteremia with Helicobacter cinaedi: case report and review of the literature. BMC Infect Dis. 2006;6:86.

50. Simons E, Spacek LA, Lederman HM, Winkelstein JA. Helicobacter cinaedi bacteremia presenting as macules in an afebrile patient with X-linked agammaglobulinemia. Infection. 2004;32(6):367–8.

51. Sullivan AK, Nelson MR, Walsh J, Gazzard BG. Recurrent Helicobacter cinaedi cellulitis and bacteraemia in a patient with HIV Infection. Int J STD AIDS. 1997;8(1):59–60.

52. Kiehlbauch JA, Tauxe RV, Baker CN, Wachsmuth IK. Evaluation of ribotyping techniques as applied to Arcobacter, Campylobacter and Helicobacter. Mol Cell Probes. 1994;8(2):109–15.

53. Burman WJ, Cohn DL, Reves RR, Wilson ML. Multifocal cellulitis and monoarticular arthritis as manifestations of Helicobacter cinaedi bacteremia. Clin Infect Dis. 1995;20(3):564–70.

54. van der Ven AJ, Kullberg BJ, Vandamme P, Meis JF. Helicobacter cinaedi bacteremia associated with localized pain but not with cellulitis. Clin Infect Dis. 1996;22(4):710–1.

Klebsiella

55. Ashour HM, El-Sharif A. Synthesis and biological evaluation of some novel polysubstituted pyrimidine derivatives as potential antimicrobial and anticancer agents. Arch Pharm (Weinheim). 2009;342(5):299–310.

56. Rodot S, Lacour JP, van Elslande L, et al. Ecthyma gangrenosum caused by Klebsiella pneumoniae. Int J Dermatol. 1995;34(3):216–7.

57. Gunnarsson GL, Brandt PB, Gad D, Struve C, Justesen US. Monomicrobial necrotizing fasciitis in a white male caused by hypermucoviscous Klebsiella pneumoniae. J Med Microbiol. 2009;58(Pt 11):1519–21.

58. DiGioia RA, Kane JG, Parker RH. Crepitant cellulitis and myonecrosis caused by Klebsiella. JAMA. 1977;237(19):2097–8.

59. Napgezek MR, Hall WH. Nonclostridial crepitant cellulitis due to Klebsiella. Minn Med. 1975;58(5):377–8.

60. Fragoulis KN, Klouvas GD, Falagas ME. Impetigo-like vegetating nasal lesions caused by Klebsiella pneumoniae. Am J Med. 2005;118(8):925–7.

61. Erbagci Z. Noma-like gangrenous cheilitis in a child with cyclic neutropenia associated with myeloperoxidase deficiency. Pediatr Dermatol. 2003;20(6):519–23.

Legionella

62. Waldor MK, Wilson B, Swartz M. Cellulitis caused by Legionella pneumophila. Clin Infect Dis. 1993;16(1):51–3.

63. Han JH, Nguyen JC, Harada S, Baddour LM, Edelstein PH. Relapsing Legionella pneumophila cellulitis: a case report and review of the literature. J Infect Chemother. 2010;16(6):439–42.

64. Ampel NM, Ruben FL, Norden CW. Cutaneous abscess caused by Legionella micdadei in an immunosuppressed patient. Ann Intern Med. 1985;102(5):630–2.

65. Kilborn JA, Manz LA, O'Brien M, et al. Necrotizing cellulitis caused by Legionella micdadei. Am J Med. 1992;92(l):104–6.

66. Chee CE, Baddour LM. Legionella maceachernii soft tissue infection. Am J Med Sci. 2007;334(5):410–3.

67. Gubler JG, Schorr M, Gaia V, Zbinden R, Altwegg M. Recurrent soft tissue abscesses caused by Legionella cincinnatiensis. J Clin Microbiol. 2001;39(12):4568–70.

68. Loridant S, Lagier JC, La Scola B. Identification of Legionella feeleii cellulitis. Emerg Infect Dis. 2011;17(1):145–6.

Morganella

69. Arranz-Caso JA, Cuadrado-Gomez LM, Romanik-Cabrera J, García-Tena J. Pyomyositis caused by Morganella morganii in a patient with AIDS. Clin Infect Dis. 1996;22(2):372–3.

70. Bagel J, Grossman ME. Hemorrhagic bullae associated with Morganella morganii septicemia. J Am Acad Dermatol. 1985;12(3):575–6.

71. Ghosh S, Bal AM, Malik I, Collier A. Fatal Morganella morganii bacteraemia in a diabetic patient with gas gangrene. J Med Microbiol. 2009;58(Pt 7):965–7.

72. Lobo I, Pinto A, Ferreira M, et al. Non-pseudomonal ecthyma gangrenosum present in diclofenac-induced agranulocytosis. Eur J Dermatol. 2008;18(3):350–1.

Pseudomonas

73. Roberts R, Tarpay MM, Marks MI, Nitschke R. Erysipelas-like lesions and hyperesthesia as manifestations of Pseudomonas aeruginosa sepsis. JAMA. 1982;248(17):2156–7.

74. Song WK, Kim YC, Park HJ, Cinn YW. Ecthyma gangrenosum without bacteraemia in a leukaemic patient. Clin Exp Dermatol. 2001;26(5):395–7.

75. Collini FJ, Spees EK, Munster A, Dufresne C, Millan J. Ecthyma gangrenosum in a kidney transplant recipient with Pseudomonas septicemia. Am J Med. 1986;80(4):729–34.

76. Huminer D, Siegman-lgra Y, Morduchowicz G, Pitlik SD. Ecthyma gangrenosum without bacteremia. Report of six cases and review of the literature. Arch Intern Med. 1987;147(2):299–301.

77. Blumenthal NC, Sood UR, Aronson PJ, Hashimoto K. Facial liberations in an immunocompromised patient. Ecthyma gangrenosum. Arch Dermatol. 1990;126(4):529–32.

78. Singh N, Devi M, Devi S. Ecthyma gangrenosum: a rare cutaneous manifestation caused by Pseudomonas aeruginosa without bacteremia in a leukemic patient. Indian J Dermatol Venereol Leprol. 2005;71(2):128–9.

79. Kusne S, Eibling DE, Yu VL, et al. Gangrenous cellulitis associated with gram-negative bacilli in pancytopenic patients: dilemma with respect to effective therapy. Am J Med. 1988;85(4):490–4.

80. Falagas ME, Pappas VD, Michalopoulos A. Gangrenous, hemorrhagic, bullous cellulitis associated with Pseudomonas aeruginosa in a patient with Waldenstrom's macroglobulinemia. Infection. 2007;35(5):370–3.

81. Koriech OM, Al-Dash FZ. Skin and bone necrosis following ecthyma gangrenosum in acute leukaemia-report of three cases. Clin Exp Dermatol. 1988;13(2):78–81.

82. Bourelly PE, Grossman ME. Subcutaneous nodule as a manifestation of Pseudomonas sepsis in an immunocompromised host. Clin Infect Dis. 1998;26(1):188–9.

83. Bagel J, Grossman ME. Subcutaneous nodules in Pseudomonas sepsis. Am J Med. 1986;80(3):528–9.

84. Berger TG, Kaveh S, Becker D, Hoffman J. Cutaneous manifestations of Pseudomonas infections in AIDS. J Am Acad Dermatol. 1995;32(2 Pt 1):279–80.

85. Kielhofner M, Atmar RL, Hamill RJ, Musher DM. Life-threatening Pseudomonas aeruginosa infections in patients with human immunodeficiency virus infection. Clin Infect Dis. 1992;14(2):403–11.

Salmonella

86. Dhanoa A, Fatt QK. Non-typhoidal Salmonella bacteraemia: epidemiology, clinical characteristics and its' association with severe immunosuppression. Ann Clin Microbiol Antimicrob. 2009;8:15.
87. Hohmann EL. Nontyphoidal salmonellosis. Clin Infect Dis. 2001;32(2):263–9.
88. Gordon MA. Salmonella infections in immunocompromised adults. J Infect. 2008;56(6):413–22.
89. Hames A, Mumford J, Hale J, Galloway A. Salmonella Michigan soft tissue infection in an immunocompromised child. J Clin Pathol. 2008;61(6):773–4.
90. Andriessen MJ, Kotsopoulos AM, Bloemers FW, Strack Van Schijndel RJ, Girbes AR. Necrotizing fasciitis caused by Salmonella enteritidis. Scand J Infect Dis. 2006;38(11–12):1106–7.
91. Rosser A, Swallow G, Swann RA, Chapman C. Salmonella enteritidis necrotising fasciitis in a multiple myeloma patient receiving bortezomib. Int J Hematol. 2010;91(1):149–51.
92. Shamiss A, Thaler M, Nussinovitch N, Zissin R, Rosenthal T. Multiple Salmonella enteritidis leg abscesses in a patient with systemic lupus erythematosus. Postgrad Med J. 1990;66(776):486–8.
93. Wolinsky S, Grossman ME, Walther RR, Silvers DN, Neu HC. Hemorrhagic bullae associated with salmonella septicemia. N Y State J Med. 1981;81(11):1639–41.

Serratia

94. Bonner MJ, Meharg Jr JG. Primary cellulitis due to Serratia marcescens. JAMA. 1983;250(17):2348–9.
95. Huang JW, Fang CT, Hung KY, et al. Necrotizing fasciitis caused by Serratia marcescens in two patients receiving corticosteroid therapy. J Formos Med Assoc. 1999;98(12):851–4.
96. Bachmeyer C, Sanguina M, Turc Y, Reynaert G, Blum L. Necrotizing fasciitis due to Serratia marcescens. Clin Exp Dermatol. 2004;29(6):673–4.
97. Langrock ML, Linde HJ, Landthaler M, Karrer S. Leg ulcers and abscesses caused by Serratia marcescens. Eur J Dermatol. 2008;18(6):705–7.
98. Friend JC, Hilligoss DM, Marguesen M, et al. Skin ulcers and disseminated abscesses are characteristic of Serratia marcescens infection in older patients with chronic granulomatous disease. J Allergy Clin Immunol. 2009;124(1):164–6.
99. Hartmann F, Gheorghiu T, Leupold H, Baer F, Diehl V. Serratia infections in patients with neutropenia. Klin Wochenschr. 1991;69(11):491–4.
100. Gössl M, Eggebrecht H. Necrotizing skin ulceration in antibiotic-induced agranulocytosis. Mayo Clin Proc. 2006;81(12):1527.
101. Muñoz-Pérez MA, Rodriguez-Pichardo A, Camacho F. Disseminated papular eruption caused by Serratia marcescens: a new cutaneous manifestation in HIV-positive patients. AIDS. 1996;10(10):1179–80.

Stenotrophomonas

102. Sakhnini E, Weissmann A, Oren I. Fulminant Stenotrophomonas maltophilia soft tissue infection in immunocompromised patients: an outbreak transmitted via tap water. Am J Med Sci. 2002;323(5):269–72.
103. Safdar A, Rolston KV. Stenotrophomonas maltophilia: changing spectrum of a serious bacterial pathogen in patients with cancer. Clin Infect Dis. 2007;45(12):1602–9.

104. Teo WY, Chan MY, Lam CM, Chong CY. Skin manifestation of Stenotrophomonas maltophilia infection—a case report and review article. Ann Acad Med Singapore. 2006;35(12):897–900.
105. Moser C, Jønsson V, Thomsen K, et al. Subcutaneous lesions and bacteraemia due to Stenotrophomonas maltophilia in three leukaemic patients with neutropenia. Br J Dermatol. 1997;136(6):949–52.
106. Smeets JG, Lowe SH, Veraart JC. Cutaneous infections with Stenotrophomonas maltophilia in patients using immunosuppressive medication. J Eur Acad Dermatol Venereol. 2007;21(9):1298–300.
107. Burns RL, Lowe L. Xanthomonas maltophilia infection presenting as erythematous nodules. J Am Acad Dermatol. 1997;37(5 Pt 2):836–8.
108. Sefcick A, Tait RC, Wood B. Stenotrophomonas maltophilia: an increasing problem in patients with acute leukaemia. Leuk Lymphoma. 1999;35(1–2):207–11.
109. Vartivarian SE, Papadakis KA, Palacios JA, Manning Jr JT, Anaissie EJ. Mucocutaneous and soft tissue infections caused by Xanthomonas maltophilia. A new spectrum. Ann Intern Med. 1994;121(12):969–73.
110. Bin Abdulhak AA, Zimmerman V, Al Beirouti BT, Baddour LM, Tleyjeh IM. Stenotrophomonas maltophilia infections of intact skin: a systematic review of the literature. Diagn Microbiol Infect Dis. 2009;63(3):330–3.
111. Son YM, Na SY, Lee HY, Baek JO, Lee JR, Roh JY. Ecthyma gangrenosum: a rare cutaneous manifestation caused by Stenotrophomonas maltophilia in a leukemic patient. Ann Dermatol. 2009;21(4):389–92.
112. Muder RR, Yu VL, Dummer JS, Vinson C, Lumish RM. Infections caused by Pseudomonas maltophilia. Expanding clinical spectrum. Arch Intern Med. 1987;147(9):1672–4.
113. Pham BN, Aractingi S, Dombret H, et al. Xanthomonas (formerly Pseudomonas) maltophilia-induced cellulitis in a neutropenic patient. Arch Dermatol. 1992;128(5):702–4.

Vibrio

114. Payinda G. Necrotizing fasciitis due to Vibrio parahaemolyticus. N Z Med J. 2008;121(1283):99–101.
115. Farina C, Luzzi I, Lorenzi N. Vibrio cholerae 02 sepsis in a patient with AIDS. Eur J Clin Microbiol Infect Dis. 1999;18(3):203–5.
116. Thodis E, Kriki P, Kakagia D, et al. Rigorous Vibrio vulnificus soft tissue infection of the lower leg in a renal transplant patient managed by vacuum therapy and autologous growth factors. J Cutan Med Surg. 2009;13(4):209–14.
117. Kuhnt-Lenz K, Krengel S, Fetscher S, Heer-Sonderhoff A, Solbach W. Sepsis with bullous necrotizing skin lesions due to vibrio vulnificus acquired through recreational activities in the Baltic Sea. Eur J Clin Microbiol Infect Dis. 2004;23(l):49–52.
118. Lee CC, Tong KL, Howe HS, Lam MS. Vibrio vulnificus infections: case reports and literature review. Ann Acad Med Singapore. 1997;26(5):705–12.
119. Iwata Y, Sato S, Murase Y, et al. Five cases of necrotizing fasciitis: lack of skin inflammatory signs as a clinical clue for the fulminant type. J Dermatol. 2008;35(11):719–25.
120. Nakafusa J, Misago N, Miura Y, et al. The importance of serum creatine phosphokinase level in the early diagnosis, and as a prognostic factor, of Vibrio vulnificus infection. Br J Dermatol. 2001;145(2):280–4.
121. Kuo Chou TN, Chao WN, Yang C, et al. Predictors of mortality in skin and soft-tissue infections caused by Vibrio vulnificus. World J Surg. 2010;34(7):1669–75.

14

Viral Related Malignancies

Between 15% and 20% of all global malignancies are attributable to an infectious agent.[1] These range from bacterial infections such as *Helicobacter pylori* (associated with stomach carcinoma and gastric lymphoma), to parasitic infections such as *Opisthorchis viverrini* (a liver fluke associated with cholangiocarcinoma) and *Schistosoma haematobium* (a blood fluke associated with bladder carcinoma), to viral infections such as the hepatitis viruses (associated with hepatocellular carcinoma), herpes viruses (associated with a range of cancers including various lymphomas and Kaposi's sarcoma), and human papillomaviruses (associated with cervical and skin cancers).[2] This chapter will focus on viral-associated malignancies with cutaneous findings that occur in immunocompromised hosts.

HUMAN PAPILLOMAVIRUS

There are a wide variety of human papillomaviruses (HPV), and the number of genotypes expands annually. Exposure to HPV can occur directly, through sexual or other contact, or indirectly, from viral particles on shared objects. Once infected, patients frequently autoinoculate additional sites. Most HPV infections result in benign warts. A subset of high-risk HPV types are involved in the development of cutaneous malignancies. High-risk HPV subtypes such as HPV-16, HPV-18, HPV-31, and HPV-35 are widely recognized as the underlying infectious agents leading to cervical dysplasia, cervical cancer, and anogenital cancer. There are currently available vaccines which protect against either two or four of the high-risk HPV strains most frequently involved in the development of cervical cancer, and given the frequency of HPV-infection-related complications in immunocompromised hosts, some have advocated for the institution of widespread HPV vaccination after transplantation.[3]

Squamous cell carcinomas (SCC) in immunosuppressed hosts behave more aggressively and impart a higher risk for development of metastatic disease.[4]

In solid organ transplant recipients, the incidence of cutaneous carcinoma reaches 40% by 10 years post-transplant, and 60–80% of those SCCs will contain HPV DNA.[5,6] Clinically these lesions resemble typical SCCs, with pink hyperkeratotic scaly plaques which may be eroded. The development of SCCs in this patient population is multifactorial and due to ultraviolet (UV) radiation, viral infection, the underlying cause of immunosuppression, and the combination and duration of immunosuppressant medications and their duration of use. Azathioprine and cyclosporine in particular may confer increased risk for secondary malignancies in organ transplant recipients.[4] The more immunosuppressive the regimen, the higher the risk of SCC, as shown by one study demonstrating an increased incidence of SCC in renal transplant recipients on cyclosporine, azathioprine, and prednisolone compared to patients on only azathioprine and prednisolone.[7] The type of transplanted organ may play a role as well. Renal transplant patients in particular appear to be at markedly increased risk. Patients status post renal transplantation have an increased risk of SCC over BCC (1.8:1), a reversal of the ratio seen in immunocompetent patients and a rate more than 30 times that of immunocompetent hosts.

Patients with cutaneous lymphoma, in particular with Sezary syndrome, have an elevated incidence of SCC. This may be due to disease-related immunosuppression or side effects of commonly used therapeutic modalities (UV light therapy, total skin electron beam radiation, topical nitrogen mustard, and chemotherapy).[8] Patients who undergo bone marrow transplantation have a 7% lifetime chance of developing a secondary solid tumor, with SCC representing about 50% of cases of

M.E. Grossman et al., *Cutaneous Manifestations of Infection in the Immunocompromised Host*,
DOI 10.1007/978-1-4419-1578-8_14, © Springer Science+Business Media, LLC 2012

secondary malignancy. Irradiation as part of the conditioning regimen for bone marrow transplant may be a risk factor for development of secondary solid tumors in this patient population.[9]

In immunocompromised patients, SCC of the nail unit is rare; however, patients with immunosuppression, particularly human immunodeficiency virus (HIV), are at increased risk for developing nail unit SCC and squamous cell carcinoma in situ (SCCis). HPV-16 is the predominant viral type associated with nail unit SCCs, although in patients with HIV other viral types have been reported, particularly HPV-26.[10] Digital SCCs rarely metastasize but have a high rate of local recurrence.

An unusual and noteworthy presentation of SCC in another immunosuppressed patient was a patient with non-scarring, subacute cutaneous lupus who developed multiple HPV-associated SCCs while being treated with prednisone and azathioprine.[11]

Verrucous carcinoma (VC) is a rare variant of squamous cell carcinoma (SCC) that is associated with both low-risk (HPV-6 and HPV-11) and high-risk (HPV-16 and HPV-18) genotypes. VC can occur in a number of anatomical locations: aerodigestive (oral florid papillomatosis or Ackerman's tumor), which may be associated with carcinogenic chemical exposures as well as high-risk HPV viral infection; anogenital (Buschke–Lowenstein tumor), which is typically associated with low-risk HPV viral types (HPV-6 and HPV-11); palmoplantar; and other cutaneous locations, which are not clearly associated with HPV infection. Although the HPV virus has been identified in verrucous carcinoma lesions and likely plays an oncogenic role, the precise mechanism remains unproven.[12-14] Clinically these lesions frequently present as massive, exuberant warty plaques and nodules, or near-confluent verrucous papules and patches. It is important to note that the histologic appearance of VC may be relatively benign. Lesions classically demonstrate a broad-based, "pushing" border of advancing "tongues" of keratinocytes with marked hyperplasia of the epidermis and frequent endophytic and exophytic growth. These lesions usually do not penetrate the basement membrane and lack abundant mitoses.

Verrucous carcinoma may behave abnormally in patients with impaired immune systems. One report of an anal Buschke–Lowenstein tumor in a patient with HIV/AIDS and a CD4 nadir of 43 progressed rapidly over a few months from a histologically benign HPV-6 and HPV-11 positive lesion to a rapidly progressive, invasive, destructive tumor which metastasized to regional nodes.[15] Verrucous carcinoma of the vulva in a woman with HIV presented as a painful, draining, obstructive vulvar mass with wide local invasion and associated reactive regional adenopathy.[16] Two reports noted the simultaneous presentation of a large verrucous carcinoma with a new diagnosis of cutaneous T-cell lymphoma.[17,18]

ANAL, VULVAR, AND PENILE CARCINOMA

Both HPV and HIV may be transmitted through sexual contact, and coinfection is common. HPV is recognized as the causative agent for cervical cancer. However, HPV can also cause premalignant and malignant epithelial tumors in noncervical tissue. Anal HPV infection is the main risk factor for the development of anal intraepithelial neoplasia (AIN) and anal cancer. HIV coinfection confers a markedly increased risk for cancer development, which increases with the severity of immunosuppression. These lesions may initially present as verrucous fleshy papules which may be grouped or confluent. More advanced intraepithelial atypia may manifest as whitish or erythematous plaques with pigmentary alteration. Women may present with a similar disease spectrum involving the vulva, ranging from vulvar intraepithelial neoplasia (VIN) of varying histologic degrees (including Bowenoid papulosis) to frank invasive vulvar carcinoma. Penile intraepithelial neoplasia and penile cancer are rare, but demonstrate a similar course and presentation.[19]

Epidermodysplasia verruciformis (EV) is a rare genetic disease inherited in an autosomal recessive pattern involving truncating mutations in *EVER1* or *EVER2*. Patients with EV may have numerous, nearly confluent lesions that resemble flat warts or tinea versicolor–like macules clinically. Histopathologic examination classically reveals a lesion resembling verruca plana with blue-gray, pale, vacuolated keratinocytes in the granular layer. These lesions frequently contain numerous HPV genotypes. HPV types 5 and 8 are most frequently associated with a diagnosis of EV. Patients with this condition frequently develop numerous actinic keratoses and 30–60% of EV patients will develop invasive SCCs in sun exposed areas, suggesting that the HPV infection and UV irradiation play a role in tumor development. In EV, HPV-5 and HPV-8 are associated with the majority of EV-associated SCCs.[14]

Immunocompromised patients, in particular those with impaired cell-mediated immunity, have recently been reported to develop an EV-like syndrome termed "acquired epidermodysplasia verruciformis (AEV)." Lesions range from tinea versicolor–like macules, to shiny, hypopigmented flat-topped warty papules, to slightly hyperkeratotic flat papules ranging from flesh colored to slightly erythematous.[20] The majority of reported patients have a history of HIV, although AEV has been reported in a renal transplant recipient on azathioprine and corticosteroids, a patient with Hodgkin's lymphoma after chemotherapy, a patient with systemic lupus erythematosus on azathioprine and prednisolone,[21] and a patient with graft versus host disease (GVHD) maintained on tacrolimus following an allogenic stem cell transplant for acute myelogenous leukemia (AML).[22] One patient developed flat wart and tinea versicolor–like lesions diffusely with a poor response to multiple therapies, and was then diagnosed with myelodysplastic syndrome seven years later.[23]

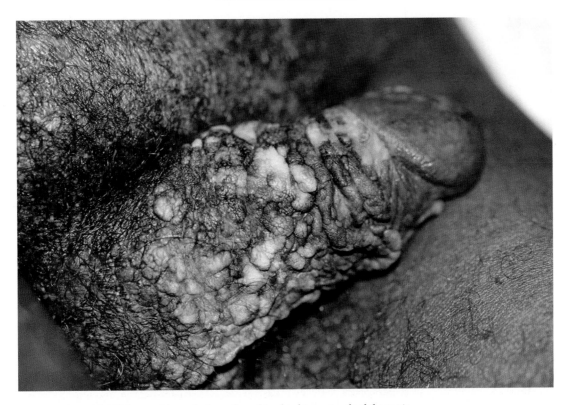

Figure 14.1. In a patient with EV, Bowenoid papulosis confirmed by skin biopsy involved the penis

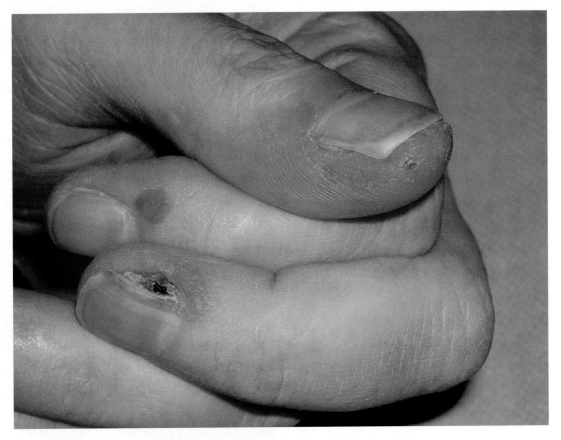

Figure 14.2. A 40-year-old HIV-positive man with multiple HPV-associated periungual squamous cell carcinomas

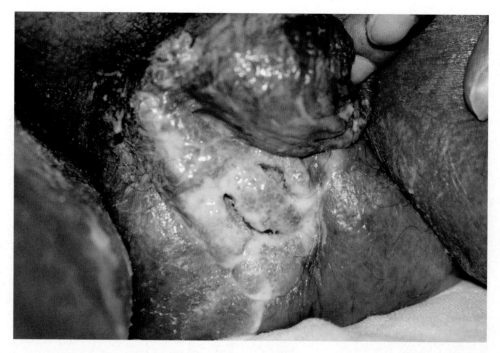

Figure 14.3. A 71-year-old HIV-positive man with extensive human papillomavirus (HPV) associated giant condyloma extending into his bladder and urothelial system with subsequent development of urinary retention, sinus tracts, and abscess formation. Low-risk HPV genotypes 6, 11, 42, 43, and 44 were positive from skin, urethra, and bladder biopsies (Courtesy of Samantha Herman, M.D.)

Figure 14.4. A 56-year-old HIV-positive man with stage IIIB anal squamous cell carcinoma. Low-risk HPV genotypes 6, 11, 42, 43, and 44 were positive, highlighting koilocytes, on anal biopsy

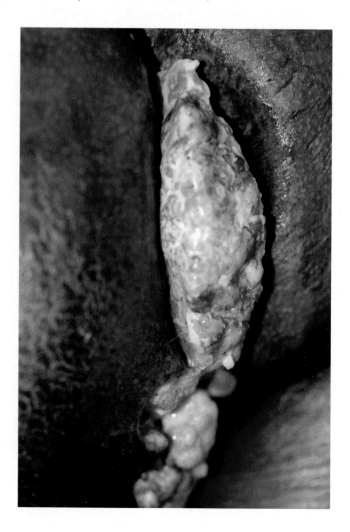

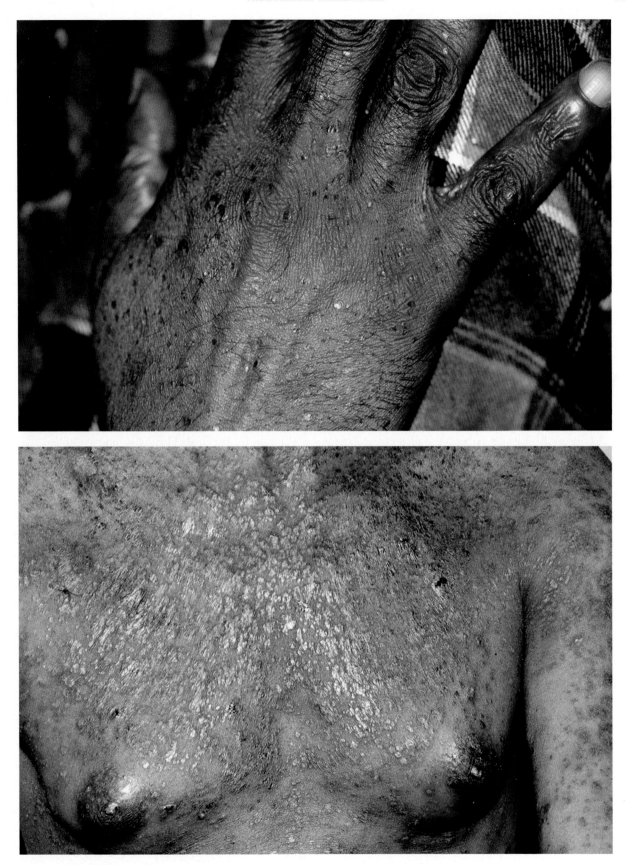

Figure 14.5. and 14.6. A 47-year-old HIV-positive man with generalized flat-topped lichenoid papules on the hands and chest of epidermodysplasia verruciformis confirmed by skin biopsy

EPSTEIN-BARR VIRUS (EBV)

Epstein-Barr virus (EBV) is associated with a number of malignancies in patients with a variety of immunosuppressive conditions. EBV can cause latent infection in B lymphocytes, transforming resting B cells into latently infected cell lines.[24,25] EBV is either involved in or associated with Burkitt's lymphoma, some Hodgkin's lymphomas, primary effusion lymphoma, NK/T-cell lymphomas, and lymphomas in transplant recipients (post-transplant lymphoproliferative disease, or PTLD). EBV has been isolated from certain gastric adenocarcinomas, salivary tumors, and nasopharyngeal carcinomas. It has been linked to some AIDS-related leiomyosarcomas. EBV was also recently linked to lymphoepithelioma-like carcinoma of the skin, a rare malignant neoplasm.[26]

Immunosuppression-related lymphoproliferative disorders (IR-LPD) include post-transplant lymphoproliferative disorders (PTLD) as well as non-transplant related immunosuppression-associated lymphoproliferative disorders (as seen in cases of iatrogenic immunosuppression or with HIV coinfection). The majority of cases of IR-LPD of B cell origin are associated with EBV infection, while T-cell driven IR-LPD is typically EBV negative, although exceptions to this rule do occur. Two to 10% of patients following organ transplantation may go on to develop PTLD, typically within the first 1–2 years following transplant while immunosuppressive regimens are strongest. The incidence of PTLD depends primarily on the type of organ transplant and nature of the immunosuppressive regimen. For example, combined heart–lung transplants and heart transplants, which require higher levels of immunosuppression, demonstrate a higher incidence of PTLD and an increased mortality. Patients on immunosuppressive regimens including either cyclosporine or the monoclonal antibody OKT3 are at the highest risk for developing PTLD. Management typically involves reducing systemic immunosuppression. Advanced cases require multimodality treatment, with the addition of antiviral therapy remaining controversial.

PTLD can manifest as a broad range of disease states, from a benign mononucleosis-like illness to a malignant non-Hodgkin's lymphoma. PTLD usually manifests with multiple tumors, often in the gastrointestinal tract, or with lymphadenopathy. Five percent of cases of PTLD involve the skin.[27] It is rare for patients with IR-LPD to present with skin lesions in the absence of systemic disease, with fewer than 30 cases reported in the literature.

Cutaneous lesions of PTLD typically resemble classic leukemia cutis, with indurated violaceous papules or plaques, or present as subcutaneous plaques, nodules, masses, or ulcerated lesions.[28,29] Purple, plum-colored papules and nodules in an immunosuppressed host may suggest PTLD. However, the spectrum of cutaneous presentations of PTLD is broad. There are descriptions of PTLD presenting as a localized erythematous maculopapular rash.[30] A 63-year-old male with a history of single lung transplant on prednisone, mycophenolate, and sirolimus developed a 1 cm × 1 cm red plaque on the left cheek over a month. It gradually enlarged, and he developed submandibular lymphadenopathy. Biopsy revealed atypical appearing cells that were CD30+ and EBV+, and he was diagnosed with EBV-related post-transplant lymphoproliferative disorder. His lesions resolved with reduction of immunosuppression.[31] One pediatric patient on immunosuppression with tacrolimus and methylprednisolone for liver and bowel transplant, in the setting of high EBV viral load, developed multiple blanchable erythematous nodules on her abdomen near her surgical scars. Biopsy was consistent with PTLD, although no tissue was sent for in situ hybridization or polymerase chain reaction (PCR) to look for EBV.[32] One review noted patients following renal transplant presenting with cutaneous signs of PTLD ranging from raised erythematous nodules on the leg and neck, to bullous lesions on the thigh, to plum-colored nodules on the legs.[27] A 64-year-old Chinese man maintained on azathioprine, cyclosporine, and prednisolone following heart transplant presented with multiple erythematous smooth-topped nodules surrounded by a patch of diffuse, indurated erythema due to EBV-positive, CD30-positive anaplastic large T-cell lymphoma.[33] Another 71-year-old male heart transplant recipient maintained on anti-thymocyte globulin, azathioprine, cyclosporine, and prednisone developed multiple reddish, ulceronecrotic cutaneous nodules and plaques on his left thigh 11 months post-transplant. He was diagnosed with primary cutaneous EBV+CD30+ post-transplant anaplastic large cell lymphoma (ALCL).[34] A 33-year-old woman 2 years status post renal transplantation for lupus nephritis, immunosuppressed with cyclosporine, prednisolone, and azathioprine developed fever and tender cutaneous lumps on the abdomen, anterior chest, back, upper extremities, and lateral thigh due to EBV-positive anaplastic large T-cell lymphoma 10 weeks after delivering a normal pregnancy.[35] A 52-year-old man 9 years status post renal transplantation for microscopic polyangiitis immunosuppressed with cyclosporine, azathioprine, and prednisolone presented with a multinodular erythematous lesion on the right upper posterior chest wall due to EBV-positive anaplastic large T-cell lymphoma.[35]

Natural killer/T-cell lymphoma (NKTL) frequently involves the nose and occurs primarily in East Asia and Latin America. It was initially known as "lethal midline granuloma" due to the aggressive nature of the tumor. More recently, EBV has been documented within lesions, and NKTL is recognized as an EBV-associated cancer. Lesions typically present with ulceration and necrosis, usually within the nasal cavity. When lesions spread they may involve the skin.[36] Classically immunosuppression is not a prerequisite for disease; however, NKTL can present in an atypical fashion in patients who are immunocompromised. NKTL has been reported in patients with AIDS, including a Spanish male with cerebral disease[37] and a

South Korean patient with unspecified clinical manifestations.[38] Another 36-year-old HIV-positive Korean man presented with an ulcerative mass on both tonsils and cervical lymphadenopathy confirmed pathologically to be NKTL.[39] EBV-associated nasal-type extranodal NKTL was reported in a renal allograft recipient presenting with left facial palsy, left cheek swelling, left tonsillitis, and intraoral aphthous ulcers.[40]

Another renal allograft recipient developed an ulceration at the posterior pharynx with cervical lymphadenopathy. He was subsequently diagnosed with EBV-associated NKTL.[41] A 62-year-old patient of unspecified ethnic background with prostate carcinoma, hepatitis C infection, and pancytopenia presented with purulent nasal discharge and periorbital swelling and edema, which progressed to a necrotic area on the right face due to NKTL.[42] The authors have seen a 47-year-old Caucasian woman on multiagent immunosuppression for systemic lupus erythematosus present with a deep calf ulcer down to muscle and simultaneous left facial swelling with a necrotic nasal mass. Biopsy specimens of both the calf and nasal cavity were consistent with EBV + NKTL.

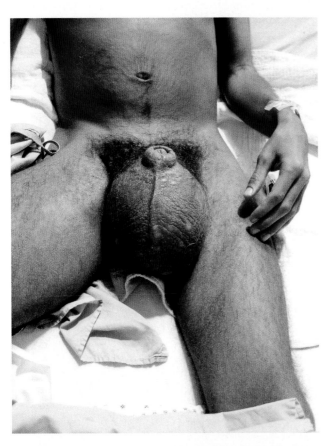

Figure 14.7. A 32-year-old man with untreated HIV/AIDS with an enlarging scrotal mass. Autopsy findings revealed Epstein-Barr virus (EBV)-positive, HIV-associated Burkitt/Burkitt-like lymphoma involving the skin, testes, lymph nodes, spleen, liver, and stomach. The patient simultaneously was found to have EBV-positive, HIV-associated classical Hodgkin's lymphoma involving the bone marrow, terminal ileum, and cecum (Courtesy of Jocelyn Lieb, M.D.)

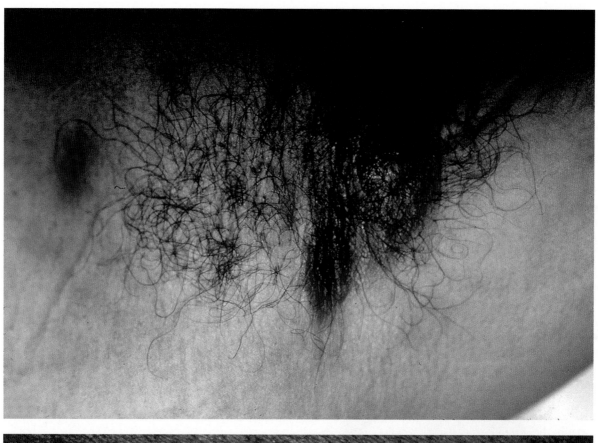

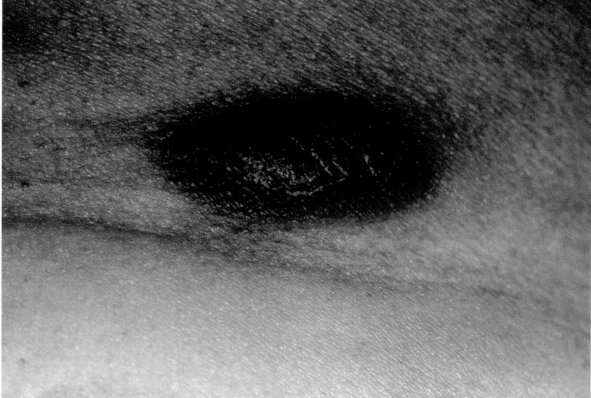

Figure 14.8. and 14.9. A 61-year-old Ecuadorian man 10 years status post renal transplant for polycystic kidney disease developed multiple pruritic red nodules on his flanks, axillae, and chest of EBV-positive post-transplant lymphoproliferative disorder (PTLD)

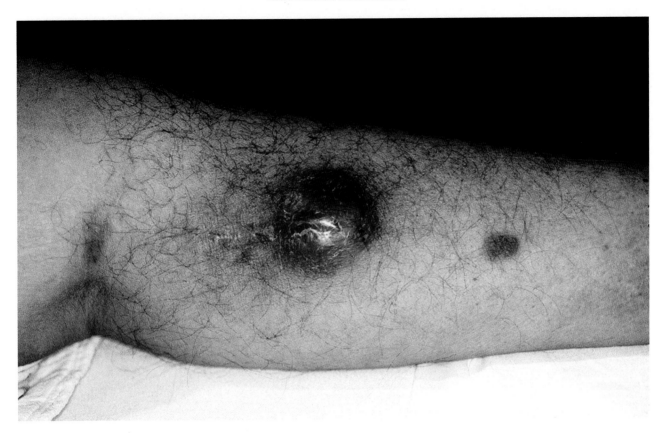

Figure 14.10. Same patient as in Figure 14.9. Two years later, recurrent purple nodules of EBV-positive PTLD

Human Herpes Virus 8 (HHV8)

Kaposi sarcoma (KS) is one of the most common malignancies associated with immunosuppression, particularly with HIV. Early in the AIDS epidemic these tumors were recognized as signs of advanced disease. It was not until more recently that researchers discovered herpes virus DNA in KS lesions and human herpes virus 8 (HHV8) was identified as the causative agent.[43] Immunosuppression-associated epidemic KS is markedly more common in patients with HIV, particularly in men who have sex with men, than in patients with iatrogenic immunosuppression. Among iatrogenically immunosuppressed patients, renal transplant patients appear to be at the highest risk. Patients on a suppression regimen that includes cyclosporine potentially are at a further increased risk while rapamycin may be somewhat protective.[44] Lesions of KS may demonstrate variable clinical morphologies, ranging from flat, purpuric patches to thicker plaques to indurated violaceous nodules. There is often involvement of the regional lymphatics and subsequent associated edema. Epidemic KS frequently involves the head and neck, mucosa, and gastrointestinal tract. Involvement may be widespread at initial presentation.

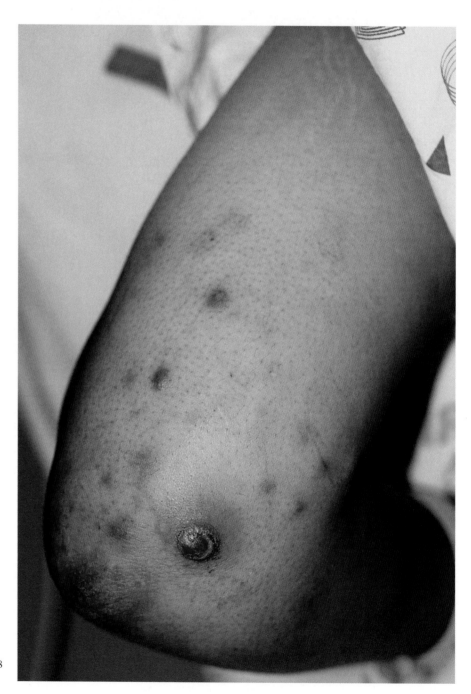

Figure 14.11. A 42-year-old man with human immunodeficiency virus/acquired immune deficiency syndrome (HIV/AIDS) with biopsy-proven lymphatic Kaposi sarcoma, and human herpes virus 8 (HHV-8)

POLYOMAVIRUS

There are now five known polyomaviruses, including the JC virus, BK virus, and Merkel cell polyomavirus. These viruses appear to be nearly ubiquitous, but cause significant disease only in immunocompromised hosts. The JC virus and BK virus are the most common polyomaviruses. The BK virus is associated with polyomavirus nephropathy and hemorrhagic cystitis, while the JC virus is associated with progressive multifocal leukoencephalopathy. While there is no clear association between either of these viruses and the development of cancer, there are reports linking viral DNA with multiple different human tumors (BK virus with brain, bladder, prostate, and various adenocarcinomas, and JC virus with mesotheliomas, lymphomas, osteosarcomas, and brain tumors).[45]

The most recently defined polyomavirus is the Merkel cell polyomavirus, which was identified from Merkel cell carcinoma (MCC).[46] MCC is a rare, aggressive tumor, far more common in immunosuppressed hosts, that classically develops as a rapidly growing red or violaceous nodule in sun exposed areas in Caucasian patients over age 50. The majority of patients with MCC are immunosuppressed, most often due to HIV, organ transplant related immunosuppression, and chronic lymphocytic leukemia.[47,48] A diagnosis of MCC should prompt clinical investigation for underlying immunoalteration, including subclinical chronic leukemias.

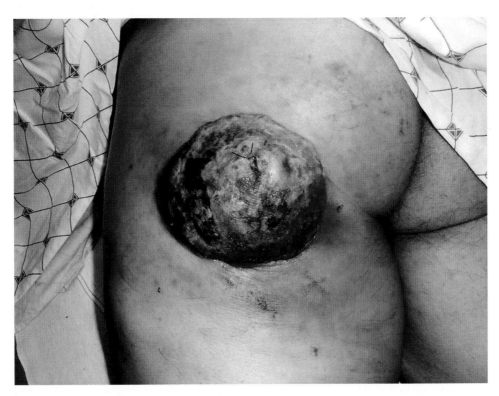

Figure 14.12. A 59-year-old diabetic man 8 years status post liver transplant for hepatitis C cirrhosis with a 4-month history of an enlarging buttock mass associated with spontaneous hemorrhage had massive inguinal, iliac, and para-aortic lymphadenopathy on positron emission tomography/computed tomography (PET/CT) scan. Surgical excision confirmed a diagnosis of Merkel cell tumor. He died in hospice care 4 months later (Courtesy of Siegrid Yu, M.D.)

Human T-Cell Lymphotrophic Virus (HTLV)

HTLV 1 and 2 are viruses endemic to Japan, South America, Africa, and the Caribbean.[1] They are transmitted vertically (e.g., breast-feeding) or through shared syringes, sexual contact, and blood transfusions. A high rate of HIV coinfection occurs in areas endemic to HTLV.

HTLV infection predisposes infected individuals to various forms of skin disease. It is the causative agent of "infective dermatitis," a form of severe childhood eczema seen in Jamaica, Brazil, Peru, and Japan.[49] HTLV-1 infection has been reported to cause acquired ichthyosis, presenting as thick, plate-like scaling on the legs, as well as less extensive forms of xerosis.[49] Patients with HTLV-1 may be coinfected with strongyloides. It has been proposed that the two infections generate opposed immunologic responses leading to decreased anti-strongyloides IgE and lack of a systemic eosinophilia, resulting in more severe and sometimes refractory strongyloides infestations.[50] Patients with HTLV-1 are at increased risk of progressing to disseminated strongyloidiasis hyperinfection, similar to patients treated with corticosteroids and other immunosuppressants, characterized by larval migration from the gastrointestinal (GI) tract leading to the secondary bacteremia, pulmonary hemorrhage, and cutaneous thumbprint purpura as detailed in Chapter 10.[51] HTLV-1 is also associated with increased incidence of scabies infestations. Crusted scabies may be the presenting sign of HTLV infection in patients from areas where HTLV is endemic.

Adult T-cell leukemia/lymphoma (ATLL) is associated with HTLV-1 infection. Affected patients may present with erythroderma that resembles the leukemic phase of mycosis fungoides (Sezary syndrome). Crusted scabies in HTLV-infected patients may suggest the development of ATLL and should prompt a search for this malignancy.[52]

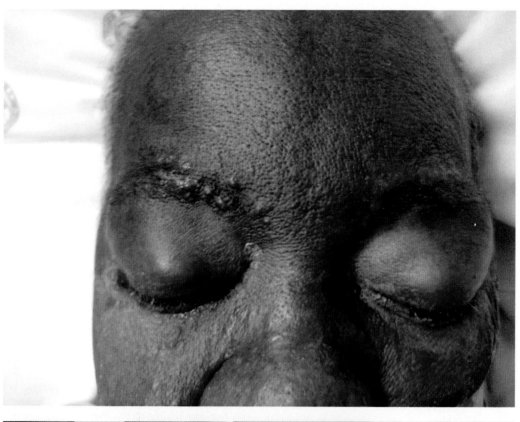

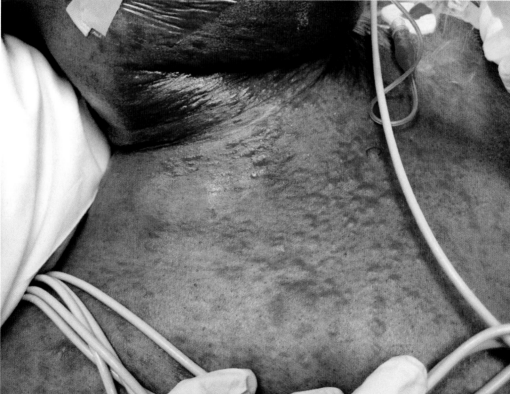

Figure 14.13. and 14.14. A 54-year-old woman with relapsed and refractory stage 4 human T-cell lymphotrophic virus type 1 (HTLV-1) associated adult T-cell lymphoma/leukemia. Skin biopsy of the patient's folliculocentric firm red papules revealed a clonal lymphoid population identical to her bone marrow biopsy. She ultimately died of her disease

HUMAN IMMUNODEFICIENCY VIRUS (HIV)

While many of the viral infections associated with malignancies discussed above occur in patients infected with HIV, patients with HIV infection alone are at risk for additional malignancies with potential for cutaneous involvement. These malignancies include lymphoma, squamous cell carcinoma, basal cell carcinoma, lung cancers, testicular cancer, and pediatric leiomyosarcomas.[53]

Cutaneous lymphoma occurs at increased rates in HIV-infected persons. CD30+ large-cell lymphoma may present as primary cutaneous disease or systemic disease with secondary skin involvement. Typical lesions include rapidly growing deep dermal nodules or indurated subcutaneous plaques, which may be single or grouped. Evidence of EBV infection is frequently present. Cutaneous T-cell lymphomas are rare but can occur in the setting of HIV infection, and may present with protean manifestations including scaly patches, thin plaques, or more advanced disease. Patients with HIV are also at risk for developing plasmablastic lymphoma, which frequently presents in the oral cavity and may demonstrate tumor-associated evidence of EBV or HHV8 viral infection.[54]

REFERENCES

1. McLaughlin-Drubin ME, Munger K. Viruses associated with human cancer. Biochim Biophys Acta. 2008;1782(3):127–50.
2. Parkin DM. The global health burden of infection-associated cancers in the year 2002. Int J Cancer. 2006;118(12):3030–44.

Human Papillomavirus

3. Tedeschi SK, Savani BN, Jagasia M, et al. Time to consider HPV vaccination after allogeneic stem cell transplantation. Biol Blood Marrow Transplant. 2010;16:1033–6.
4. Espana A, Redondo P, Fernandez AL, et al. Skin cancer in heart transplant recipients. J Am Acad Dermatol. 1995;32:458–65.
5. Shamanin V, zur Hausen H, Lavergne D, et al. Human papillomavirus infections in nonmelanoma skin cancers from renal transplant recipients and nonimmunosuppressed patients. J Natl Cancer Inst. 1996;88:802–11.
6. Berkhout RJ, Tieben LM, Smits HL, et al. Nested PCR approach for detection and typing of epidermodysplasia verruciformis-associated human papillomavirus types in cutaneous cancers from renal transplant recipients. J Clin Microbiol. 1995;33:690–5.
7. Glover MT, Deeks JJ, Raftery MJ, Cunningham J, Leigh IM. Immunosuppression and risk of non-melanoma skin cancer in renal transplant recipients. Lancet. 1997;349:398.
8. Vidulich KA, Rady PL, He Q, Tyring S, Duvic M. Detection of high-risk human papillomaviruses in verrucae of patients with mycosis fungoides and Sezary syndrome: a case series. Int J Dermatol. 2009;48:598–602.
9. Curtis RE, Rowlings PA, Deeg HJ, et al. Solid cancer after bone marrow transplantation. New Engl J Med. 1997;336:897–904.
10. Handisurya A, Rieger A, Bankier A, et al. Human papillomavirus type 26 infection causing multiple invasive squamous cell carcinomas of the fingernails in an AIDS patient under highly active antiretroviral therapy. Br J Dermatol. 2007;157:788–94.

11. Cohen LM, Tyring SK, Rady P, Callen JP. Human papillomavirus type 11 in multiple squamous cell carcinomas in a patient with subacute cutaneous lupus erythematosus. J Am Acad Dermatol. 1992;26:840–5.
12. Schwartz RA. Verrucous carcinoma of the skin and mucosa. J Am Acad Dermatol. 1995;32:1–21.
13. Lubbe J, Kormann A, Adams V, et al. HPV-11 and HPV-16-associated oral verrucous carcinoma. Dermatology. 1996;192:217–21.
14. Dubina M, Goldenberg G. Viral-associated nonmelanoma skin cancers: a review. Am J Dermatopathol. 2009;31:561–73.
15. Handisurya A, Rieger A, Bago-Horvath Z, et al. Rapid progression of an anal Buschke-Lowenstein tumour into a metastasizing squamous cell carcinoma in an HIV-infected patient. Sex Transm Infect. 2009;85:261–3.
16. Massad LS, Ahuja J, Bitterman P. Verrucous carcinoma of the vulva in a patient infected with the human immunodeficiency virus. Gynecol Oncol. 1999;73:315–8.
17. Chung SD, Huang KH, Lai YH, et al. Synchronous advanced scrotal verrucous carcinoma with peripheral T-cell lymphoma. Urology. 2007;69:184.e5–7.
18. Parsons AC, Sheehan DJ, Sangueza OP. Synchronous verrucous carcinoma and cutaneous T-cell lymphoma. J Am Acad Dermatol. 2008;58:S124–5.
19. Gormely RH, Kovarik CL. Dermatologic manifestations of HPV in HIV-infected individuals. Curr HIV/AIDS Rep. 2009;6:130–8.
20. Rogers HD, MacGregor JL, Nord KM, et al. Acquired epidermodysplasia verruciformis. J Am Acad Dermatol. 2009;60:315–20.
21. Holmes C, Chong AH, Tabrizi SN, Downes N, Nindl I. Epidermodysplasia verruciformis-like syndrome in association with systemic lupus erythematosus. Australas J Dermatol. 2009;50:44–7.
22. Kunishige JH, Hymes SR, Madkan V, et al. Epidermodysplasia verruciformis in the setting of graft-versus–host disease. J Am Acad Dermaol. 2007;57:S78–80.
23. Oliveira WR, Ferreira GN, Rady PL, Festa C, Tyring SK. Epidermodysplasia verruciformis associated with myelodysplastic syndrome: an intriguing association. J Cutan Med Surg. 2009;13:317–20.

Epstein-Barr Virus

24. Ferreri AJM, Ernberg I, Copie-Bergman C. Infectious agents and lymphoma development: molecular and clinical aspects. J Intern Med. 2009;265:421–38.
25. Tao Q, Young LS, Woodman CBJ, Murray PG. Epstein-Barr virus (EBV) and its associated human cancers – genetics, epigenetics, pathobiology and novel therapeutics. Front Biosci. 2006;11:2672–713.
26. Aoki R, Mitsui H, Harada K, et al. A case of lymphoepithelioma-like carcinoma of the skin associated with Epstein-Barr virus infection. J Am Acad Dermatol. 2008;62:681–4.
27. Salama S, Todd S, Cina DP, Margetts P. Cutaneous presentation of post-renal transplant lymphoproliferative disorder: a series of four cases. J Cutan Pathol. 2010;37:641–53.
28. Capaldi L, Robinson-Bostom L, Kerr P, Gohh R. Localized cutaneous posttransplant Epstein-Barr virus-associated lymphoproliferative disorder. J Am Acad Dermatol. 2004;51:778–80.
29. Schumann KW, Oriba HA, Bergfeld WF, et al. Cutaneous presentation of posttransplant lymphoproliferative disorder. J Am Acad Dermatol. 2000;42:923–6.
30. Chai C, White WL, Shea CR, Prieto VG. Epstein Barr virus-associated lymphoproliferative-disorders primarily involving the skin. J Cutan Pathol. 1999;26:242–7.
31. Snavely NR, Sonabend M, Rosen T. Posttransplant Epstein-Barr virus related lymphoproliferative disorder with a primary cutaneous presentation. Dermatol Online J. 2007;13:7.

32. Hernandez C, Cetner AS, Wiley EL. Cutaneous presentation of plasmablastic post-transplant lymphoproliferative disorder in a 14-month-old. Pediatr Dermatol. 2009;26:713–6.

33. Chiu LS, Choi PCL, Luk NM, Chang M, Tang WYM. Spontaneous regression of primary cutaneous Epstein-Barr virus-positive, CD30-positive anaplastic large T-cell lymphoma in a heart transplant recipient. Clin Exp Dermatol. 2009;34:e21–4.

34. Lucioni M, Ippoliti G, Campana C, et al. EMV positive primary cutaneous CD30+ large T-cell lymphoma in a heart transplanted patient: case report. Am J Transplant. 2004;4:1915–20.

35. Coyne JD, Banerjee SS, Bromley M, et al. Post-transplant T-cell lymphoproliferative disorder/T-cell lymphoma: a report of three cases of T-anaplastic large-cell lymphoma with cutaneous presentation and a review of the literature. Histopathology. 2004;44:387–93.

36. Harabuchi Y, Takahara M, Kishibe K, et al. Nasal natural killer (NK)/T-cell lymphoma: clinical, histological, virological, and genetic features. Int J Clin Oncol. 2009;14:181–90.

37. Cobo F, Talavera P, Busguier H, Concha A. CNK/T-cell brain lymphoma associated with Epstein-Barr virus in a patient with AIDS. Neuropathology. 2007;27:396–402.

38. Kim JS, Kim SJ, Kim JS, et al. Report of AIDS-related lymphoma in South Korea. Jpn J Clin Oncol. 2008;38:134–9.

39. Oh SC, Choi CW, Kim BS, et al. NK/T-cell lymphoma associated with Epstein-Barr virus in a patient infected with human immunodeficiency virus: an autopsy case. Int J Hematol. 2004;79:480–3.

40. Momose A, Mizuno H, Kajihara S, et al. EBV-associated nasal-type NK/T-cell lymphoma of the nasal cavity/paranasal sinus in a renal allograft recipient. Nephrol Dial Transplant. 2006;21:1413–6.

41. Stadlmann S, Fend F, Moser P, et al. Epstein-Barr virus-associated extranodal NK/T-cell lymphoma, nasal type of the hypopharynx, in a renal allograft recipient: case report and review of the literature. Human Pathol. 2001;32:1264–8.

42. Jia H, Sun T. Extranodal NK/T-cell lymphoma mimicking cellulitis. Leuk Lymphoma. 2004;45:1467–70.

Human Herpes Virus 8 (HHV8)

43. Chang Y, Cesarman E, Pessin MS, et al. Identification of herpesvirus-like DNA sequences in AIDS-associated Kaposi's sarcoma. Science. 1994;266:1865–9.

44. Wen KW, Damania B. Kaposi sarcoma-associated herpesvirus (KSHV): Molecular biology and oncogenesis. Cancer Lett. 2010;28:140–50.

Polyomavirus

45. Jiang M, Abend JR, Johnson SF, Imperiale MJ. The role of polyomaviruses in human disease. Virology. 2009;384:266–73.

46. Feng H, Shuda M, Chang Y, et al. Clonal integration of a polyomavirus in human Merkel cell carcinoma. Science. 2008;319:1096–100.

47. Rockville Merkel Cell Carcinoma Group. Merkel cell carcinoma: recent progress and current priorities on etiology, pathogenesis, and clinical management. J Clin Oncol. 2009;27:4021–6.

48. Heath M, Jaimes N, Lemos B, et al. Clinical characteristics of Merkel cell carcinoma at diagnosis in 195 patients: the AEIOU features. J Am Acad Dermatol. 2008;58:375–81.

Human T-Cell Lymphotrophic Virus (HTLV)

49. Nobre V, Guedes AC, Martins ML, et al. Dermatological findings in 3 generations of a family with a high prevalence of human T cell lymphotropic virus type 1 infection in Brazil. Clin Inf Dis. 2006;43:1257–63.

50. Arch EL, Schaefer JT, Dahiya A. Cutaneous manifestation of disseminated strongyloidiasis in a patient coinfected with HTLV-1. Dermatol Online J. 2008;14(12):6.

51. Montes M, Sanchez C, Verdonck K, et al. Regulatory T cell expansion in HTLV-1 and strongyloidiasis co-infection is associated with reduced IL-5 responses to *Strongyloides stercoralis* antigen. PLoS Negl Trop Dis. 2009;3:1–8.

52. del Giudice P, Sainte Marie D, Gérard Y, Couppié P, Pradinaud R. Is crusted (Norwegian) scabies a marker of adult T cell leukemia/lymphoma in human T lymphotropic virus type I-seropositive patients? J Infect Dis. 1997;176(4):1090–2.

Human Immunodeficiency Virus (HIV)

53. Wilkins K, Turner R, Dolev JC, et al. Cutaneous malignancy and human immunodeficiency virus disease. J Am Acad Dermatol. 2006;54:189–206.

54. Castillo J, Dezube BJ, Pantanowitz L. Plasmablastic lymphoma in HIV: a review of 131 cases. J Clin Oncol. 2008;26:abstr 19519.

15

Clues to the Diagnosis of Skin Lesions in the Immunocompromised Host

When the skin is involved by an infection in the immuno-compromised host, the astute clinician must immediately use all available clues to find its cause.

1. The presence of symptoms other than the rash may localize or aid identification of the source of infection or the extent of involvement. The acquired immune deficiency syndrome (AIDS) patient with fever, cough, or pulmonary infiltrates and rash has disseminated histoplasmosis unless the skin lesion is in the ear, in which case it may be *Pneumocystis*. The AIDS patient with fever, headache, and rash has disseminated cryptococcosis. The constellation of fever, erythematous papules, and myalgias in the neutropenic leukemic patient means disseminated candidiasis. If the papules become centrally necrotic, *Fusarium* becomes a consideration. Diffuse cutaneous lesions with polyarticular arthritis, particularly involving the joints of the hands and wrists, may be the presenting signs of disseminated sporotrichosis.

2. Recognize the clinical setting in which the skin lesions are occurring. The transplant patient with a subcutaneous nodule probably has disseminated *Cryptococcus* unless hospital demolition, renovation, or construction is ongoing. Then, *Aspergillus* is more likely. Cellulitis or hemorrhagic bullae developing in an acute febrile illness after exposure to a marine (salt water) environment suggests *Vibrio vulnificus* infection, while fresh water contamination implicates *Aeromonas* infection in the immunocompromised patient. The immunosuppressed patient at a hospital undergoing construction or renovation may be part of a cluster of patients with skin lesions due to invasive aspergillosis.

3. Determine the host factors that predispose to certain infections: diabetic ketoacidosis, organ transplantation, HIV infection, acute leukemia, multiple myeloma, chronic lymphocytic leukemia, solid tumors, systemic steroids, chemotherapy (cytotoxic or immunosuppressant), tumor necrosis factor (TNF) alpha inhibitors, graft versus host disease, or neutropenia.

4. The timing of the skin infection may offer some clues as to its etiology. In the transplant recipient each phase of the transplantation process is characterized by specific defects in the host defense and is associated with a specific group of infections. The patterns of infection are similar for all forms of solid organ transplantation which follow almost a consistent time table of occurrence after transplantation. In newly diagnosed leukemic patients and patients with myeloma, bacterial infections (streptococcal and staphylococcal) are more likely than disseminated fungal infections.

5. Evaluate the recent treatment of the underlying disorder. Neutropenia from cytotoxic or myelosuppressive drugs, particularly a rapidly dropping neutrophil count, can place the patient at maximum risk of infection from gram-negative bacteria and opportunistic fungi. Acral, axillary, or perianal hemorrhagic bullae in the acutely ill, febrile, neutropenic patient indicate gram-negative sepsis.

6. In neutropenic patients, the classic findings of swelling and fluctuance appear late in the course of infection or not at all. There may be scant or no pus formation. Erythema is the most reliable clue to the presence of infection irrespective of the absolute white blood cell count.

7. Avoid excluding laboratory "contaminants" which actually are pathogens such as *Penicillium* or *Acremonium*. Communicate with the clinical microbiology laboratory. Precise identification of all isolates recovered from clinically significant specimens is essential because of the continuously expanding list of pathogens in the immunocompromised patient.

M.E. Grossman et al., *Cutaneous Manifestations of Infection in the Immunocompromised Host*, DOI 10.1007/978-1-4419-1578-8_15, © Springer Science+Business Media, LLC 2012

8. The profoundly immunosuppressed patient is susceptible to multiple, synchronous infections and unusual infections. The finding of one bacterial, viral, or fungal pathogen does not preclude a second or third. Complete staining and culture studies should be performed on all specimens, especially if clinical resolution has not occurred with the appropriate therapy.

9. One must be alert to common pathogens with unusual or bizarre clinical presentations and unusual pathogens producing routine appearing skin lesions.

   Common skin infections may occur in unexpected locations: condyloma acuminata in the mouth, herpes simplex on the scalp or finger, or molluscum contagiosum in extragenital locations. Usually minor skin infections may be severe: condyloma acuminata so florid as to cause anal blockage, herpes simplex infection leading to necrotizing ulceration of the digit, and scabies producing an exfoliative erythroderma. Atypical appearances of routine infections in the immunocompromised host may be seen: giant molluscum contagiosum may look like keratoacanthomas or cutaneous staphylococcal infection may progress to botryomycosis.

   Unusual pathogens and organisms in the past considered uncommon or non-pathogenic may produce routine appearing skin infections: pustules due to protothecosis, cellulitis from *Mycobacterium haemophilum* or *Cunninghamella*, or a purulent draining nodule of *Acanthamoeba*.

10. Inquire about geographic, nosocomial, occupational, or behavioral exposures for a clue to the etiology of infection in the immunocompromised patient.

11. A travel history or residence in an endemic region may be a clue to the origin of a skin lesion. Reactivation of an endogenous or latent infection because of immunosuppression may produce a recognizable pattern of disease: a diagnosis of hyperinfection *Strongyloides* may be made from periumbilical purpura in a patient from Kentucky or the Caribbean; *Penicillium marneffei* may be diagnosed from molluscum contagiosum-like lesions in a patient from Southeast Asia or Coccidioidomycosis from facial papules in a patient from the San Joaquin valley. Truncal reddish-brown crusted papules in immigrants from Asia or India may be a clue to disseminated *Mycobacterium tuberculosis*.

12. Many emerging or opportunistic infections exhibit geographic restrictions. *Fusarium* infections are more frequently reported in medical centers in the southern United States and South America and *Scedosporium* infections more often in Spain.

13. Inquire about animal contacts: pets or exposure to cats, pigeons, or contaminated bat caves, which may lead to a diagnosis of bacillary angiomatosis, cryptococcosis, or histoplasmosis.

14. New, re-emerging, and neglected infections acquired from animals should be considered as sources of infection. These pathogens may be acquired from recreational or sporting activities (hunting and tularemia, brucellosis, or leptospirosis), companion animals (cats and toxoplasmosis, or cat scratch disease; dogs and methicillin resistant staphylococcus aureus), exotic pets (prairie dogs and monkey pox), tourism or unusual holiday destinations.

15. Be aware of the medical procedures that damage the anatomic barriers of the skin and mucous membranes and predispose to opportunistic infection in the compromised host. Erythematous or purpuric bullae or nodules with necrosis at the site of taping for intravenous administration in the leukemic patient are probably primary inoculation aspergillosis, possibly *Trichoderma*. An erythematous plaque with superficial pustules at the site of application of elastic (Elastoplast, Beiersdorf UK Limited, Birmingham, United Kingdom) dressings may be due to cutaneous *Rhizopus* infection.

16. The appearance of the skin lesion and its location even in the immunocompromised host may be diagnostic. Any periorificial ulceration in an immunocompromised patient is herpes simplex until proven otherwise. The combination of nasal lesions and facial cellulitis in a neutropenic leukemic patient is likely to be rhinocerebral mucormycosis. Onychomycosis of the toenails and red-purple nodules of the feet and lower legs is probably invasive dermatophyte.

17. Persistent genital or perianal ulceration despite treatment for herpes simplex virus in a patient with AIDS, especially with retinitis, colitis, esophagitis, or pneumonitis should alert the clinician to the diagnosis of cytomegalovirus (CMV).

18. The source of a disseminated fungal infection may be at your feet. Longstanding onychomycosis, paronychia, or toeweb ulceration may be the origin of a systemic infection due to *Fusarium*, *Paecilomyces*, or *Scopulariopsis*. All patients with intertrigo or onychomycosis should have cultures of nail scrapings obtained so that appropriate antifungal therapy can be initiated.

19. When the skin is involved by an opportunistic infection, the clinical lesions may be nondescript and not allow diagnosis by observation alone. The differential diagnosis of a particular type of skin lesion in the immunocompromised host is extensive because the variety of organisms that can cause infection is all inclusive and the inflammatory response to the infection may be altered by the underlying disease or its treatment. For all of these reasons, skin biopsy should be performed for histology and culture to establish a definitive diagnosis.

20. Any chronic or unexplained skin lesion in the immunocompromised host should be suspicious and biopsied at an early stage for fungal, viral, bacterial, and protozoal causes.

21. Despite an unimpressive or absent inflammatory infiltrate on skin biopsy specimen, the pathologist should not be fooled and an infectious process should be considered. If the pathologist diagnoses a panniculitis or a vasculitis on

a skin biopsy from an immunocompromised host, the clinician must consider an infectious panniculitis or a septic vasculitis and request special stains and cultures.

22. In organ transplant recipients or AIDS patients with sterile cutaneous ulcers, pustules, or subcutaneous nodules particularly if a skin biopsy only demonstrated "macrophages or histiocyte-like cells amid necrotic debris" and the patient also had sinusitis, seizures, or central nervous system (CNS) disease (diagnosed as toxoplasmosis despite negative serology or head computed tomography (CT) scan with infarct or hemorrhage), search for *Acanthamoeba*. Special stains are not necessary, only special thought.

16

Differential Diagnoses

ACRAL HEMORRHAGIC BULLAE

1. Aspergillosis (J Am Acad Dermatol 1985;12:313)
2. *Fusarium* (J Am Acad Dermatol 1990;23:393)
3. *Trichosporon* (Mayo Clin Proc 1983;58:684)
4. Herpes simplex
5. Herpes zoster
6. *Clostridium septicum* (N Engl J Med 1990;323:1406)
7. *Bacillus cereus* (Southeast Asian J Trop Med Public Health 1987;18:112)
8. *Pseudomonas aeruginosa* (Pediatr Dermatol 1987;4:18)
9. *Citrobacter* (J Am Acad Dermatol 1981;5:613)
10. *Enterobacter* (J Am Acad Dermatol 1992;27:637)
11. *Klebsiella*
12. *Morganella* (J Am Acad Dermatol 1985;12:575)
13. *Escherichia coli* (Arch Dermatol 1974;110:105)
14. *Vibrio vulnificus* (Ann Intern Med 1988;109:318)
15. *Pseudallescheria boydii* (Arch Dermatol 1996 Apr;132(4): 382)
16. *Scedosporium apiospermum* (Cutis 2009;84:275)

BLACK NECROTIC ULCER OF PALATE

1. Aspergillosis
2. Mucormycosis (J Oral Maxillofac Surg. 2006 Feb;64(2): 326)
3. *Trichosporon beigelii* (Cancer 1981;48:2163)
4. *Fusarium* (Cancer 1986;57:2141)
5. *Mycobacterium avium-intracellulare* (Oral Surg Oral Med Oral Pathol 1985;60:567)
6. *Pseudomonas* (Ann Plast Surg. 1981 Feb;6(2):138)

CELLULITIS

1. Aspergillosis (J Am Acad Dermatol 1985;12:313)
2. *Cryptococcus neoformans* (J Am Acad Dermatol 1987;17: 469)
3. Histoplasmosis (Cutis 1980;25:152)
4. Mucormycosis (Am J Med Sci. 2007 Feb;333(2):122)
5. *Cunninghamella* (Am J Clin Pathol 1983;80:98)
6. *Fusarium* (Clin Infect Dis 2007;44:1220)
7. *Paecilomyces* (Arch Dermatol 1986;122:1169)
8. Trichosporonosis (Mayo Clin Proc 1983;58:684)
9. Protothecosis (Lab Invest 1981;44:81A)
10. *Mycobacterium avium-intracellulare* (J Am Acad Dermatol 1989;21:574)
11. *Mycobacterium chelonae* (J Infect Dis 1992;l66:4O5)
12. *Mycobacterium haemophilum* (J Am Acad Dermatol 1994;30:804)
13. *Mycobacterium kansasii* (Arch Dermatol 1980;116:207)
14. *Mycobacterium marinum* (South Med J 1990;83:471)
15. *Mycobacterium szulgai* (Am Rev Respir Dis 1977;115: 695)
16. *Staphylococcus epidermidis* (Arch Dermatol 1984;120: 1099)
17. Group G *Streptococcus* (Arch Dermatol 1982;118:934)
18. *Streptococcus pneumoniae* (Am J Med 1975;59:293)
19. *Clostridium septicum* (Rev Infect Dis 1991;13(3):525)
20. Nocardiosis (Rev Infect Dis 1981;3:492)
21. *Pseudomonas aeruginosa* (JAMA 1982;248:2156)
22. *Escherichia coli* (Clin Pediatr 1987;26:592)
23. *Aeromonas hydrophila* (Infection 2001;29:109)
24. *Vibrio vulnificus* (Ann Intern Med 1988;109:318)
25. *Serratia marcescens* (Int J Infect Dis 1998;3:36)

M.E. Grossman et al., *Cutaneous Manifestations of Infection in the Immunocompromised Host*, DOI 10.1007/978-1-4419-1578-8_16, © Springer Science+Business Media, LLC 2012

26. *Xanthomonas maltophilia* (Arch Dermatol 1992;128:702)
27. *Rhizopus arrhizus* (Arch Surg 1976;111:532)
28. *Legionella micdadei* (Ann Intern Med 1985;102:630)
29. *Haemophilus influenzae* (Am J Med 1977;63:449)
30. *Heliobacter cinaedi* (Ann Intern Med 1994;121:90)
31. Candidiasis
32. *Coccidioidomycosis* (Am J Med. 1987 Nov;83(5):949)
33. Sporotrichosis (J Am Acad Dermatol 1999;40:272)
34. *Leclercia adecarboxylata* (Pediatr Dermatol 2011;28:162–164)

Ecthyma Gangrenosum

1. *Aspergillus* species (Am J Clin Pathol 1979;72:230)
2. Disseminated candidiasis (Am J Med 1981;70:1133)
3. Mucormycosis (JAMA 1973;225:737)
4. *Exserohilum rostratum* (Pediatr Infect Dis 1986;5:380)
5. *Fusarium* (Eur J Clin Microbiol Infect Dis 1992;11:1160)
6. *Staphylococcus aureus* (Arch Intern Med 1981;141:689)
7. *Pseudomonas aeruginosa* (Arch Intern Med 1971;128:591)
8. *Pseudomonas cepacia* (Arch Dermatol 1977;113:199)
9. *Escherichia coli* (J Clin Gastroenterol 1982;4:145)
10. *Aeromonas hydrophila* (N Y State J Med 1982;82:1461)
11. *Vibrio* species (Rev Infect Dis 1980;2:854)
12. *Serratia marcescens*
13. *Klebsiella pneumonia* (Int J Dermatol 1995;34:216)
14. *Cirtobacter freundii* (J Am Acad Dermatol 2004;50:S114)
15. *Stenotrophomonas maltophilia* (Ann Dermatol 2009;21:389)

Molluscum Contagiosum-Like

1. Aspergillosis (Arch Dermatol 1982;128:1229)
2. Cryptococcosis (Arch Dermatol 1985;121:901)
3. Histoplasmosis (Arch Dermatol Venereol 1983:110:715)
4. *Alternaria alternata* (Am J Clin Pathol 1976;66:565)
5. *Penicillium marneffei* (Clin Infect Dis 1992;14:871)
6. *Mycobacterium tuberculosis* (J Am Acad Dermatol 1992;26: 356)
7. *Pneumocystis carinii* (Arch Dermatol 1991;127:1699)
8. Sporotrichosis (AIDS 1991;5:1243)
9. *Cladosporium carrionii* (Fitzpatrick TB, et al. Dermatology in general medicine. 4th ed. New York: McGraw-Hill; 1993:1523)
10. *Paecilomyces* (J Am Acad Dermatol 1998;39:401)

Necrotic Skin Lesions

1. *Saksenaea vasiformis* (Am J Clin Pathol 1981;76:116)
2. Aspergillosis (J Am Acad Dermatol 1980;3:397)
3. Candidiasis (Arch Intern Med 1986; 146:385)
4. Histoplasmosis (Br J Dermatol 1985;113:345)
5. Mucormycosis (Arch Dermatol 1977;113:1075)
6. *Bipolaris* (Arch Dermatol 1977;113:813)
7. *Fusarium* (South Med J 1986;79:513)

8. Cytomegalovirus (Am J Dermatol Pathol 1988;10:524)
9. *Citrobacter* (N Engl J Med 1969;280:1286)
10. *Scopulariopsis brevicaulis* (Diagn Microbiol Infect Dis 1989:12:429)
11. *Trichosporon asahii* (Eur J Clin Microbiol Infect Dis 2002; 21:892)
12. *Pseudomonas* (Clin Exp Dermatol 1988;13:78)
13. *E. coli* (Cutis 2009 Nov;84(5):261)
14. *Stenotrophomonas maltophilia* (Ann Dermatol. 2009;21(4): 389)
15. *Prototbecosis* (Mykosen 1983; 26:455)
16. *Scedosporium apiospermum* (Int J Dermatol. 1997 Sep; 36(9):684)
17. *Scedosporium prolificans* (Med Pediatr Oncol. 2001 Aug; 37(2):122)

Pustules

1. Aspergillosis (J Am Acad Dermatol 1985;12:313)
2. Blastomycosis (Medicine (Baltimore) 1993;72:311)
3. Candidiasis (J Am Acad Dermatol 1985;121:898)
4. Coccidioidomycosis (Cutis 1987;39:203)
5. Cryptococcosis (J Infect Dis 1957;28:159)
6. Histoplasmosis (JAMA 1979;242:456)
7. Alternariosis (Mycopathologia 1986;96:3)
8. *Exophiala spinifera* (Sabouraudia 1984;22:493)
9. *Fusarium* (Arch Dermatol 1986;122:1171)
10. *Penicillium marneffei* (J Acquir Immune Defic Syndr 1993;6:466)
11. Trichosporonosis (Medicine (Baltimore) 1986;65:268)
12. Dermatophytosis (Mycoses. 2007;50 Suppl 2:31)
13. *Pityrosporum orbiculare* (Cutis 1985;35:536)
14. Prototbecosis (Arch Dermatol 1971;104:490)
15. *Mycobacterium bovis* (J Am Acad Dermatol 1993;28:264)
16. *Mycobacterium chelonae* (Arch Dermatol 1990;126:1064)
17. *Mycobacterium haemophilum* (J Am Acad Dermatol 1993; 28:264)
18. *Mycobacterium kansasii* (Arch Dermatol 1980;116:207)
19. Herpes simplex
20. Herpes zoster
21. Nocardiosis(J Am Acad Dermatol 1989;20:889)
22. *Corynebacterium jeikeium* (Am J Med 1987;82:132)
23. *Citrobacter* (J Am Acad Dermatol 1981;5:613)
24. *Staphylococcus aureus*
25. *Acanthamoeba* (Transplant Inf Dis 2010;12: 529–537)
26. *Pseudallescheria boydii* (Mycoses 1995 Sep-Oct;38(9–10):369)

Sporotrichoid Lesions

1. *Cryptococcus neoformans* (Br J Dermatol 1989;120:683)
2. *Sporothrix schenckii*
3. Trichosporonosis (Ann Intern Med 1988;108:772)
4. *Mycobacterium avium-intracellulare* (Arch Dermatol 1993; 129:1343)

5. *Mycobacterium chelonae* (Australas J Dermatol 1990; 31:105)
6. *Mycobacterium kansasii* (Penneys NS. Skin manifestations of AIDS. Philadelphia: JB Lippincott; 1990:43)
7. *Mycobacterium marinum* (Ann Intern Med 1981;94:486)
8. *Leishmania tropica*
9. *Staphylococcus aureus* (Arch Intern Med 1987;147:793)
10. *Nocardia asteroides* (Int J Dermatol 1992;31:178)
11. *Nocardia brasiliensis* (Arch Dermatol 1986;122:1180)
12. *Nocardia caviae* (J Am Acad Dermatol 1993;29:639)
13. *Fusarium* (Arch Derm 1995;131:1329)
14. *Paecilomyces* (J Drugs Dermatol 2007;6:436)
15. *Acanthamoeba* (Int J Dermatol 2006;45:942)
16. Phaeohyphomycosis (*Alternaria infectoria*). (Br J Dermatol 2001;154:484)
17. Aspergillosis (Pediatr Dermatol. 2009 Sep-Oct;26(5):592–6)
18. *Scedosporium marinum* (J Clin Pathol. 1999 Nov; 52(11):846)

SUBCUTANEOUS NODULES

1. Aspergillosis (Cleve Clin J Med 1990;57:92)
2. Candidiasis (J Cutan Pathol 1989;16:183)
3. Coccidioidomycosis
4. Cryptococcosis (JAMA 1978;240:2460)
5. Histoplasmosis (Ann Intern Med 1977;86:586)
6. *Bipolaris* (Medicine (Baltimore) 1986;65:203)
7. *Exophiala jeanselmei* (Clin Infect Dis 1994;19:339)
8. Sporotrichosis (Ann Intem Med 1970;73:23)
9. *Fusarium* (Int J Dermatol 1988;27:698)
10. *Paecilomyces* (J Infect Dis 1992;24:191)
11. *Trichophyton rubrum* (Am J Med 1987;82:321)
12. Prototheceosis (Arch Dermatol 1985;121:1066)
13. *Mycobacterium tuberculosis* (Medicine (Baltimore) 1981; 60:95)
14. *Mycobacterium chelonae* (J Infect Dis 1992;166:405)
15. *Mycobacterium fortuitum* (Medicine (Baltimore) 1981;60:95)
16. *Mycobacterium intracellulare* (Arch Pathol Lab Med 1982;106:112)
17. *Mycobacterium kansasii* (Arch Intern Med 1982; 142:888)
18. *Mycobacterium marinum* (Ann Intern Med 1981;94:486)
19. Bacillary angiomatosis
20. Nocardiosis(Mayo Clin Proc 1975;50:657)
21. *Pseudomonas aeruginosa* (Am J Med 1986;80:528)
22. *Mycobacterium haemophilum* (Ann Intern Med 1982; 97:723)
23. *Phialophora richardsiae* (J Am Acad Dermatol 1988;19:478)
24. *Staphylococcus aureus*
25. *Acanthamoeba* (J Cutan Pathol. 2001 Jul;28(6):307)
26. *E. coli* (Am J Dermatopathol 1998;20:185)
27. *Stenotrophomonas* (J Eur Acad Dermatol Venereol 2007;21:1298)
28. Blastomycosis (Semin Respir Infect 1997 Sep;12(3):243)
29. Phaeohyphomycosis (Alternaria alternata) (J Dermatol Treat 2008;19:246)

30. Phaeohyphomycosis (*Cladophialophora bantiana*) (J Burn Care Rehabil 2005;26:285)
31. *Scedosporium apiospermum* (Acta Derm Venereol. 1999 Sep;79(5):402)
32. *Pseudallescheria boydii* (Br J Dermatol. 1995 Mar;132(3): 456)

ULCERS

1. Aspergillosis (Cancer 1975;36:2271)
2. Candidiasis (Clin Exp Dermatol 1989;14:295)
3. Coccidioidomycosis
4. Paracoccidioidomycosis (J Am Acad Dermatol 1989;20:854)
5. Cryptococcosis (J Am Acad Dermatol 1981;5:32)
6. Mucormycosis (J Am Acad Dermatol 1989;21:1232)
7. Sporotrichosis (Arch Dermatol 1986;122:691)
8. Histoplasmosis
9. *Exserohilum rostratum* (Pediatr Infect Dis 1986;5:380)
10. Prototheceosis (Arch Dermatol 2000;136:1263)
11. *Mycobacterium tuberculosis* (Rev Infect Dis 1991;13:265)
12. *Mycobacterium haemophilum* (Rev Infect Dis 1991;13:906)
13. Chronic herpes simplex (Am J Med 1986;80:486)
14. Chronic varicella-zoster (J Am Acad Dermatol 1988;18:584)
15. Cytomegalovirus (J Am Acad Dermatol 1998;38:349)
16. *Acanthamoeba* (J Am Acad Dermatol 1992;26:352)
17. Nocardiosis (Int J Dermatol 1991;30:804)
18. *Citrobacter* (N Engl J Med 1969;280:1286)
19. *Trichoderma* (Med Mycol 2009;47:207)
20. *Pseudomonas* (Arch Dermatol 1990;126:527)
21. *Serratia* (Eur J Dermatol 2008;18:705)
22. *Stenotrophomonas* (Am J Med Sci 2002;323:269)
23. Leishmaniasis (Lancet Infect Dis. 2008 Mar;8(3):191)
24. *Entamoeba histolytica* (J Am Acad Dermatol. 2009;60(6): 897)

VESICLES OR BULLAE

1. Cryptococcosis (Arch Dermatol 1976;112:1734)
2. *Fusarium* (Eur J Clin Microbiol Infect Dis 1992;11:1160)
3. Prototheceosis (Int J Dermatol 1986; 25:54.)
4. Herpes simplex
5. Herpes zoster
6. Cytomegalovirus (J Am Acad Dermatol 1984;11:743)
7. *Staphylococcus aureus*
8. *Bacillus cereus* (Arch Dermatol 1991;127:543)
9. *Pseudomonas aeruginosa*
10. *Klebsiella*
11. *Escherichia coli* (Arch Dermatol 1974;110:105)
12. *Aeromonas hydrophila*
13. *Vibrio* species
14. *Enterobacter* (J Am Acad Dermatol 1992;27:637)
15. *Morganella* (J Am Acad Dermatol 1985;12:575)
16. *Stenotrophomonas* (Am J Med Sci 2002;323:269)
17. Dermatophytosis (Mycoses. 2007;50 Suppl 2:31)

Index

Page numbers in *italics* denote figures

M.E. Grossman et al., *Cutaneous Manifestations of Infection in the Immunocompromised Host*,
DOI 10.1007/978-1-4419-1578-8, © Springer Science+Business Media, LLC 2012